Psychiatric Consultation in Long-Term Care

Psychiatric Consultation in Long-Term Care

A Guide for Health Care Professionals

Abhilash K. Desai, M.D., FAPA
Associate Professor and Director of the Center for Healthy Brain Aging

and

George T. Grossberg, M.D.
Samuel W. Fordyce Professor and Director

Division of Geriatric Psychiatry,
Department of Neurology and Psychiatry
Saint Louis University School of Medicine
Saint Louis, Missouri

The Johns Hopkins University Press
Baltimore

© 2010 The Johns Hopkins University Press
All rights reserved. Published 2010
Printed in the United States of America on acid-free paper
9 8 7 6 5 4 3 2 1

The Johns Hopkins University Press
2715 North Charles Street
Baltimore, Maryland 21218-4363
www.press.jhu.edu

Library of Congress Cataloging-in-Publication Data
Desai, Abhilash K.
    Psychiatric consultation in long-term care : a guide for health care professionals / Abhilash K. Desai and George T. Grossberg.
        p.   ;   cm.
    Includes bibliographical references and index.
    ISBN-13: 978-0-8018-9386-5 (hardcover : alk. paper)
    ISBN-10: 0-8018-9386-0 (hardcover : alk. paper)
    1. Geriatric psychiatry. 2. Nursing home patients—Mental health services. I. Grossberg, George T. II. Title.
    [DNLM: 1. Aged—psychology. 2. Long-Term Care—psychology. 3. Assisted Living Facilities.
4. Homes for the Aged. 5. Mental Disorders—therapy. 6. Nursing Homes. WT 150 D441p 2010]
    RC451.4.A5.D485 2010
    618.97'689—dc22   2009048411

A catalog record for this book is available from the British Library.

Special discounts are available for bulk purchases of this book. For more information, please contact Special Sales at 410-516-6936 or specialsales@press.jhu.edu.

The Johns Hopkins University Press uses environmentally friendly book materials, including recycled text paper that is composed of at least 30 percent post-consumer waste, whenever possible. All of our book papers are acid-free, and our jackets and covers are printed on paper with recycled content.

Contents

Preface

A coauthored text such as this, unlike edited texts, gives the authors a unique opportunity to present state-of-the-art information regarding biopsychosocial and environmental interventions in long-term care (LTC) together with our philosophy of caring for older adults who live in LTC settings. Our philosophy of care is that "there is life in the nursing home" and other LTC facilities and that health care professionals in many disciplines—physicians, nurses, administrators, nurse aides, social workers, various rehabilitative therapists, pharmacists, psychologists, clergy, recreational therapists, music therapists, and others—all have a lot to offer in improving the quality of life for LTC residents and their families. Every health care provider has an important role to play as a member of the health care team.

Our philosophy of care places the needs and dignity of the LTC resident at its center. It promotes the notion that, to some degree, we can help every LTC resident and his or her family. A caring attitude on the part of all health care professionals in LTC is vital in meeting this goal. Our philosophy sees the LTC environment as warm, nurturing, and supportive. For residents, it is their extended family, or, at times, their only family.

Achieving excellence in the care of LTC residents will require physicians not only to be responsible to each individual resident, but also to promote the well-being of family members and other professional caregivers, as well as to understand the systems of care. This means a team approach—in addition to individual assessments—to determine what intervention strategies are most effective, to standardize care where possible, and to eliminate errors.

Our philosophy of care promulgates the use not only of biological therapies, when appropriate, but also of psychosocial, behavioral, and environmental interventions. In fact, one of the longest chapters in this text is devoted to psychosocial-environmental (i.e., nonpharmacologic) treatments of behavioral problems in LTC.

This guide is written to be user-friendly and is targeted to physicians, physician assistants, nurse practitioners, nurses, social workers, administrators, and other health care professionals involved or interested in behavioral and psychosocial issues in LTC. It can also be useful for students and trainees who desire to learn more about behavior, aging, and LTC. We hope our book will further education and training regarding LTC by providing evidence-based, state-of-the-science approaches to improving the well-being of all residents in LTC.

We would like to thank our spouses and families for their support of this project. We also appreciate the high-quality editorial work of Ms. Wendy Harris of the Johns Hopkins University Press. Without her unfailing support, this project would not have been realized. Lastly, we have learned a great deal from our patients, their families, and the staff of the outstanding LTC facilities with which we have been affiliated.

We hope you enjoy reading this book and find it helpful in your work with LTC residents.

Psychiatric Consultation in Long-Term Care

CHAPTER 1

Introduction and Epidemiology

Long-term care (LTC) is one of the fastest-growing segments of health care in the United States and is an important setting in which to prevent, identify, and treat behavioral and psychological symptoms the residents experience. LTC facilities include both nursing homes and alternatives to nursing homes (primarily assisted living facilities). The spectrum of LTC also may include people living in subacute care, special care units, and hospice, as well as people in retirement communities who receive assistance with activities of daily living (ADLs) or whose medications are monitored.

Psychiatric disorders are prevalent in elderly people, and this prevalence (especially of dementia, delirium, and depression) increases considerably with age (Martens et al. 2007). The presence of dementia, delirium, depressive disorders, anxiety disorders, psychotic disorders, and sleep disorders in LTC is so high (40%–100%) that many consider LTC facilities to be psychiatric institutions. The relative rates of these disorders depend on a person's age and the severity of coexisting medical illnesses. Although psychiatric disorders have a major impact on disability, mortality, care needs, and care costs, they are underrecognized and undertreated. There is growing evidence that mental health care is efficacious for residents in LTC facilities, and data is accumulating from both randomized clinical trials and the outcomes of real-life care that treatment can improve daily functioning.

Psychiatric morbidity and the prevalence of dementia are increasing in LTC facilities. In fact, LTC facilities are becoming places primarily for individuals who have advanced dementia. Of those with dementia, 30 percent are cared for in an LTC facility and 70 percent reside in the community, either in their own homes or in retirement communities (also called residential care communities) (Caselli et al. 2006). Between 70 and 90 percent of all people with dementia eventually develop one or more behavioral symptoms. Yet the intensity of the services required for residents of LTC facilities is significantly greater than that for community-dwelling older adults, with the former using twice the number of prescriptions and accounting for four times the total overall amount of health care spending (Stefanacci 2006). These numbers underscore the urgency of improving the psychosocial well-being and quality of life for all residents in LTC facilities, as well as for their families and professional caregivers.

The residents' characteristics (acuity, prevalence of dementia, etc.) and the services provided to them vary considerably from one LTC facility to another and from one state to another. Although the regulation of assisted living facilities also differs greatly from one state to another, all nursing homes are regulated by the federal government. Nonetheless, the differences between some assisted living facilities and nursing homes are vague and ill defined, with a certain number of assisted living facilities providing a mix of services once reserved for nursing home residents. On the whole, LTC facilities are more different than similar. Thus, across all community and facility settings, more consistency is needed in the information collected on the characteristics of the settings and the services offered, as well as on the characteristics of residents, so that analyses can identify factors associated with the choice of setting, transitions between settings, and outcomes.

Demographics of Residents in Long-Term Care Facilities

In term of demographics, residents of LTC facilities are becoming older and increasingly female (table 1.1), with the women older than the men (mean age 83 versus 76). According to a recent American Community Survey, 1,834,880 people were living in LTC facilities (U.S. Census Bureau 2007). The majority were women (69.2%), and 42.8 percent of all residents were 85 years of age or older. The median age was 83.2 years. Additionally, 83.9 percent were white, 12.8 percent were black, 3.8 percent were Hispanic or Latino, 1.2 percent were Asian, and 0.5 percent were American Indian or Alaskan native. All of those surveyed reported not living with a marital partner. About 17.9 percent said they were married but living separately from the spouse, 1.4 percent were separated, 10.7 percent were divorced, 54.1 percent were widowed, and 15.8 percent had never married. The average per capita income of those surveyed was $12,251. Some 58.8 percent had completed high school or had some college education, and 9.8 percent had received a

TABLE 1.1
*Demographics of residents in long-term care
facilities (in percentages)*

Age distribution	
Less than 65 years old	0–9
65–74 years old	0–16
75–84 years old	30–40
85+ years old	40–60
Gender	
Male	20–30
Female	70–80
Marital status	
Single, never married	10–14
Married	12–20
Divorced or separated	4–8
Widowed	60–70
Race	
White	80–95
Black	10–14
Hispanic	1–5
Other minorities	0–1

Sources: Data from National Institute on Aging and
Duke University 2004; National Center for Health
Statistics 2009.

bachelor's degree or higher. Some 13.6 percent were veterans living in LTC facilities. Ninety-four percent were born in the United States. The survey also reported that 90 percent of the respondents spoke only English in their place of residence, 9.8 percent spoke a language other than English, and 4.7 percent said they spoke English "less than very well."

According to the National Nursing Home Survey and the National Long-Term Care Survey, the United States has about 16,000 certified nursing homes with 1.68 million beds and 1.4–1.45 million residents on any given day and 2.8 million discharges over the course of the year (National Institute on Aging and Duke University 2004; White 2005; National Center for Health Statistics 2009). The estimates also indicate that about 1 million residents live in alternative residential care settings, with the majority in assisted living facilities . These numbers do not include persons living in settings for special populations, such as those who have a mental illness or mental retardation. (The difference between the figures obtained by the National Nursing Home Survey and the National Long-Term Care Survey are due in large part to differences in definitions of assisted living facilities.) These numbers are expected to increase substantially in the next few decades because of the aging of the baby boom generation and a dramatic increase in the prevalence of dementia among elderly people. As many as 12 million Americans are expected to need LTC by the year 2020 (*Lancet* 2003).

Nearly 25 percent of older adults will spend some time in a nursing facility. The majority will subsequently return home, but a significant number (5%–7%) are likely to require continued care in either a nursing home or an assisted living facility. Some 20 percent of the nursing home population stay for less than 30 days, 24.2 percent for three to 12 months, 30.3 percent for one to three years, and 25.6 percent for three years or more. Some 17.2 percent of the residents are in a nursing home for rehabilitation. Fifty to 60 percent of residents receiving rehabilitation are cognitively intact, are there primarily for rehabilitation after hospitalization, and will be discharged home. Admission to LTC is strongly associated with age, even after adjusting for disability. Approximately 60–70 percent of elderly people with impairments in five or more ADLs will be admitted to an LTC facility. Although the public perception is that no one likes living in an LTC facility, the truth is that many residents prefer the reassurance of medical care, socialization, and a safe environment and find that the experience is positive.

In the United States, 67 percent of nursing homes are for-profit, 26 percent are nonprofit, and 7 percent are governmental entities. Fifty-six percent of nursing homes are affiliated with other nursing homes, through chain ownership. Most nursing homes (62%) are located in a metropolitan statistical area. Most have between 50 and 199 beds, and only 8 percent have more than 200 beds. The average size of a nursing home is 107 beds. There are generally from 67 to 81 staff members per 100 residents: administrative/medical, 5–6; registered nurses (RNs), 8–10; licensed practical nurses (LPNs), 12; certified nursing assistants (CNAs), 20–25; and all others, 22–28.

Nursing Homes

With the introduction of Medicaid funding in 1965, nursing homes became the most common institutional settings for persons with disabilities, particularly elderly people. Nursing homes provide services to those needing two distinct types of service: (1) long-term custodial stays, primarily financed by the residents' own resources and Medicaid (the joint federal and state safety net program for individuals who have a low income and few assets), and (2) a short-term postacute rehabilitation stay (after at least three days of hospitalization) to recover from an acute episode, such as a hip fracture or pneumonia, primarily financed by Medicare at higher reimbursement rates. Medicaid is the largest source of financing for nursing homes (43%), followed by individual and family resources (28%) and Medicare (14%). Although Medicaid finances 43 percent of nursing home revenues, 65 percent of the residents at any time have Medicaid as their primary source of payment. This difference occurs because Medicaid payment rates tend to be lower than those of other sources of financing, so they do not contribute as much to nursing home revenue as the number of residents might suggest, and because Medicaid requires unmarried nursing home residents to contribute nearly all of their income toward the cost of care, while Medicaid picks up the remainder.

Nursing home residents usually have a much higher prevalence of psychiatric disorders (70%–100%) than residents in assisted living facilities, where the prevalence is comparatively lower (40%–100%). Many residents, especially in nursing homes, have two or more psychiatric disorders.

Family caregivers' reasons for placing someone in a nursing home include the resident's dementia-related behaviors (most common); the caregivers' health; and the resident's incontinence, need for more skilled care, and need for more assistance. These factors are usually evident in the year before admission. When the person has Parkinson disease, psychotic symptoms are the leading reason for admission to LTC (Miyasaki et al. 2006). In the skilled nursing section of LTC, admission is primarily for rehabilitation from an acute illness or after hospitalization and surgery. In recent years, trends in care for those who have a disability, particularly elderly people, point to a shift from nursing homes to alternative residential care settings (predominantly assisted living facilities).

Alternative Residential Care Settings

Alternative residential care settings encompass a variety of places and care arrangements that provide both housing and services outside of a nursing facility for those who are unable or unwilling to live independently. Hallmark services usually include assistance with independent living activities, such as meals and housekeeping, and with personal care activities, such as bathing, dressing, mobility, toileting, and eating. Beyond that broad description, there appears to be no consensus on the criteria for identifying or distinguishing between these settings. They include such places as small foster care homes, board and care or personal care homes, congregate housing, and assisted living facilities.

The terms *board and care* and *assisted living* have been used both popularly and in state licensure to refer to a range of settings, from small supervised homes serving a largely Medicaid-funded clientele in private or shared rooms to large luxury facilities serving a well-to-do, privately paying clientele in private apartments. Assisted living appears to have become the more popular term, supplanting board and care as a blanket term for alternative residential care. Nevertheless, some, including the assisted living industry and its trade associations, believe that the term should be reserved for settings adhering to a specific model with a consumer-centered philosophy that emphasizes independence, dignity, privacy, decision making, and autonomy. Assisted living can be defined as facilities that provide 24-hour supervision, oversight of personal and supportive services, health-related services, social services, recreational activities, meals, housekeeping and laundry, and transportation. The assisted living setting is the fastest-growing segment of elder care in the United States (Vance 2008).

Assisted Living Facilities

The idea that assisted living facilities are primarily for people who have physical problems or who can, for the most part, look after themselves has become a myth. Today's assisted living resident is the nursing home resident of yesteryear. The *Overview of Assisted Living* demonstrates the increasing number of acutely ill among assisted living residents (Assisted Living Federation of America 2006). The number of people with dementia is growing, and physicians have recommended that they move into an assisted living facility for one or more of the following reasons: safety (administration of medications, regular intake of meals), medical problems (incontinence), and psychosocial issues (socialization to address loneliness, meaningful activities to address boredom, insomnia, and agitation). Many other older adults move to assisted living because of frailty, a stroke, or other serious medical conditions. A third category is the increasing numbers of older adults who move to assisted living facilities from nursing homes. These older adults most likely had been hospitalized for surgery or another medical challenge, were discharged from the hospital to a skilled nursing facility for rehabilitation, were able to improve enough (ambulate, reduce their need for help with ADLs) to no longer need the level of care provided by a nursing home, but still had sufficient disability not to be able to move back home. Conversely, residents with psychiatric disorders (e.g., advancing dementia, depression, psychotic symptoms, and severe agitation) are at increased risk of being discharged from assisted living to a nursing home. Thus improved management of psychiatric disorders in assisted living facilities may support the concept of aging in place.

The newest trend is for couples to become residents of assisted living facilities in instances where there is some compromised health, but where the spouse can no longer provide the needed care. Some of these couples have been married for 40, 50, or more years and have never been without each other. For the cognitively impaired spouse, psychosocial approaches would focus on how to prevent further decline, and for the healthier spouse, professional caregivers should help the person cope with loss, grief, stress, and situational depression.

People in assisted living facilities live with each other in close settings 24 hours a day, seven days a week. They have their own apartments but come together for meals, socializing, activities, and entertainment. These are small, intense communities, and professional caregivers will need to manage the associated conflicts and disputes by conflict resolution in order to maintain the residents' autonomy yet keep control of the situation. These challenges are different from those just 10 to 20 years ago.

Long-Term Care Facilities That Specialize in Dementia Care

Assisted living facilities and nursing homes that specialize in dementia care occupy a unique position in LTC that is distinct from home care and from traditional assisted living facilities and nursing homes. Primarily due to increasing care needs, most residents in specialized assisted living facilities relocate to a nursing home after a median stay of 11 months (Kopetz et al. 2000). Residents who have dementia and major medical care needs have a high rate of hospitalizations and may do better in a nursing home setting, where more aggressive medical care can be provided, thus avoiding some hospitalizations (Sloane et al. 2005).

The Epidemiology of Psychiatric Conditions

Much more data regarding the epidemiology of psychiatric conditions are available for the nursing home population than for the assisted living population (table 1.2). Cognitive impairment is high in LTC residents. Small assisted living facilities (≤ 15 beds) have a higher prevalence of dementia (81%) than larger facilities (63%), and the mean score on the Mini-Mental State Examination (MMSE) across all residents in small assisted living facilities was 13, compared with almost 20 in large facilities (Leroi et al. 2007). The prevalence of cognitive impairment is even higher in nursing homes than in assisted living. Lifetime delirium (or acute confusion) in nursing home residents is 60

TABLE 1.2
Some characteristics of residents in long-term care facilities

Condition	Residents (%)
Psychiatric condition	
Depression (major and minor depression)	20–40
Dementia	60–90
Cognitive impairment but no dementia	5–30
Delirium	6–16
Delirium in a postacute setting or a skilled nursing facility	5–30
Psychotic symptoms	8–12
Severe mental illness (e.g., schizophrenia)	0.2–5
Behavioral symptoms occurring at least once a week	30–35
Behavioral symptoms affecting others	15–22
Aggressive behavior once a week	13–20
Aggressive behavior injuring staff	3–6
Abnormal circadian rhythms	90–99
Nonaggressive behavioral symptoms once a week	20–30
Frequent screaming	10–20
Daytime sleeping	65–75
Disturbed nighttime sleep	55–65
Resistance to taking medications	13–15
Resistance to activities of daily living	13–15
Self-injurious behavior (pinching or scratching oneself)	20–25
Restraints (geri-chair, bedrails)	7–10
Residents who spend most of the time in a bed and/or chair	4–16
Psychotropic medication prescriptions	30–60
Antipsychotic use in the absence of a psychotic condition	16–22
Dependency	
Dependent for ambulation	20–40
Dependent for transfers	14–34
Dependent for bathing	46–100
Dependent for dressing	56–100
Dependent for toileting	37–77
Dependent for feeding	20–60
Medical conditions	
A fall	45–70
Two or more falls	30–40
Serious injury after a fall	10–12
Catheter	5–8
Contracture	25–35
Urinary incontinence	50–60
Bowel incontinence	20–50
Pressure ulcer	5–10
Tube feeding	0–10
Significant weight loss	8–14
Annual fracture incidence	5–10
Dehydration	10–20
Any intensity of pain	40–80
Moderate to severe pain	10–40
Nine or more medications	40–80
Potentially inappropriate medication prescriptions	5–15
Mobility limitation	75–90
Nighttime oxygen desaturation	30–50
Urinary tract infection	8–11
Vision impairments	20–40
Hearing impairments	70–90
Arthritis	20–40

continued

TABLE 1.2 *continued*

Condition	Residents (%)
Obesity	5–40
Obesity in new residents	20–25
Obesity in residents younger than 65	20–40
Infection	5–15
Taking antibiotics	0–8

Sources: Data from Fox, Raina, and Jadad 1999; Mulsant and Ganguli 1999; Magaziner et al. 2000; Mechanic and McAlpine 2000; Paulsen et al. 2000; House Committee on Government Reform 2001; Margallo-Lana et al. 2001; Mathews and Dening 2002; Ostling and Skoog 2002; Payne et al. 2002; Grossberg and Desai 2003b; R. Jones, Marcantonio, and Rabinowitz 2003; Blazer, Hybels, and Hays 2004; Burns, Gallagley, and Byrne 2004; Gruber-Baldini et al. 2004; Rosenblatt et al. 2004; Sloane et al. 2005; Smoyak 2005; Cowles 2006; Lyons 2006; Martin et al. 2006; Stefanacci 2006; D. Thomas and Morley 2006; L. Watson et al. 2006; Zanni 2006; Leroi et al. 2007; Levin et al. 2007; U.S. Census Bureau 2007; Zuidema et al. 2007; National Center for Health Statistics 2009; American Health Care Association, *OSCAR Data Reports: Patient Characteristics for June 2005*, www.ahcancal.org/research_data/oscar_data/; Centers for Medicare & Medicaid Services Web site, www.cms.hhs.gov/MDSPubQIandResRep/ [accessed February 4, 2008]; Centers for Medicare and Medicaid Services, *National Health Expenditure Data: Tables*, www.cms .gov/NationalHealthExpendData/downloads/tables.pdf; Lewin Group tabulations, 2004 National Nursing Home Survey current resident file, www.cdc.gov/nchs/nnhs.htm.

percent (Burns, Gallagley, and Byrne 2004). Nursing home residents who are transferred there from a hospital have a high point prevalence of delirium (10%–60%), especially after surgery to repair a hip fracture. Hospitals tend to discharge patients to skilled nursing facilities for rehabilitative services relatively soon after surgery or other medical challenges. Thus the prevalence of delirium in nursing homes may be increasing as a result of pressure to reduce the patients' length of stay in the hospital.

Depression (both major and minor) is frequent in LTC residents, with a higher prevalence in nursing homes than in assisted living facilities. Major (or clinical) depression in nursing homes occurs in 6–10 percent of the population with dementia and 20–25 percent of those without dementia, with some 4.3 percent of the residents developing new-onset major depression within one year. The prevalence of minor (or low-grade) depression is 25–33 percent. Up to 7.4 percent of the residents may develop new minor depression over a one-year period, and up to 23.5 percent may have their minor depression escalate to major depression within that time frame. Up to 38 percent of newly admitted residents in nursing homes may develop depressive symptoms by day 14. On average, only 34 percent of the residents have a reduction in depressive symptoms by day 60. Less than half of the residents who do not improve have changes in their treatment. More than half of the residents who have major depression continue to have major depression, and almost one-third of those who have minor depression still have minor depression one year later. Thus depression is undertreated in LTC populations. Although we have made strides in recognizing depression in LTC populations, it is underrecognized in many subgroups, especially in African American residents, the oldest old residents, and residents with cognitive impairments.

Psychotic disorders affect from 8 to 12 percent of LTC residents, compared with 0.2 to 5.7 percent of community-dwelling older adults. In individuals aged 85 or older who do not have dementia, the prevalence of psychotic symptoms may be as high as 10 percent (Ostling and Skoog 2002). More than 50 percent of the people with Alzheimer disease have some form of psychosis at some point during the course of that illness (Paulsen et al. 2000). The prevalence of severe and persistent mental illness ranges from 0.2 to 2.5 percent in LTC facilities and is much higher in some government-owned nursing homes. Older persons with schizophrenia make up the majority of these residents.

One study analyzed data from 2000–2001 and detected the highest level of use of antipsychotic medications in nursing homes in more than a decade (Briesacher et al. 2005). The same study found that more than half (58.2%) of the nursing home residents who received antipsychotic medication took doses exceeding the maximum levels, received duplicative therapy, or had inappropriate indications according to nursing home guideline requirements. Other researchers have also shown that there are considerable gaps between the medications clinical evidence recommends and the medications clinical practice delivers (Lau et al. 2004). The use of antidepressants by LTC residents with dementia has risen dramatically, from 28 percent in 2000 to 40 percent in 2006 (Teigland 2007). Up to 40 percent of nursing home residents resist taking medication. The proportion of nursing home residents with serious behavioral problems has grown, from 29 percent in 1995 to 31 percent in 1999 (Office of the Inspector General 2001). More than 30 percent of the nursing homes in the United States were cited for abuse violations that had the potential for significant harm to residents (House Committee on Government Reform 2001). The most frequent legal allegations of malpractice against nursing homes involve falls, negligent care, pressure ulcers, lack of care, abuse/assault, dehydration/malnutrition, and elopement/wandering.

Resident-to-resident aggression is ubiquitous in LTC facilities (T. Rosen et al. 2008). Up to 700,000 of the nation's 5 million elderly people who have dementia become physically violent each year. Self-injurious behaviors (pinching or scratching oneself, banging one's fist against an object) are often seen in residents who are immobile.

The psychosocial well-being of many residents in LTC facilities depends considerably on the well-being of family and professional caregivers. As many as 44 million Americans care for aging mothers, fathers, spouses, aunts, in-laws, and other elderly relatives. Many of the caregivers continue to carry a substantial burden of caregiving even after admission of the loved one to an LTC facility. Caring for a loved one who resides in an LTC facility can be rewarding, but also overwhelming at times. Factors that are stressful for family caregivers of LTC residents are different in many ways from those for family caregivers of elderly people living in the community. The job of professional caregivers for LTC residents is also uniquely challenging and stressful, due to their daily exposure to verbal and physical aggression, the burden of caring for "too many" residents, and low salaries. Nursing assistants in LTC facilities—who often experience harassment, threats, and assaults from residents—have the highest incidence of workplace assault among all workers (Bureau of Labor Statistics 2008). A substantial proportion (60%–80%) of aggressive incidents in LTC facilities goes unreported. One of the major problems for high-quality mental health care for LTC residents is the high rate of staff turnover (American Health Care Association 2002). In the United States, CNA turnover rates exceed 60 percent in 65 percent of the states, exceed 80 percent in 37 percent of the states, and are above 100 percent in 20 percent of the states. Also, the psychosocial well-being of family and professional caregivers needs to be routinely addressed, along with the psychosocial well-being of residents. This goal creates not only additional challenges of working in LTC, but also additional opportunities to enhance the quality of life for both residents and caregivers.

The Epidemiology of Disability

The residents' psychosocial well-being depends to a considerable extent on their functional abilities. Approximately 40–45 percent of assisted living residents have at least one disability in the basic activities of daily living, as do some 84–97 percent of nursing home residents. On average, some 21.2 percent of the nursing home population needs assistance for three to four ADLs, and 65.1 percent needs assistance for five to six ADLs. The functional status of most residents in LTC facilities usually declines with time. Improvement or maintenance of function, or slowing functional decline, rather than cure of the disease, is the major goal for LTC residents.

The Epidemiology of Physical Conditions

Almost 80 percent of the patients hospitalized for a stroke and 65 percent of the patients hospitalized for a hip fracture are discharged to skilled nursing facilities for rehabilitation services (Hoverman et al. 2008). The psychosocial well-being of LTC residents is also significantly influenced by comorbid physical conditions (table 1.2). Sensory deficits, urinary tract infections, dehydration, constipation, musculoskeletal pain, electrolyte imbalance, falls, and the psychotropic side effects of commonly prescribed drugs are some of the most common treatable physical conditions encountered in LTC populations. Gross hearing impairments and vision impairments are underdetected in a substantial number of LTC residents. Arthritis and osteoporosis are also underdetected and undertreated. Frequently, the work-up for infection is inadequate, and in 25–75 percent of the cases the antibiotics chosen are inappropriate. Untreated medical comorbidity contributes to reduced psychosocial well-being, increases the physical burden on the staff, decreases a resident's functional capacity, and interferes with that resident's ability to age in place. Thus both residents and staff can benefit from better diagnosis of, intervention in, and education regarding these commonly occurring and treatable conditions.

Trends in the Characteristics of Long-Term Care Residents

Over the past 20 years, financing changes, policy changes, and innovation in the private sector and the government have fundamentally altered the system of long-term care supports. Today's LTC residents differ from those admitted just 10 years ago, and residents 10 years from now will be different from today's residents. While the population aged 65 or older increased by 29 percent between 1985 and 2005, the number of older adults in nursing homes increased by only 10 percent. As a result, the use of nursing homes as a long-term residence for older adults with disabilities declined from 4.2 percent in 1985 to 3.6 percent in 2004. The use of nursing homes by the oldest old—those age 85 or older—declined even more sharply, from 21 percent in 1985 to 14 percent in 2004 (National Center for Health Statistics 2009). More than half of the decline in the rates of nursing home use among those age 85 or older occurred during the past six years. Possible reasons include new alternatives to nursing homes (e.g., assisted living facilities), less disability, improved financial resources of the oldest old, and alterations in the pattern of nursing home care.

LTC populations and their health care providers are changing on several other fronts: race, ethnicity, and sexual orientation. The first step is to recognize that the cultures of both the resident and the health care provider influence clinical care. The psychosocial needs of residents from ethnic minority and gay/lesbian groups may be considerably different from those of others. Health care providers need to keep pace with this diversifying population, understand their psychosocial needs, and ensure that the care delivered to them is culturally sensitive.

There are also changes in the patterns of nursing home use. The use of postacute short-term rehabilitation stays has increased (in response to changes in Medicare reimbursement and other forces), resulting in a decline in the average length of stay from 2.9 years in 1985 to 2.4 years in 2004, and in the median length of stay from 1.7 years to about 1.3 years. The proportion of stays paid for by Medicare increased from 1.5 percent in 1985 to 12.9 percent in 2005 (Cowles 2006). Those in nursing homes for long-term stays became frailer and more likely to have cognitive impairments. The proportion of residents needing assistance with five or six basic ADLs increased from one-half to almost two-thirds between 1985 and 2004. The combination of greater frailty and increased postacute stays results in nursing homes serving individuals with more acute and more complex medical needs.

The older population in alternative residential care is increasing rapidly, either as a substitute for or a precursor to traditional nursing homes. Over the last decade, (1) residential facilities, such as assisted living, that provide alternatives to nursing homes grew substantially; and (2) more home-based services became available through state-funded and Medicaid waiver programs for home- and community-based services targeting those at risk of nursing home entry. Families have also continued their significant role in providing unpaid care for frail and disabled older adults. Assisted living beds are increasing at a much higher rate than nursing home beds. From 1990 to 2002, the number of nursing home beds per 10,000 people declined, while assisted living beds increased.

The number of residents in LTC facilities who use wheelchairs or who have contractures has increased over the last 10 years. However, the single characteristic that evidences the greatest shift is the percentage of residents taking psychoactive drugs (antidepressants, antipsychotics, antianxiety drugs). Residents with dementia have dramatically increased to 50–100 percent (Zanni 2006). Ostomy care has also risen significantly in nursing homes, as has bowel and bladder incontinence. The number of dedicated long-term beds has expanded for dialysis, dementia, and ventilator needs, but it has decreased for AIDS, hospice care, and rehabilitation. There is also an improvement in service delivery trends, as LTC facilities may increase specialized services, such as hospice care, without creating separate units. The gender ratio has risen toward more women residents than men (3 to 1 currently), although there is a growing number of men in LTC, and they adapt differently from women.

Approximately 10 percent of all adults 65 or older now own an LTC insurance policy, which provides a small group of policy holders with the resources to choose where they want to receive care. Many states have tried to reduce the number of Medicaid recipients in nursing homes by providing more home- and community-based services, along with implementing preadmission screening or single-entry-point systems to divert people away from nursing homes. Measuring and improving the quality of care at all LTC facilities—not just nursing homes—is becoming a bigger issue for regulators.

The baby boom generation will have twice as many older adults in 2030 as today's cohort of older adults. While the number of LTC residents will invariably increase as a result of the aging of the baby boom generation, the use rate of LTC facilities (especially nursing homes, but also assisted living facilities) may continue to decline as innovative strategies are implemented to keep the elderly disabled population at home.

With longevity increasing, a growing emphasis on strategies promoting healthy aging, and an exponential growth in medical advances, the identity of LTC has changed and will continue to change. The current population shift is undoubtedly not the last. Population and its driving forces are not static, and the skills of health care providers should not be, either. More residents will be divorced, have stepchildren, come from different cultural backgrounds, and believe in active aging. Also, the children and spouses of residents may be more active, assertive, and involved, want to micromanage, and be more vigilant. There may be more choices and more frequent changes in LTC due to family dissatisfaction.

Conclusion
Our health care system is currently failing the nation's elderly population in long-term care when it comes to meeting their mental health needs, which are substantially underdetected and undertreated. This is happening despite increasing evidence that residents who receive treatment for mental health problems typically benefit considerably. Unfortunately, underdetection and undertreatment of mental health needs leads to profound social, economic, emotional, and medical costs. Greater effort needs to be devoted at all levels (academic centers, governmental [local, state, and federal], organizational,

individual, and societal [in terms of eliminating ageism]) to increasing the availability, accessibility, and affordability of mental health services for LTC populations. Failure to do so will risk a crisis in geriatric mental health in this most vulnerable elderly population, given the impending growth of the aging population and future projections of an increased prevalence of mental disorders.

CHAPTER 2

The Assessment Process

Regular screening, comprehensive assessment, and evidence-based, state-of-the-science treatment of mental disorders are central to high-quality care of residents in a long-term care facility. A comprehensive assessment process for initial evaluation involves a thorough history (from the resident, the family, and professional caregivers and by reviewing previous records); pertinent physical and neurological exams; a detailed mental status examination; standardized assessment scales; pertinent laboratory tests and brain imaging, if indicated; and good documentation. A good follow-up assessment involves pertinent information from the resident, the staff, and the resident's family; a focused mental status examination; assessment of the resident's response to treatment; and modification of the treatment plan as necessary. For all residents, the clinician should ask screening questions to identify any abuse or uncontrolled pain (table 2.1). The clinician should ask the resident at least one of the screening questions during each visit.

Although the initial interview focuses on gathering data to understand the etiology of the resident's behavioral and psychological symptoms in order to arrive at an accurate diagnosis and formulate a treatment plan, other equally important goals are to build a therapeutic relationship, instill hope in the resident and the family, sustain the resident's sense of self-worth, emphasize his or her strengths at the end of the interview, and review his or her past coping skills/successes. The primary reason for psychiatric consultation is to reduce behavioral and psychological symptoms, but mental health professionals also use this opportunity not only to address the particular symptoms that have triggered the assessment, but also to screen for any abuse and identify any overlooked excess disability (table 2.2). Mental health care providers

TABLE 2.1
Screening questions to assess abuse and pain

Abuse
   Is the staff treating you well?
   Is anyone bothering you?
   Are your needs being addressed?
   Is anyone trying to hurt you?
   Has anyone hurt you physically?
   Has anyone mistreated you?
Pain
   Are you in pain?
   Are you hurting anywhere?
   Do you have any aches or pains?
   Do you have a tingling or burning sensation anywhere on your body?

TABLE 2.2
Excess disability

Undercorrected vision or hearing impairments

Undercorrected pain

Untreated cognitive, behavioral, or psychological symptoms of dementia

Potentially inappropriate medication prescriptions[a]

Unnecessary medication (such as statins for a resident with advanced dementia, aspirin for a resident in hospice, proton pump inhibitors for a resident who does not have gastroesophageal reflux disease or another justifying medical condition)

Undercorrected medical problems (e.g., anemia, pressure ulcers, diabetes mellitus, congestive heart failure, obstructive sleep apnea)

Overcorrected medical problems (e.g., hypothyroidism, diabetes mellitus)

Limited mobility

Ill-fitting dentures

also have an opportunity to address the needs and concerns of the family and staff. Thus the assessment process should incorporate the well-being of the resident, the family, and professional caregivers. In addition, mental health care providers use each consultation as an opportunity to address environmental issues (e.g., adequate lighting of the facility) and cultural issues (e.g., negative attitude toward aging and disability, myths such as people with advanced dementia do not experience pain) that impose additional psychosocial stress on residents.

The etiology of behavioral and psychological symptoms involves four elements: predisposing, precipitating, perpetuating, and protective factors. Psychiatric symptoms should be conceptualized as an expression of the resident's unmet biological, psychosocial, and environmental needs (table 2.3), as any of these factors could be predisposing, precipitating, or perpetuating causes. For the majority of residents, behavioral and psychological symptoms are multifactorial. Thus even when the clinician identifies one factor (e.g., uncontrolled pain), he or she should look for other contributing factors (e.g., depression, an inappropriate medication prescription, untreated dementia). Assessments should also cover factors that may reduce the potential for behavioral and psychological symptoms. Behavioral and psychological symptoms, and the risk factors for them, are prevalent in LTC populations, so an assessment of these symptoms should occur regularly (e.g., on admission, at each quarterly review, when there is a significant change in the resident's condition, and whenever the clinician suspects behavioral or psychological symptoms) (table 2.4).

Strategies for Improving the Residents' Experience of the Assessment

For the initial and subsequent interviews or therapeutic sessions, we recommend a quiet, private place that is free from distraction, the presence of a trusted family member or staff member when possible, the use of the same place for each encounter, and sensitivity to the need for confidentiality. For residents receiving individual therapy or who wish to be interviewed alone, the clinician may dispense with the presence of family or staff members. For residents who are incapable of making medical decisions but who wish to be interviewed alone, the clinician would talk to the resident alone and then later consult with the family or with staff members about any medical decisions that would need to be made. For many residents (e.g., a resident who becomes agitated when moved to a different place or a resident who has lost the ability to communicate verbally), it may be appropriate to conduct a follow-up assessment interview in the same place where they were at the time of the initial visit (e.g., in the television room or in front of the nurses' station) rather than move them to a quiet room. For a thorough initial assessment, most residents need far more time and patience than a typical evaluation of a young adult that takes place in the clinician's office. The clinician should sit down for the initial assessment, but if the resident is being treated for certain infections (e.g., due to methicillin-resistant *Staphylococcus aureus* [MRSA] or *Clostridium difficile*), the clinician should avoid sitting on the resident's bed. It is important to be at eye level with the resident, with the clinician's face in clear view of the resident. The clinician may need to repeat information and ask the resident to verify what he or she heard the clinician say. If the clinician suspects uncorrected or undercorrected hearing or vision deficits, he or she should consider referring the resident to an audiologist or ophthalmologist before the next visit. For some residents (e.g., those who become easily

TABLE 2.3
Biological, psychosocial, and environmental needs of long-term care residents

Biological needs
  Food and water
  Clothing (for protection from cold, heat, sun, insects)
  Comfortable positioning (in a chair, in bed, etc.)
  Sexual needs
  Optimal vision and hearing
  Freedom from physical pain
  Treatment of medical conditions and medication-induced behavioral and psychological symptoms
  Treatment of behavioral and psychological symptoms of dementia
  Treatment of behavioral and psychological symptoms due to a preexisting severe and persistent mental illness (schizophrenia, bipolar disorder, other psychotic disorders)
  Treatment of behavioral and psychological symptoms due to other preexisting psychiatric disorders (major depression [single episode or recurrent], obsessive-compulsive disorder, panic disorder, social phobia, generalized anxiety disorder, personality disorder, etc.)
Psychosocial needs
  To be treated with dignity (to be respected, honored, valued, acknowledged)
  To be useful
  To engage in meaningful (purposeful) activities
  To be free from boredom
  To have companionship
  To have opportunities for creative expression
  To have opportunities for spiritual expression (including religious rituals)
  To be appreciated
  To be found attractive
  To be liked
  To be part of the community
  To be able to have a pet
  To be able to interact with children regularly
  To be close to nature
Cultural needs (language, ethnic food, ethnic clothing, celebration of ethnic festivals)
Environmental needs
  Physical environment
    Adequate natural light and artificial lighting
    Freedom from excessive noise
    A clean and pleasant-smelling environment
    Esthetics (paintings, sculpture, well-designed architecture that addresses the residents' unique cognitive, emotional, and spiritual needs, etc.)
    The ability to walk and wander safely
    Nature and natural surroundings
    Other safety needs (carpeting, etc.)
  Caregiving environment (includes professional caregivers [staff-resident interactions], family caregivers [family-resident interactions], other residents [resident-resident interactions], and volunteers [volunteer/visitor–resident interactions])
    The caregiver is not argumentative with the resident and does not frequently correct the resident's impaired memory
    The caregiver does not ignore the resident's nonverbal communications (e.g., caregiver is not too busy to realize that a resident has decreased his or her social interaction dramatically in the last few days)
    The caregiver does not ignore the resident's verbal communications (e.g., caregiver does not walk past a resident who is calling out "Help me, help me")
    The caregiver's expectations are not beyond the resident's capacity (due to cognitive or functional deficits)
    The caregiver does not perform a functional activity (e.g., bathing) that the resident can do on his or her own (if given time, props, and assistance)

continued

TABLE 2.3 *continued*

The caregiver does not provide too much stimulation or too many activities for the resident
The same caregiver provides consistent care (low staff turnover)
An adequate number of supervisory staff are present at mealtimes
Staff members, family, other residents, volunteers, and visitors treat all residents with dignity

TABLE 2.4
Key factors that may protect the resident from severe behavioral and psychological symptoms

Well-trained staff
An adequate number of staff members
Consistent staffing (staff caring for the same residents each day)
High staff satisfaction
Low staff turnover
Knowledgeable family members
Good social support
A continuous activity program
An intimate, homelike setting
A clean environment with plenty of natural light
A path to allow safe wandering or pacing
Planned admission to a long-term care facility
Experience with an adult day program before moving into a long-term care facility
Person-centered care strategies (e.g., dementia care mapping)
The availability of mental health care providers with geriatric expertise for routine rounds and consultation
Antidementia drugs for residents with dementia
The use of technology to reduce medication errors and inappropriate medication prescriptions
Palliative care programs

tired, frustrated, or agitated), two visits (either on the same day or on separate days) may be needed to complete the initial assessment.

The clinician should make sure that a resident who has impaired vision has eyeglasses and uses them, and that a resident who has impaired hearing has hearing aids and wears them (adjusted properly with the batteries in working condition). The clinician should also sit close to a resident who has a significant hearing impairment, speak into a particular ear if the resident prefers, and speak in a slow, clear voice with a low pitch. Some residents read lips to help them understand what is being said, so the clinician should sit where the resident can see his or her face. For residents with a visual impairment, verbal and physical (touch) communication may be more important than visual communication (e.g., facial expression, gestures). If the clinician needs to speak loudly, he or she should bear confidentiality in mind and avoid disturbing nearby residents. Some residents with dementia may become discouraged if the clinician's questions force them to acknowledge their cognitive deficit again and again. In such a situation, it is prudent to avoid detailed cognitive testing, at least until a rapport is established over time. Alternatively, the clinician may request that another trained member of the care team (e.g., another staff member) perform a standardized cognitive test.

A resident who has difficulty walking may have trouble meeting the clinician far from his or her own room. The clinician may need to arrange for a staff person to bring the resident in a wheelchair; alternatively, the clinician can wheel the resident. Residents who have chronic pain may find it difficult to sit comfortably in one position for more than a short time, so the clinician should offer breaks for repositioning. A resident who needs to use the restroom is likely to have difficulty concentrating, so the clinician should be aware of this need. The clinician should also pay attention to the temperature of the interview room, as it may be warmer or cooler than is comfortable for the resident. This needs to be addressed at the onset of the interview. Providing a comfortable chair for the resident, having a beverage available, keeping a box of tissues handy, and commenting on any memorabilia or pictures of family/friends in the room may enhance the resident's comfort level for the interview.

Changes in the body due to aging can leave residents feeling unattractive and untouchable. Thus holding a hand, touching the person gently on the arm, rubbing the person's back, commenting on his or her nice clothes, or giving the person a hug may be a rare and welcome connection for many residents, and the clinician should integrate touch and praise in the initial and follow-up encounters, as appropriate (both culturally and based on the resident's personal preferences). Many residents may view mental illness as a personal defect or as shameful and thus may not comply with an interview. It might be worthwhile for the clinician to anticipate this, have a friendly attitude, and consider sharing something from his or her own life to gain the resident's trust and put the person at ease so the interview can proceed. In fact, older adults may benefit from (indeed, may expect) a higher degree of personal disclosure than younger adults, especially in an LTC setting. For a resident who is skeptical about mental health treatment, actions such as sharing information about the clinician's training and experience, quoting research and support from reputable organizations, and requesting that the resident give the clinician a chance may help overcome the barriers to a mental health assessment. Understanding the resident's values, beliefs, and interactional styles, as well as the expectations of diverse cultures, is also important for establishing a therapeutic alliance.

Some other strategies to enhance the resident's experience and the quality of the assessment include limiting or eliminating extraneous noise (television, radio, trolleys), using short simple sentences, speaking slowly and clearly, giving the resident time to understand each short sentence, giving the resident time to reply (up to 20 seconds), writing down simple questions if the resident's hearing is severely impaired (or using preprinted cards with routine questions in large print), writing down simple questions if the resident has difficulty comprehending spoken language but not written language, pointing to objects or people as you mention them, being literal and avoiding the use of metaphors, breaking down commands into a series of individual steps (task segmentation), having the staff or family members repeat the questions if necessary (especially if the clinician is from a different cultural or ethnic heritage), and coming back at a later time if the resident is agitated, eating, or sleeping.

For residents who speak limited or no English, the presence of a family or staff member who speaks the resident's language is necessary. In many cultures, there may be a lack of understanding about dementia and the potential benefits of psychiatric intervention. Thus the clinician may need to educate the resident and his or her family members before starting the assessment process.

The Process Itself

The assessment process includes how psychiatric consultation is initiated, the initial evaluation, follow-up assessments, and documentation.

Who Initiates Psychiatric Consultation?

The most common process involves the staff recognizing the need for psychiatric consultation because they suspect a resident is depressed (e.g., is frequently tearful, is losing weight), agitated (persistent yelling, sexually inappropriate behavior), or aggressive (verbal and physical aggression) and the staff are unable to manage with psychosocial interventions. Often the resident's family requests a psychiatric consultation because they suspect the person is depressed or anxious, especially if the person has a past history of psychiatric illness or if there is a family history of psychiatric illness. Occasionally, the primary care provider (physician, nurse practitioner, or physician's assistant) initiates a psychiatric consultation, either because the resident continues to be psychiatrically ill (resistant depression, persistent aggression) despite treatment with psychiatric medications, or because of the health care provider's reluctance to give antipsychotic medications due to recent warnings by the U.S. Food and Drug Administration (FDA) concerning increased mortality and cerebrovascular events. For residents in nursing homes that receive federal funding, the presence of preexisting severe and persistent mental illness requires an evaluation by a psychiatrist. An ombudsperson may recommend psychiatric assessment if he or she suspects abuse or neglect.

Any other team member (e.g., pharmacist, dietician) may also initiate a psychiatric consultation. Managers (e.g., directors of nursing, assistant directors of nursing) should empower all staff members to initiate a psychiatric consultation, with the help of the resident's primary nurse. Referral to a pharmacist to review the resident's medications before a psychiatric consultation (especially if the resident is taking several medications) is also good practice, as the pharmacist can play a crucial role in identifying drug-induced cognitive and other psychiatric symptoms, correcting dosages of psychotropic medications because of the resident's liver and/or kidney impairment, spotting potentially inappropriate medications, and noticing potential adverse interactions between psychotropic and nonpsychotropic medications. Documented consent from the resident or the surrogate health care decision maker (or both) for an interview to assess behavioral and psychological symptoms is necessary. A formal order for psychiatric consultation from the resident's primary care physician should be in the resident's record before the assessment.

Initial Evaluation

HISTORY   A thorough history is the crucial first step in the assessment process. The clinician obtains this history from the family member and the staff member (typically the CNA primarily assigned to the resident) who are most familiar with the resident, as in most (but not all) situations the resident may not be able to give a reliable history, due to dementia or other impairments (e.g., aphasia, dysarthria, severe hearing deficits). It may be useful to consult with family members and significant others to elicit any family history of psychiatric illness (e.g., dementia, depression, psychoses) and prior psychotic or affective episodes. It is also important to assess the context in which the resident's psychiatric problems are arising. For example, a resident may be agitated because of a roommate problem. Although this concern needs to be addressed specifically, it might be worthwhile inquiring whether the resident has had difficulty reaching out to others in a constructive way in the past.

HISTORY OF THE PRESENT ILLNESS   It should be mentioned from the start in the notes whether the history is obtained primarily from the resident, the family, or a professional caregiver. The history of the present illness should elicit details about the chief complaint (a description, its frequency, its intensity, the context in which it occurs, triggers, relieving factors), other symptoms accompanying the chief complaint, and psychiatric symptoms (anxiety, depressive, psychotic, sleep, impulse control [aggressive, sexual], appetite). The clinician should look for predisposing and precipitating factors. Is excessive demand or stress placed on the resident? Is there a balance between sensory-stimulating and sensory-calming activities? Is there sufficient human interaction for this particular resident?

How the resident, the family, and the staff rate the resident's quality of life can give valuable insights into the severity and nature of the problem. A resident's poor ratings for his or her quality of life usually indicate symptoms of depression, anxiety, or pain. Poor ratings by the staff usually indicate that the resident has behavioral problems (Hancock, Livingston, and Orrell 2006).

It is important for the clinician to inquire into the reason for the resident's admission to LTC and whether the admission was planned or not. Planned admission usually helps reduce agitation and depression after admission. Also, admission to LTC due to behavioral and psychological symptoms related to dementia or a stroke gives some indication of the seriousness and chronicity of the behavioral and psychological symptoms. Behavioral and psychological symptoms in the context of being in the LTC facility for only a few days or a few weeks may indicate that the resident is still adjusting to the loss of his or her previous home and the stress of living with strangers.

It is important to inquire about potential triggers for the agitated behaviors. Caregivers may report that a problem behavior occurred out of the blue, but a detailed analysis of problematic behavior often indicates a specific trigger. For example, analysis of an occasion in which a resident resists bathing and becomes physically aggressive during bathing may indicate that the behavior happened after a specific event, such as a Hoyer lift moving upward, a whirlpool motor being turned on, the shock of skin first touching water, or the resident being unable to see the caregiver during the bath.

Withdrawal, restlessness, procrastination, and escapism (such as watching television all day) may suggest depression. Many residents are unlikely to express their feelings of sadness or hopelessness. Grumbling about head-aches, backaches, or other physical complaints may be other signs of depression and a reaction to multiple loses (e.g., loss of independence, loss of a reason to live, loss of a spouse, loss of home, loss of the ability to drive, lack of adequate opportunities for sexual expression).

The analysis of the person's symptoms (anxiety, depression, pain, etc.) should be detailed, but it can be short. In addition to documenting symptoms, the initial assessment should include the effectiveness of previous efforts to relieve these symptoms, the resident's, family's, and staff's satisfaction with current symptom management, and other diagnoses or comorbidity that may contribute to the symptoms. This helps develop and implement an individualized care plan.

To encourage reporting, it is important for the clinician to ask about behavioral and psychological symptoms in different ways. For example, the clinician could ask "Are you feeling down?" or "Are you feeling 'blah'?" or "Are you happy?" or "If you had one wish, what would it be?" The response to the last question may often give a glimpse into what losses the resident is dealing with currently. Some common answers to this question include "I wish to go home," "I wish I could walk," "I wish I could remember." Behavioral and psychological symptoms are often nonspecific. Many residents, including some who do not have a cognitive impairment, cannot readily report or describe behavioral and psychological symptoms in terms of their duration, their severity, their onset, precipitating and perpetuating factors, factors that relieve symptoms, or any responses to previous treatments. Thus it is necessary to seek as much objective information as possible to distinguish various causes, as the treatment alters with the cause.

The clinician should differentiate verbal and physical agitation (such as repetitive questioning, pacing) from resistance to care (resistance to assistance with ADLs, eating, taking medications), as they are distinct behavioral problems that require different management strategies.

Assessment of Specific Behavioral and Psychological Symptoms
This includes an assessment of suicidality and violence, sexually inappropriate behavior, and sleep disturbances.

ASSESSMENT OF SUICIDALITY AND VIOLENCE   Suicidality is one of the most serious clinical concerns in LTC residents. Demographic factors (older age, male gender, white race), the presence of a mood disorder (most notably depression), physical health factors (e.g., high medical comorbidity), and social factors (e.g., stressful life events, low social interaction) increase the risk of suicidality. A past history of suicide attempts is one of the most important risk factors for future suicidality. Most studies have not associated dementia with suicidality (Conwell et al. 2002).

With residents who are cognitively intact, the clinician should ask about any history of the person expressing suicidal or self-harming thoughts, plans, behaviors, or intent; whether the resident has considered specific methods for suicide, their lethality, and the resident's expectation about lethality, as well as the resident's accessibility to means (firearms, hoarding medications, use of a cord round the neck, etc.); evidence of hopelessness, impulsiveness, agitation, anxiety, or aggression; the resident's reasons for living and plans for the future; current use of alcohol; thoughts, plans, or intentions of violence toward others; and overt behaviors indicating suicidal gestures, attempts, or intentional aggression toward others (staff, residents, visitors) outside of the context of personal care. The clinician also needs to assess previous suicide attempts, other self-harming behaviors, a family history of suicide, previous or current medical diagnoses (especially severe pain, visual impairments, neurological disorders, and malignancy) and the resident's psychosocial situation (acute crises/losses, chronic stressors [financial, interpersonal conflicts, etc.], support system, cultural and religious beliefs about death or suicide). Finally, the clinician should inquire into individual strengths and vulnerabilities (coping skills, personality traits [high rigidity, low openness to experience], past responses to stress, capacity for reality testing, ability to tolerate psychological pain and satisfy psychological needs). To assess physical aggression, the clinician should look into various predisposing factors. The severity of a cognitive impairment is the most significant predisposing factor for aggressive behavior among older adults in LTC facilities. Physical and chemical restraints are also associated with aggressive behavior. Orbitofrontal injury due to stroke, head injury, and the like is strongly correlated with impulsive aggression.

ASSESSMENT OF SEXUALLY INAPPROPRIATE BEHAVIOR   The clinician should inquire about details of sexually inappropriate behavior (the setting, the context, an exact description of the behavior, its frequency, the staff's approach, the outcome of the staff's approach) so that he or she can differentiate between true sexually inappropriate behavior (e.g., a resident masturbating during personal care) and pseudosexually inappropriate behavior (e.g., a resident disrobing due to feeling hot). The clinician should inquire about residents who display sexually aggressive behavior (e.g., repeatedly grabbing the private parts of staff), have a past history of sexually inappropriate behavior, have a past history of sexually abusive behavior toward a spouse or partner, or have a legal history (e.g., for pedophilia). Is the staff approach therapeutic? Does the staff support an appropriate expression of the resident's sexual needs (e.g., give the resident an opportunity to masturbate in his or her room with the door closed)? Does the staff ignore inappropriate behavior and thereby inadvertently give a wrong message that the behavior is acceptable? To understand and treat sexually inappropriate behavior, the clinician needs to ask all of these questions.

ASSESSMENT OF SLEEP DISTURBANCES   The clinician should inquire about excessive daytime sleepiness, nighttime snoring, complaints of leg discomfort, crossing the legs repeatedly, rubbing the legs, pacing, flexing the legs, general restlessness, constant movement of the legs at night, and the presence of any strange behavior in the middle of the night in residents with insomnia, in order to identify a variety of sleep disorders such as obstructive sleep apnea (OSA), restless leg syndrome (RLS), periodic limb movement disorder, and rapid eye movement (REM) sleep behavior disorder. Does the resident get enough exercise in the daytime (e.g., a program of walking)? Is the resident exposed to natural sunlight or enough bright light during the day? At night, are any loud noises or bright lights disturbing the resident? Is the resident taking several naps during the day? Does the resident go to bed at the same time and wake up at the same time? Could any medications or foods (e.g., caffeine-containing drinks and food items) be causing the sleep problems? Are there any medical issues (e.g., pain, frequent urination at night) that could be causing sleep problems? These questions help identify the causes of sleep problems and their potential remedies. The clinician should evaluate any resident for sleep disorders whose depression has been treated but who has residual symptoms of depression, such as insomnia.

Allergies

The clinician should note allergies to medications and differentiate them from adverse effects. Many adverse effects can be managed, but an allergic reaction means that the person should not take that drug in the future.

Current Medications

The clinician should thoroughly review all medications the resident is taking, both on a routine basis and on an as-needed basis. The clinician should ask about the frequency of the resident's use of as-needed medications and the response to these medications. To clarify the possibility of medication-induced (or medication-withdrawal-related) behavioral and psychological symptoms, the clinician should inquire into any recent reduction or discontinuation of psychoactive drugs. The clinician should specifically inquire about any use of over-the-counter medications, vitamins, herbal remedies, and nonherbal supplements, because some cognitively intact residents and some family members may administer such medications without the knowledge of the staff. The clinician should also look for any correlation between the onset of behavioral and psychological symptoms and the start of a new medication (e.g., onset of behavioral and psychological symptoms after starting an antibiotic or a steroid medication).

Past Psychiatric History

The clinician should inquire about any past history of clinically significant psychiatric symptoms (depression [may be expressed as "nervous breakdown," "postpartum nervous breakdown," etc.], long-standing anxiety [expressed as "I have always been a worrier," "he/she has always been hyper, easily stressed"], psychotic symptoms [expressed as "nervous breakdown"]), their treatment (with psychotropic medications, counseling, electroconvulsive therapy ["shock treatment"], hospitalization in an inpatient psychiatric unit), and the person's response to treatment.

Use of Street Drugs, Tobacco, Prescription Drugs, or Alcohol

The clinician should ask about alcohol use, as many residents continue to drink alcohol on a daily basis after moving into an LTC facility. One or two alcoholic drinks may not have been a problem for most of a resident's life, but with the development of dementia or other serious medical conditions, the same amount may be sufficient to cause significant cognitive, behavioral, affective, or psychotic symptoms or symptoms of anxiety. The clinician should also inquire into the use and abuse of prescription drugs (e.g., benzodiazepines, opiates), caffeinated drinks, tobacco (smoking, chewing), street drugs (marijuana, cocaine, etc.). The clinician should request information about any recent cessation or resumption of cigarette smoking, because of the potential for chronic smoking (using nicotine) to induce cytochrome P450 1A2 isoenzymes, which in turn may affect drug levels of certain psychotropic medications (e.g., clozapine, olanzapine, fluvoxamine) metabolized by 1A2 isoenzymes.

Medical History

An assessment of behavioral and psychological symptoms includes inquiring about potentially undiagnosed current medical conditions, as well as a review of preexisting medical conditions. Table 2.5 lists common medical conditions that are often the primary cause of or exacerbate behavioral and psychological symptoms in LTC populations. For residents with a severe cognitive/intellectual impairment (e.g., advanced dementia, aphasia, severe mental retardation), psychiatric symptoms such as agitation may be the first or only manifestation of an underlying medical disease. The clinician should use nonverbal behaviors, vocalizations, changes in function, and caregiver reports to assess pain in residents who are unable to report pain due, to severe cognitive impairments. Aggressiveness and resistance to care, for example, may be attempts to guard against pain caused by movement. Auditory behaviors that suggest pain include moaning, growling, and an increased loudness

TABLE 2.5
Common medical causes of behavioral and psychological symptoms in the long-term care population

Medication-induced
Hearing and/or vision impairment
Urinary tract infection
Constipation
Fecal impaction
Pain (acute or chronic)
Pressure ulcers
Dry skin
Dehydration
Malnutrition
Electrolyte imbalance
Urinary retention
Congestive heart failure
Acute renal failure
Pneumonia
Gastroesophageal reflux disease
Obstructive sleep apnea
Severe anemia
Other (intestinal obstruction, skin rash, bedsores, gallstones, etc.)

of vocalizations. Resistance to mobility may be due to arthritic pain rather than depression.

Failure to recognize physical health conditions as underlying cause(s) of behavioral and psychological symptoms may result in the inappropriate administration of psychiatric medications that may further obscure an underlying medical condition, sometimes with fatal consequences. If a resident needs an antipsychotic medication, the clinician should assess cardiovascular and cerebrovascular risk so that he or she can compare the individualized risk of stroke, sudden cardiac death, and mortality associated with the use of antipsychotic medication to its potential benefits before initiating any short- or long-term administration of antipsychotic medications. Residents with a history of incontinence may show problem behaviors as a consequence of incontinence, so the clinician should inquire whether a toileting schedule and prompted voiding has been implemented.

A resident who has vision problems and needs eyeglasses may not be actively using the glasses for a variety of reasons (e.g., the resident is too cognitively impaired to request them, the glasses are broken or misplaced, the staff is not aware that the resident uses glasses, or the prescription is no longer sufficient to correct vision problems). The clinician should inquire whether the glasses are labeled, whether the resident has an extra pair, and whether the resident is receiving an annual or biennial eye exam. A resident who has hearing problems and needs hearing aids may not be actively using the hearing aids for similar reasons. In addition, the hearing aids may need new batteries, the resident may be too cognitively impaired to know how to use them or may often misplace them, the hearing aids do not fit well or hurt, or the hearing aids were not functioning well. Furthermore, the staff may not have received training in the use and maintenance of hearing aids. Also, there is often no delegation of responsibility for managing the resident's hearing, and family members are frequently expected to maintain hearing aids.

Is the resident dehydrated? The resident may say "No" when asked "Are you thirsty?" because normal aging decreases the sensation of thirst. Pain is another vital sign, and the clinician should inquire about pain during any evaluation of behavioral and psychological symptoms. When a resident with a cognitive impairment reports pain, the clinician should believe it. Residents who have dementia but retain the capacity to communicate may not be able to give all the details of their pain, but they often are able to give important information regarding the presence of pain, its intensity, and its location. The assessment of a resident's pain should always involve input from caregivers. Frequently a resident denies pain during the interview, but caregivers are able to give a detailed description of the resident's verbalizations and behaviors that strongly indicate the presence of significant pain. For example, many residents with gastroesophageal reflux disease (GERD) may not have typical symptoms, such as heartburn, abdominal pain, and indigestion. In contrast, other symptoms, such as weight loss, anorexia, and anemia, may be the only manifestation of GERD. Although the typical features of OSA are snoring and daytime sleepiness, its presentation with neuropsychiatric symptoms (e.g., confusion in the daytime and hallucinations at night in a resident who is overweight and has hypertension) is not uncommon.

The clinician should also inquire about any past history of hospitalization or a stay in an intensive care unit. For many people with dementia or who are frail, hospitalization is extremely stressful. Repeated or prolonged hospitalization is associated with serious psychiatric sequelae, such as delirium, depression, agitation, and anxiety.

Social, Spiritual, and Developmental History

The clinician should ask questions to elucidate a premorbid personality (personality characteristics before the onset of dementia). For example, "agreeableness" as a personality trait is associated with less agitation after one develops dementia. Hostile, antisocial, or paranoid characteristics can make it difficult to establish a therapeutic alliance. A resident who has always been timid, passive, and dependent may have difficulty being assertive with the staff or expressing ideas or concerns. It is important to distinguish between characterological features that are part of the resident's premorbid nature and those that emerged as a consequence of dementia, a stroke, or another neurological disorder. Statements from family members—such as "He was never as short-tempered as he is now" or "Ever since I've known him, he has been pessimistic"—help the clinician understand a resident's personality problems.

Because a person's spiritual beliefs may be an important source of strength and comfort, the clinician should assess the degree to which the resident relies on spiritual beliefs to cope with life's difficulties. An assessment of spirituality may include questions such as Is spirituality important for the resident? How does the resident express and experience spirituality? Has the resident been actively religious throughout life? What spiritual/religious rituals did the resident engage in before living in an LTC facility? The clinician should also obtain information regarding the resident's occupational history, the extent of his or her education, previous traumatic events (if any, and the resident's ability to cope with those events), previous losses, hobbies and interests, and what the resident has been passionate about. Some inquiry into whether the resident had an abusive or exceptionally difficult childhood may help the clinician and staff develop compassion for the resident who is behaving in an abusive manner.

Legal History

A past history of felony due to violence, incarceration due to sexually abusive behavior toward children, or driving under the influence of drugs or alcohol are some of the many situations that the clinician should inquire into if any of these are indicated from current behavioral problems and other historical information. Although most residents who engage in sexually inappropriate touching do not have any past history of pedophilia, residents who engage in sexually violent behavior may have such a past history; family members may not have been forthcoming with this information but may acknowledge it if specifically asked.

Assessment of Caregivers

A resident's behavior can be substantially influenced by the caregiver's (family and professional) attitude, emotions, and behavior. An assessment of the family and staff's beliefs about aging, disability, life in an LTC facility, and death is an important part of the assessment process, especially during end-of-life care. Family and/or professional caregivers (staff) who feel uncomfortable about issues of loss of control, who are anxious about physical illness or death, or who are anxious about "losing one's mind" in the context of dementia may see the residents' suffering and depression as an unavoidable and normal part of aging. Family and/or staff may believe that residents are not interested in sexual activity or in expressing sexuality. Thus they may neglect residents' sexual needs and fail to understand the residents' suffering in relation to this. Family and/or staff may doubt that mental health treatment can be of any benefit to a resident with advanced dementia and may not be forthcoming in their input during the assessment process. Family and/or staff may be reinforcing a resident's dependency by doing things that that person is capable of doing. Family relationships that have been poor for many years may inhibit progress by dredging up old conflicts that undo gains the mental health treatment may make in a resident's mood and attitude. Family members may be experiencing significant emotional distress (e.g., anxiety over a loss of control, guilt, grief), which in turn may lead to unrealistic expectations from the treatment team and even to hostile interactions with members of the team. Also, if the family or staff caregiver is overburdened, he or she may have little motivation to cooperate with the clinician's recommendations, which may further increase stress and the risk of caregiver burnout and breakdown.

Family and staff members are an important resource in the accurate assessment of behavioral and psychological symptoms and in implementing a treatment plan. The clinician should assess and acknowledge the strengths of family and staff in the initial and subsequent encounters. Building a therapeutic bond with the family is important not only in achieving a family member's well-being, but also in partnering with that person to improve the resident's quality of life.

Examination of Previous Records

Because of diagnostic complexities, the clinician should review all previous diagnostic evaluations (psychiatric and medical). This is especially helpful with residents who have a psychiatric illness that existed before the disability caused by dementia, a stroke, or other disabling conditions that precipitated functional decline and admission to LTC. Examining previous psychiatric records will help in the differential diagnosis, as will soliciting direct input from previous mental health care providers. In complex cases, it may be worthwhile to review all previous diagnostic evaluations and consider consulting with the resident's nonpsychiatric care providers. Many elderly persons carry "labels" of problems and take medications for years, only to realize later that they never had the problem in the first place or perhaps that no one thought to discontinue the medication. Clinicians need to recognize that valuable information is often omitted during the transition from a hospital to an LTC facility (and vice versa). Use of the Universal Transfer Form (www.amda.com/tools/) can facilitate the transfer of necessary patient information between care settings.

Reviewing the Minimum Data Set

The Minimum Data Set (MDS) is part of the federally mandated Resident Assessment Instrument developed as a primary assessment tool for residents in skilled nursing facilities. Items in the MDS include demographics and patient history, functional capabilities, cognitive and mood/behavior patterns, psychosocial well-being, the use of medication, continence, nutritional and dental status, activity patterns, and potential for discharge. The MDS helps LTC staff identify health problems on admission, and quarterly thereafter, to create a comprehensive care plan for each resident. The MDS can give the clinician significant information and thus make further information gathering and assessment easier.

Elucidating Residents' Existing Strengths and Skills

Inquiring about a resident's current strengths and skills is as important as inquiring about the etiology of current behavioral and psychological symptoms (table 2.6). Even in the moderate stages of dementia, residents retain the ability to recognize new images. They may maintain appropriate social behavior in a one-on-one interaction in the face of extreme cognitive difficulties, which suggests that basic responses to social cues are retained throughout the course of the illness.

Pertinent Physical and Neurological Examinations

If the clinician suspects delirium, infection, or an exacerbation of underlying medical conditions (congestive heart failure, chronic obstructive pulmonary disease [COPD], etc.), he or she should measure the resident's vital signs. If the resident is complaining of pain in a limb or another site, we recommend a brief examination of the site during the initial psychiatric evaluation. If the resident grimaces, moans, or pulls away when the limb is moved, he or she could be experiencing pain. Physical examination should focus on the potential etiology of pain. The clinician should pay specific attention to a neurologic examination for paresthesia, hyperesthesia, numbness, or allodynia, and to the muscular system for signs of tenderness, inflammation, deformity, or trigger points. If the resident is not moving any limb, the clinician should assess whether this is part of the resident's baseline deficit or a new problem. We also recommend a routine assessment of posture and movement for all residents who may need antipsychotic medications. Does the resident have a stooped posture, an unsteady gait, or involuntary movements (tremors, akathisia, tardive dyskinesias, myoclonic jerks)?

　　If the clinician suspects abuse, he or she should look for lesions that do not appear to be organically caused (bruises under the breast, in the armpit, or behind the knee) and for patterns of injury (e.g., two black eyes without scratches or injuries to the nose, indicating that the black eyes were not due to a fall). We recommend a physical examination to assess signs of dehydration. Poor turgor of the central skin (tenting of the skin over the forehead,

TABLE 2.6
Assessment of strengths and skills

Language	Vision
Cognition	Hearing
Social/interpersonal	Gardening
Ambulation	Spirituality
Physical strength	Self-care
Sense of humor	Altruism
Cooking	Reading
Musical abilities	

sternum, thigh, or subclavian area) is a better indicator of hydration status in elderly individuals than turgor of peripheral skin (tenting of the skin over the dorsum of the hand, which may occur with normal age-related loss of subcutaneous tissue). Some residents who say they are not thirsty may enthusiastically drink an entire glass or two of water or other liquid (all at once or in frequent small sips) when it is offered.

Detailed Mental Status Examination

A detailed mental status examination involves:

Alertness: Is the individual awake and alert, or drowsy, sleepy, oversedated?

Orientation: Is the individual oriented to time, place, and person?

Attention: Is the individual attentive, inattentive, or distractible?

Appearance: Is the individual well-groomed or unkempt, disheveled; does the resident look the stated age or older or younger?

Eye contact: Does the individual make eye contact, or instead look down during the interview (taking into account impaired vision or hearing)?

Attitude: Is the individual cooperative, or defensive, taciturn, distrustful, or hostile?

Behavior: Does the individual show normal psychomotor activity, or exhibit restlessness (increased psychomotor activity) or have psychomotor retardation? Is the resident calm, or yelling or showing other signs of agitation?

Mood (subjective emotional state): Does the individual voice a depressed or anxious mood, a fearful mood, an apathetic mood?

Affect (objective emotional state at the time of the interview): Does the individual look sad, depressed? Is the individual tearful, anxious, fearful, perplexed? Does the individual have a bright and cheerful affect or an euthymic and broad affect?

Speech: Does the individual have language deficits orally, in writing, in reading, or globally (deficits in comprehension [receptive aphasia], or expression [expressive aphasia], or both [global aphasia])? Does the individual have difficulty finding words? Does the individual have slurred speech or other forms of dysarthria? Is the individual's speech normal in tone and volume, or loud? Is the individual's flow of speech rapid and difficult to interrupt (pressure of speech) or slow (slowness in thinking or bradyphrenia)?

Thought processes: Are the individual's thought processes coherent and logical or incoherent, illogical, difficult to follow, tangential? Does the individual show perseveration (giving the same answer to a different question)? Does the individual show flight of ideas (jumping from one topic to another rapidly, with the topics related somehow)?

Thought content: Does the individual have paranoid ideas/delusions (e.g., others are stealing his or her belongings), other delusions (grandiosity, jealousy, infidelity, persecution, somatic complaints, delusional mis-identification)? Does the individual have ideas of hopelessness, helplessness, guilt, and worthlessness? Does the individual have suicidal or homicidal ideas, intentions, or plans?

Memory: Does the individual have impaired short- or long-term memory?

Insight: Does the individual have good insight into his or her illness and disability? Does the individual have intellectual but not emotional insight? Is the individual in denial?

Judgment: Assess judgment by asking the individual what he would do if he found a stamped and addressed envelope on a road. Most residents may not need their judgment formally tested because of a significant cognitive impairment or obvious evidence of impaired judgment during the interview process. Assess social judgment by observing the individual's verbal and physical behavior during social interactions and in social settings. Does the individual show normal test and social judgment? Does the individual show impaired social judgment (e.g., by sexually disinhibited behavior)?

Standardized Assessment Scales

Table 2.7 lists recommended scales for standardized assessments of cognition, function, behavioral and psychological symptoms, pain, and caregiver grief. Although standardized assessment scales may require an additional two to ten minutes to complete, their routine use (at least in complicated or

TABLE 2.7
Recommended standardized assessment scales

Cognitive assessment scales
  Mini-Mental State Examination (MMSE)
  Saint Louis University Mental State (SLUMS) examination
  Tests for executive function: Trail Making Test-Oral Version (TMT-Oral) and Controlled Oral Word
    Association Test (COWAT)
  Test to detect delirium: Confusion Assessment Method (CAM)
Functional assessment scales
  To measure instrumental activities of daily living (IADLs): Functional Activity Questionnaire (FAQ)
  To measure basic activities of daily living (ADLs): Physical Self-Maintenance Scale (PSMS), Katz
    Index of Independence in Activities of Daily Living, and Barthel Inventory
Behavioral and psychological symptoms assessment scales
  For depression: Geriatric Depression Scale (GDS) and Cornell Scale for Depression in Dementia
    (CSDD)
  For agitation: Behavioral Symptoms in Alzheimer's Disease (BEHAVE-AD), Cohen-Mansfield
    Agitation Inventory (CMAI), and Neuropsychiatric Inventory-Nursing Home Version
    (NPI-NH)
Pain assessment scales
  Visual analog scale
  Iowa Pain Thermometer
  McGill Pain Questionnaire
  Pain Assessment in Advanced Dementia (PAINAD)
  Doloplus–2
Caregiver grief assessment scales
  Zarit Burden Inventory (ZBI)
  Marwit-Meuser Caregiver Grief Inventory (MM-CGI)

treatment-resistant cases) can help the clinician avoid (or discontinue) futile treatments and measure the resident's response to each new intervention. Staff training to administer most of the standardized assessment scales can greatly improve the clinician's assessment process and the staff's understanding of the problems. Although the majority of the recommended scales have not been rigorously researched regarding their reliability (inter-rater and intrarater) and their validity and ease of clinical use in LTC settings, they are clinically important tools. In assessing behavioral and psychological symptoms, standardized screening and assessments of the risk of falls, nutritional status, dehydration, and frailty may also be necessary for many residents.

Cognitive Assessment Scales

MINI-MENTAL STATE EXAMINATION   The Mini-Mental State Examination is commonly used as a screening tool for cognitive function in LTC. In the MMSE, residents are asked to respond to a ten-minute, 30-point questionnaire that assesses memory, orientation skills (e.g., time, place, naming), reading/writing, and the ability to follow a three-stage command. The MMSE is scored from 0 to 30 points; the lower the score, the greater the cognitive impairment. Individuals with dementia usually score no higher than 24 points. Although MMSE scores on average may decline by three to four points per year in people with Alzheimer disease, there is usually a substantial variability in the rates of decline among residents with dementia. The MMSE is a highly sensitive screening tool for moderate to severe dementia and thus is ideally suited for LTC residents, because most residents with dementia are within this range. Many residents (especially highly educated residents) with mild dementia do not score below 24 (the generally accepted cutoff score). If the clinician has a high index of suspicion based on the individual's history, neuropsychological testing can confirm the diagnosis of dementia.

The MMSE can also be used for staging dementia in Alzheimer disease (Perneczky et al. 2006). MMSE scores range from 21 to 24 for mild, 11 to 20 for moderate, and 0 to 10 for severe dementia. Clinical use of the MMSE became more expensive since Psychological Assessment Resources purchased its copyright, and photocopying and Internet downloads of the form without permission are no longer allowed. To print a copy of the MMSE test form and to purchase the MMSE, go to www.minimental.com.

SAINT LOUIS UNIVERSITY MENTAL STATE EXAM   The Saint Louis University Mental State (SLUMS) examination, developed by the Division of Geriatrics at the Veterans Affairs Medical Center and Saint Louis University, is another tool that can be used to screen for dementia in LTC populations (http://aging.slu.edu/). Its advantage over the MMSE includes no copyright restrictions (i.e., it is freely available) and it may be better at detecting residents with mild dementia and those with mild cognitive impairment (MCI) (Tariq et al. 2006).

COGNITIVE PERFORMANCE SCALE   The Cognitive Performance Scale (CPS) was generated from five MDS items: comatose status, short-term memory, daily decision making about tasks or ADLs, the ability to communicate, and self-performance in eating. The CPS is used to assign residents in nursing homes to easily understood categories of cognitive and functional performance.

ASSESSMENT OF EXECUTIVE DYSFUNCTION   Executive dysfunction refers to deficits in initiating, planning, and modifying goal-directed behavior (Elliot 2003). Assessing executive function can help determine a resident's capacity to execute health care decisions and discharge-planning decisions. With impaired executive functioning, the resident's capacity to exercise command and self-control and to direct others to provide care becomes diminished. The oral version of the Trail Making Test (TMT-Oral), is a simple bedside screening test for executive dysfunction. This test elicits mental flexibility, which is impaired in people with executive dysfunction. The TMT-Oral requires the individual to count from 1 to 26 and then recite the 26 letters of the alphabet. For testing, the resident is asked to pair numbers with letters in sequence (e.g., 1-A, 2-B, 3-C, etc.) until he or she reaches the pair 13-M. More than two errors in 13 pairings are considered impairment (Ricker and Axelrod 1994).

The Controlled Oral Word Association Test (COWAT) is another simple test that assesses working memory (attention-concentration), which is impaired in people with executive dysfunction. With categories beginning with the letter *F*, then *A*, then *S*, the COWAT requires individuals to fill each category by providing words composed of three or more letters. For example, correct responses to the category cue *F* would include "fish," "foul," "fact," and the like. Individuals who do not have executive dysfunction will produce 10 words in each category within one minute (Spreen and Benton 1977). We also recommend an assessment of executive dysfunction for residents who are significantly impaired in the ADLs but have minimal or only mild impairment on the MMSE.

TESTS TO DETECT DELIRIUM   One effective instrument for diagnosing delirium is the Confusion Assessment Method (CAM) (Inouye et al. 1990). CAM is used primarily to detect delirium in a hospital setting, but it may be used for LTC populations, especially with residents who have just been transferred from the hospital.

Functional Assessment Scales

Functional impairment is a key criterion for the diagnosis of dementia. A functional assessment helps determine an individual's ability to perform the basic ADLs needed for personal care as well as the more complex tasks needed for independent living (instrumental activities of daily living, or IADLs). We recommend the Functional Activity Questionnaire (FAQ) (Pfeffer et al. 1992) to assess IADLs and the Physical Self-Maintenance Scale (PSMS), the Katz Index of Independence in Activities of Daily Living (S. Katz et al. 1970), or the Barthel Inventory (Mahoney and Barthel 1965) to assess basic ADLs. The severity of dementia correlates closely with a progressive loss of function. The least complex ADL is eating and the most complex is bathing. Hence it is not surprising that bathing is the ADL most commonly associated with severe behavioral consequences.

Behavioral and Psychological Symptoms Assessment Scales

For an assessment of depression in LTC residents, we recommend the Geriatric Depression Scale (GDS) (15- and 30-item versions) for residents who have an MMSE equal to or greater than 15 and the Cornell Scale for Depression in Dementia (CSDD) for residents with an MMSE of less than 15 (Yesavage et al. 1983; Alexopoulos et al. 1988). For assessing behavioral and psychological symptoms, we recommend one of the following measurement tools: the Behavioral Symptoms in Alzheimer's Disease (BEHAVE-AD) (Reisberg et al. 1987), the Cohen-Mansfield Agitation Inventory (CMAI) (Cohen-Mansfield, Marx, and Rosenthal 1989), and the Neuropsychiatric Inventory-Nursing Home version (NPI-NH) (Wood et al. 2000). These measures can be used to establish a baseline and assess responses to treatment. These measures also help the clinician decide not to reduce or to discontinue antipsychotic medications for some residents (residents with continued moderate scores in these measures) and to try reducing or discontinuing antipsychotic doses for others (e.g., residents who have low scores on these measures).

The BEHAVE-AD test involves asking the individual questions covering behaviors over the most recent two weeks in seven domains: paranoid and delusional ideation, hallucinations, activity disturbances, aggressiveness, a disturbance of diurnal rhythms, affective disturbances, and anxieties and phobias. There are 25 questions with answers rated from 0 to 3. The staff is then asked to assign a global rating from 0 (not at all troubling to the caregiver or dangerous to the patient) to 3 (severely troubling or dangerous). The CMAI rates 14 areas of distressed behavior, including hitting, verbal aggression, grabbing, constant requests for attention, repetitive sentences, weird laughter, and hiding or hoarding things. The frequency of these behaviors is tabulated on a five-point scale, from never to a few times per hour. The NPI-NH is a 12-item scale that measures the frequency and severity of behavioral and psychological symptoms such as agitation, anxiety, apathy, irritability, and disinhibition over the preceding four weeks. The staff provide information regarding the resident's behavior and associated caregiver stress. If the symptom has been present, the rater answers yes, rating the frequency and severity, and then caregiver distress, on five-point scales. Scores range from 0 to 144, with higher scores indicating greater disturbance.

Pain Assessment Scales

For individuals who are relatively cognitively intact and those with mild to moderate dementia, a visual analog scale is quick and reliable (Scherder and Bouma 2000). A visual analog scale documents the intensity of pain on a simple scale of 0 to 10 (0 being no pain and 10 being the worst pain). Other scales, such as the Iowa Pain Thermometer and the McGill Pain Questionnaire, may also be used (Herr et al. 2007). We recommend observational/ behavioral scales, such as the Pain Assessment in Advanced Dementia (PAINAD) scale or the Doloplus-2 scale, for residents with moderate to severe cognitive impairment or who are uncommunicative (Lefebvre-Chapiro and Doloplus-2 Group 2001; Warden, Hurley, and Volicer 2003; Tait and Chibnall 2008). The clinician may also consider facial expression scales for residents with impaired communication (Herr et al. 1998).

Assessment of Caregiver Burden and Grief

We recommend the Zarit Burden Inventory (ZBI) and the Marwit-Meuser Caregiver Grief Inventory (MM-CGI) to identify issues of caregiver burden, grief, and loss in the family caregivers of residents (Zarit, Reever, and Bach-Peterson 1980; Marwit and Meuser 2002). The ZBI is a 22-item questionnaire, with each item scored from 0 to 4. The total score ranges from 0 to 88, and a high score correlates with a higher level of burden. The clinician may also consider administering a 12-item short version and a 4-item screening version to assess caregiver burden (Bedard et al. 2001). The MM-CGI, an 18-item inventory filled out by family caregivers, allows the psychiatrist to target specific interventions such as support groups, respite, stress management, and coping with grief.

Laboratory Tests

If tests for liver function (serum bilirubin, liver enzymes, and serum albumin) and kidney function (serum blood urea nitrogen [BUN] and serum creatinine levels) have not been done in the last three months, the clinician should order them. More recent tests may be needed if there has been a significant recent change in the resident's physical functioning. Due to recent reports of sudden cardiac death associated with the use of antipsychotic drugs, the clinician should obtain a baseline electrocardiogram (EKG) before initiating such drugs. For residents in a hospice or in the terminal stage of dementia, these baseline blood tests may not need to be ordered. Additional tests include a basic metabolic panel (including serum levels of sodium, potassium, BUN, and serum creatinine) to detect electrolyte imbalance and renal insufficiency, urine analysis (and culture and sensitivity if indicated) to detect a urinary tract infection (UTI), thyroid-stimulating hormone (TSH) levels to detect thyroid disorders, and vitamin B_{12}, folate, and vitamin D levels to assess the etiology of new-onset or resistant behavioral and psychological symptoms.

If the clinician suspects infection (such as pneumonia), a complete blood count (CBC) may be added, although frail LTC residents may not have the elevated white blood cell count typically seen in community-dwelling healthy adults who have pneumonia. The clinician should also consider subtle seizure disorder in the differential diagnosis of new-onset or atypical psychiatric syndromes, and he or she may order an electroencephalogram (EEG) and referral to a neurologist. The clinician should consider ordering free testosterone levels for male residents with a suspected androgen deficiency syndrome, manifesting as fatigue, depression, weight loss, cognitive impairment, and sarcopenia (muscle cell loss). In some situations, the clinician may need to order a polysomnogram or a nocturnal pulse-oximetry to evaluate the resident for sleep disorders, such as OSA, RLS, periodic limb movement disorder, and REM sleep behavior disorder.

Neuroimaging

The clinician should consider neuroimaging for residents who have a suspected new stroke or a fall with a head injury and for residents who have a dementia that has not been evaluated in order to identify its cause, unless the resident is in the severe or the terminal stage of dementia, or the terminal stage of any other condition, or in a hospice. Computed tomography (CT) of the brain is the neuroimaging of choice for residents who have advanced dementia and residents who require urgent neuroimaging, as it takes less time and is less affected by motion artifacts than magnetic resonance imaging (MRI).

Assessment of Residents with Severe and Persistent
Mental Illness

Severe and persistent mental illness includes schizophrenia, schizoaffective disorder, and bipolar disorder. The MDS is not a suitable rating instrument to evaluate the symptoms and functional characteristics of LTC residents with severe and persistent mental illness (Bowie, Fallon, and Harvey 2006). A mental health care provider should perform a thorough assessment and review previous records for all residents with severe and persistent mental illness.

Screening Tests

No screening test should be used in isolation. Nor should screening be based on chronological age; but it should instead be targeted to a high-risk group. We recommend screening all residents for dementia on admission to LTC (if not formally diagnosed) and every six months after that. Screening tests for dementia include the MMSE and SLUMS. Mandatory screening for depression in LTC facilities can improve treatment rates (C. Cohen, Hyland, and Kimhy 2003). We recommend screening for depression using the GDS or CSDD. The nine-item depression scale of the Patient Health Questionnaire (PHQ-9) has been validated for depression screening in primary care (Spitzer, Kroenke, and Williams 1999). A study found that the PHQ-9 was more reliable and efficient than the GDS screen and took less time to complete (Saliba 2008). The MDS 2.0 scale is not reliable for detecting depression in nursing home residents. Screening for depression should take place two to four weeks after admission to an LTC facility and be repeated at least every six months (American Geriatrics Society and American Association for Geriatric Psychiatry 2003b). New onset or a worsening of symptoms should prompt an assessment that includes psychological, situational, and medical evaluations. The clinician should refer residents with suicidal ideas, those with psychotic symptoms, and those who have not responded to six or more weeks of treatment to a mental health care provider.

We recommend screening residents for pressure ulcers using the Braden Risk Assessment Scale, ideally within eight hours of admission, and implementing preventive actions in the first 24 hours for those identified as being at risk (Braden and Bergstrom 1989). We also recommend screening hospice care residents with a limited life expectancy (e.g., those with severe and terminal-stage dementia, or end-stage congestive heart failure and COPD, or those who are completely dependent on the staff for basic ADLs). Although no specific screening tools have been devised to identify residents in need of hospice care, any resident who has an MMSE of two or less, is fully dependent on caregivers for all ADLs, is unable to recognize family members, and has an acute decline in health should be referred to a hospice for evaluation. We also recommend screening residents for pain on admission and then every one to four weeks. The clinician may also consider periodically screening for fall risk, dehydration, malnutrition, and frailty. Screening guidelines should take into account the potential benefit versus the burden and, most importantly, the resident's preferences. The clinician may discontinue futile medical screening tests such as a colonoscopy, breast clinical and self-examinations, mammography, and tests for lipid levels for residents with a limited life expectancy (e.g., less than five years), which would be the majority of LTC residents. Futile testing may cause considerable psychosocial stress in LTC populations.

Developing an Individualized Care Plan and Implementing and Coordinating Treatment

The clinician should work with the resident, the family, and the staff to develop and implement an individualized care plan for behavioral and psychological symptoms. We recommend figuring out which interventions are realistic and then monitoring (and documenting) the response to the interventions. The clinician should try to anticipate adverse events (e.g., constipation with pain medication) and plan interventions for them. It is not enough for the clinician to be ready to assess and manage behavioral and psychological symptoms among LTC residents; the rest of the staff has to be trained to assess such symptoms, monitor interventions, and document their findings. This training should also be aimed at overcoming any biases or misconceptions about behavioral and psychological symptoms. For example, in the case of opiates for pain management, some certified nursing assistants may not understand the differences among tolerance, physical dependence, and addiction. Educating the staff will improve resident care as well as the facility's performance on surveys. Coordinating care with the hospice when the resident is receiving hospice care is also important, as the LTC facility is still responsible for any uncontrolled behavioral and psychological symptoms and pain.

While the patient's self-report contains important information, an additional direct examination is needed to help the clinician identify the characteristics and possible causes of behavioral and psychological symptoms. Therefore, a self-report should not be the sole basis for discussing behavioral and psychological symptoms with a clinician or for initiating treatment. It is important to seek a cause for behavioral and psychological symptoms. However, it is also reasonable to try to address behavioral and psychological symptoms even if the cause is unknown—although this should be done carefully.

Behavioral and psychological symptoms need to be managed one step at a time. Often a serial trial of different interventions is needed before the clinician identifies a final group of interventions (psychosocial-environmental and pharmacological) that are effective.

During the development of a treatment plan, the first concern to be addressed is whether the resident's behavioral and psychological symptoms are so severe that they cannot be safely managed in the LTC facility and may require transferring that individual to an inpatient psychiatric unit (preferably a geropsychiatric unit) in a hospital.

Follow-Up Assessments

Follow-up assessments are usually much shorter than the initial assessment, although with complicated cases or with the emergence of new problems, follow-up assessments may take considerable time. Follow-up encounters with family members to address palliative care and other treatment concerns also require a longer time. During follow-up, the clinician should assess all residents for adequate pain management, signs of abuse, sleep patterns, nutritional status (Are they eating well? Are they losing weight?), and, if ambulatory, whether they have been experiencing falls or have an unsteady gait. At some point during the follow-up for all residents (and during the initial assessment for residents in the terminal stage of dementia or another medical condition), we recommend a discussion with the resident and the family regarding palliative care goals, when to forgo life-prolonging treatments, and when to consider hospice care. For residents with advanced cognitive impairment, we recommend some simple questions (table 2.8). Even if a resident with moderate dementia does not accurately report whether he or she slept

TABLE 2.8
*Some questions to ask during follow-up with residents
who have moderate to severe dementia*

Moderate dementia (open-ended questions)
How are you doing?
Do you have any complaints?
Are you hurting anywhere?
Did you sleep well last night?
Do you like the food?
Are you nervous?
Are you tired?
If you had one wish, what would it be?

Severe dementia (primarily simple yes or no questions)
Are you hurting?
Are you in pain?
Are you hungry?
Are you thirsty?

well or is eating well, the answers to these questions may reflect that person's current subjective emotional state (positive answers indicate subjective well-being and negative answers indicate a lack of well-being at that moment).

Assessment Pearls

The assessment process in LTC populations is as much an art as a science, especially for residents with severe cognitive impairments. The typical questions to assess depression (e.g., "Over the past two weeks, have you [has the resident] felt down, depressed, or hopeless?" or "Over the past two weeks, have you [has the resident] felt little interest or pleasure in doing things?") are useful, especially for residents who are cognitively intact, but they often do not identify depression, due to a resident's cognitive impairment or to cultural issues (many aged residents associate feeling depressed with a lack of inner strength [or personal failure] and thus say "No" to feeling depressed). Statements such as "I am a burden" or "I wish I were dead" and suicidal ideas, plans, and attempts are obvious signs of depression. Table 2.9 lists some assessment pearls for LTC residents.

Documentation

The goal of good documentation is to record what was done, the findings of the assessment, the diagnosis, and the treatment plan. Such a document helps all members of the treatment team have access to and understand the outcome of the assessment. Thorough and accurate documentation is crucial to a high-quality assessment process and for medicolegal purposes; it can also serve as a good teaching tool for new staff members. The documentation can be handwritten (if the writing is legible) or dictated (especially for an initial evaluation or, if one's handwriting is not legible, even for follow-up notes) or typed. Some nursing homes have implemented electronic medical records, and the clinician may document the assessment directly in the electronic record. The clinician may use preprinted templates for the resident's history and physical examination and for follow-up notes, but adequate individualized information is necessary for this documentation to be clinically useful.

LTC facilities should have a system in place to formally carry out the recommendations of a mental health consultant. This usually involves informing the primary care physician, who then authorizes the consultant's recommendations after the resident or surrogate legal decision maker expresses agreement with these recommendations. In some situations, the mental health consultant is given the privilege of (or is expected to take responsibility

TABLE 2.9
Assessment pearls

Depression in residents with moderate cognitive impairment
Multiple somatic complains
Irritability and verbally abusive behavior
Procrastination
Escapism (e.g., watching television all the time)
Avoidance of socialization
Pain not improving with standard treatment

Depression in residents with severe cognitive impairments
Depressed affect (tearfulness, looks sad)
"Help me, help me" statements
Persistent yelling
Restlessness
Verbal and or physical aggression
Resistance to care with activities of daily living

Delirium
Acute (one to five days) change in mental status (certified nursing assistant or housekeeping staff
reports that the resident is not acting like him- or herself)
Acute onset of disorientation (in a resident who is generally at least partially oriented to time and
place), distractibility, disorganization in thinking and/or speech
Acute onset (over one to five days) of depression
Acute onset (over one to five days) of not eating
Acute onset (over one to five days) of agitation
Sudden exacerbation of previously well-controlled behavioral and psychological symptoms
Frequent napping, but can be aroused
New onset of an inability to repeat a five-digit number

Psychoses
Ask if the resident feels safe in the long-term care facility
Ask if the resident believes the food is poisoned
Ask if the resident believes people are talking about him or her
Resident yells at imaginary people
Resident shows verbal and or physical aggression
Resident engages in sexually aggressive behavior
Resident complains of a strange smell in the room or to food

---

for) direct management of the resident's behavioral and psychological symptoms, writing the recommendations as orders directly in the resident's chart; the primary care physician and the resident or surrogate legal decision maker are then informed about these orders. The privileges, expectations, and roles of the mental health consultant should be clarified before he or she begins routine rounds for the psychiatric care of residents. Usually the original document is kept in the resident's chart in the LTC facility and a copy is placed in the resident's chart in the consultant's office. Any changes made to the treatment plan or any specific test result that is not being addressed should be documented, and the reason for what is done or not done should be stated. Such notes must conform to standard billing codes.

Enhancing the Efficiency of Psychiatric Rounds in Long-Term Care Facilities

We recommend assigning a specific staff person (e.g., nurse or social worker) to accompany and thus improve the efficiency of rounds by the mental health care provider. This staff person can be titled a *mental health navigator*. The mental health navigator is available for two to six hours during rounds days; maintains a "mailbox" for the mental health care provider where the staff can leave messages (often a notebook for writing specific resident concerns); is responsible for preparing a list of residents to be seen, involving family members in the assessment and treatment process (informing the family about the visit and the results of the assessment and encouraging their active participation), keeping the charts and documentation ready on the day of the rounds, and locating residents and having them ready when they are to be seen (if necessary, with the help of the CNA and/or charge nurse); and acts as a liaison between team members and consultants. The mental health navigator could also become the facility's mental health expert through hands-on coaching (on the assessment of behavioral and psychological symptoms and on problem solving) taught by the mental health care provider during rounds. The mental health navigator can become the mental health care provider's eyes and ears, be able to think like the mental health care provider, and help the facility solve problems even before the mental health care provider does an assessment.

In complex or treatment-resistant cases, we recommend a mini-huddle in which team members gather for a few minutes to problem solve, identify potential etiological factors for behavioral and psychological symptoms, and discuss both treatment strategies that have been tried and failed and those that need to be tried. We recommend that the team adopt the BEST approach: identify the biological, environmental, social/psychological, and treatment-related factors that are contributing to continued behavioral and psychological symptoms. For example, the mini-huddle can quickly identify biological factors (medications, medical condition), social and psychological factors (lack of companionship, boredom), environmental factors (overstimulation of a resident, a new caregiver who needs more training because the caregiver is telling the cognitively impaired resident [who is looking for his or her mother] that the mother could not possibly be alive), and treatment factors (which of the previous recommendations were carried out, barriers to the implementation of previous treatment [e.g., lack of confidence by the staff or the resident's family regarding aromatherapy as an effective intervention; overexpectation from the staff or the family that medications will "fix" the problem], identifying treatment recommendations that are impractical or unsustainable [such as staff members staying one-on-one with the resident]).

Conclusion

Behavioral and psychological symptoms of long-term care residents are among the most challenging to assess and manage. No known intervention—whether psychosocial-environmental or pharmacologic—is invariably effective. Therefore, it is essential to follow a systematic process to evaluate and manage behavioral and psychological symptoms. Good intentions must be combined with clinical knowledge, skill, and creativity.

CHAPTER 3

Dementia

Dementia is a progressive impairment in cognition and the ability to reason, which substantially interferes with one's abilities to perform daily activities and live independently and may eventually cause death. Cognition is a combination of skills, including attention, learning, memory, language, praxis, recognition, and executive functions such as decision making, goal setting, planning, and judgment (Grossberg and Desai 2006). Recent estimates indicate that more than 5 million Americans have Alzheimer disease (AD) and related dementias (Alzheimer's Association 2009). The report notes that between 200,000 and 500,000 people younger than 65 have some form of early-onset (young-onset) dementia. This includes frontotemporal dementias (FTDs) and rare forms of AD that affect people in their 30s, 40s, or 50s.

Approximately 30 percent of all individuals with dementia are cared for in a long-term care facility; the other 70 percent live in their homes or in the community (Caselli et al. 2006). A high proportion (80%–90%) of people with dementia eventually require admission to an LTC facility. Approximately 66–80 percent of LTC residents have dementia (Tariot et al. 1993; Magaziner et al. 2000; Rosenblatt et al. 2004), and some assisted living facilities and nursing homes are designed for and care exclusively for people with dementia. As many as 90 percent of the residents with dementia have behavioral and psychological symptoms. The average length of stay in a nursing home for people with dementia is two to three years, because many of them first go to an assisted living facility; by the time they move to a nursing home, they are in more advanced stages of dementia. However, with the availability of hospice care for people with terminal dementia who have an acute decline, many assisted living residents spend their last years entirely in the assisted living facility. On average, LTC residents with dementia require 229 more hours of care annually than residents who do not have dementia (O'Brien and Caro 2001). An accurate diagnosis of dementia, finding its cause, and instituting appropriate treatment for residents with cognitive impairments is critical for improving their quality of life.

Causes of Dementia

There are many causes of dementia (table 3.1), 90 percent of which result in progressive, irreversible dementias. The relative frequencies of AD and vascular dementia (VaD) increase with age, whereas the relative frequencies of FTD and dementia with Lewy bodies (DLB) decline with age. Males predominate among those with DLB, whereas females predominate among those with AD where the age of onset is over 70 (Grossberg and Desai 2003a).

Probable Alzheimer Disease

AD is an age-related irreversible dementia that develops over a period of several years. It is the most common cause of dementia in people aged 65 or

TABLE 3.1
Causes of dementia

Progressive irreversible dementia
    Common irreversible dementias
        Alzheimer disease
        Dementia with Lewy bodies
        Vascular dementia
        Parkinson disease dementia (includes Parkinson disease-plus syndromes)
        Frontotemporal dementia (includes the frontal lobe variant of frontotemporal dementia,
            progressive nonfluent aphasia, semantic dementia, and amyotrophic lateral sclerosis-
            associated dementia)
    Irreversible dementia in a high-risk population (e.g., intravenous drug abusers)
        HIV-associated dementia
    Rare causes of irreversible dementia
        Huntington disease
        Creutzfeld-Jakob disease
Potentially reversible dementia (acronym: DEMENTIAS)
    D: Depression
    E: Endocrine problems (thyroid disorders, adrenal gland disorders)
    M: Medications (prescription and over-the-counter)
    E: Epilepsy (status complex partial epilepsy)
    N: Nutritional (chronic malnutrition [due to celiac disease, other causes], vitamin deficiencies
        [B_{12}, folate, thiamine]), normal pressure hydrocephalus, and obstructive hydrocephalus
    T: Tumor (brain, paraneoplastic limbic encephalitis), toxicants (such as pesticides)
    I: Infections (syphilis, Lyme disease, sequelae of encephalitis), inflammation (central nervous
        system vasculitis due to autoimmune disorders [such as systemic lupus erythematosus]
        and other causes)
    A: Alcohol and street drugs
    S: Subdural hematomas and sleep apnea (especially obstructive sleep apnea)

older, accounting for 60–75 percent of all causes of dementia (Grossberg and Desai 2003b). Insidious onset and a slow but relentless decline in cognition that impairs one's ability to perform daily activities are the most striking features of AD. There is no cure. It is estimated that 2–5 percent of people over the age of 65 and up to 33 percent of those over 85 have the disease. More women than men have AD, and the longer life span of women may be the key factor in this preponderance (Baum 2005). Other contributing factors for women may be a lower burden of cerebrovascular disease, the loss of the protective effects of estrogen, and less testosterone in women than in men. A definitive diagnosis of AD is possible after death (during brain autopsy), when the plaques and tangles of the disease can be seen under the microscope in specific areas of the brain and correlated with clinical manifestations of AD.

The typical clinical syndrome of AD includes an amnestic type of memory defect with difficulty learning and recalling new information, and progressive language disorder, beginning with anomia and progressing to fluent aphasia (Cummings and Cole 2002). Short-term memory deficits are classic, with the individual's remote memory remaining intact until the severe stages of AD. Some people with incipient memory loss are aware of their declining abilities, but most never acknowledge that they have significant memory dysfunctions. It becomes obvious over time to family and friends that persons with incipient dementia routinely forget recent events and conversations and repeat themselves. Behind a forgetfulness that appears benign may be more serious mistakes, such as forgotten bills, missed appointments, improperly taken medications, and misdirected travels.

Deficits in executive function and disturbances of visuospatial skills (manifested by environmental disorientation) are usually absent or mild in early AD but become evident in the more advanced stages. Sometimes, anomia or visual agnosia can be nearly as prominent as anterograde amnesia in AD. People with Down syndrome have a high risk of developing AD by the time they are in their 40s or 50s. The clinician should interview a knowledgeable informant, because genuine memory failure should be evident to those who are close to the individual.

Criteria for Probable Alzheimer Disease
The diagnosis of AD is made by using criteria established by various authorities, such as the National Institute of Neurological and Communicative Disorders and Stroke and the *Diagnostic and Statistical Manual of Mental Disorders*,

fourth edition, text revision, or DSM-IV-TR (American Psychiatric Association 2004). Probable AD is determined when a person has

- dementia confirmed by a clinical and/or a neuropsychological examination;
- problems in at least two areas of cognitive functioning (memory, language [aphasia], praxis [apraxia], recognition [agnosia], and executive function [e.g., impaired judgment]);
- progressive worsening of memory and other cognitive functions;
- no disturbance of consciousness; and
- no other disorders that might account for the dementia.

Other typical areas of cognitive impairment besides memory in people with AD or other dementias include aphasia, agnosia, apraxia, and executive dysfunction.

APHASIA   Aphasia (called *dysphasia* if mild) is a loss of language ability. Expressive aphasia is a loss of the ability to convey oral or written information to others. Anomia, or difficulty finding words, is a common form of expressive aphasia in mild AD. A loss of verbal fluency is profound in individuals with moderate and severe AD, although, unlike those who have some types of FTD (especially progressive nonfluent aphasia), mutism is rare. Receptive aphasia is the loss of one's ability to understand the meaning of oral and written language. Comprehension breaks down in those with moderate to severe AD, and both literal and semantic paraphrases are prominent. Examples include not understanding questions or instructions and not being able to express what one wants to say. The clinician may consider referral to a speech therapist for residents with mild dementia and significant expressive aphasia.

AGNOSIA   Agnosia is the inability to recognize familiar objects by sight (visual agnosia), touch (tactile agnosia), sound (auditory agnosia), smell (olfactory agnosia), or taste (gustatory agnosia). Examples include not recognizing one's favorite chair (hence family or staff should avoid rearranging the furniture in the resident's room), not recognizing one's home, and eventually not recognizing one's family and friends. Frequent if brief visits may help delay the loss of recognition of family and friends.

APRAXIA   Apraxia (called *dyspraxia* if mild) is characterized by a loss of the ability to execute or carry out skilled movements and gestures, despite having the desire and the physical ability to perform them. Apraxia results from a dysfunction of the parietal lobe. Examples of apraxia often seen in residents with dementia include ideational apraxia (the inability to coordinate activities with multiple, sequential movements, such as dressing, bathing, and eating) and constructional apraxia (the inability to copy, draw, or construct simple figures).

EXECUTIVE DYSFUNCTION   Executive function is an interrelated set of abilities that includes cognitive flexibility, concept formation, and self-monitoring. Executive dysfunction results in impairments in decision making, goal setting, planning, and exercising good judgment. Assessing executive function can help determine a resident's capacity to make health care decisions. It is seen early in FTD, in some people with major (clinical) depression, and in the advanced stages of other degenerative dementias (e.g., AD and DLB). It is also seen in people who have had a stroke involving the frontal lobe (especially the dorsolateral prefrontal area) and its projections from the basal ganglia.

The Five Stages of Alzheimer Disease

There are five stages of AD: preclinical, mild, moderate, severe, and terminal. The clinical stages (mild, moderate, severe, and terminal) span five to eight years on average (with an overall range of two to 20 years) after diagnosis. The length of survival depends on one's age at the onset of symptoms (the younger the age, the longer the survival) and comorbid conditions (especially cerebrovascular disease). For residents older than 85, survival after the onset of dementia may be much shorter, three years on average (Wolfson et al. 2001).

Preclinical

AD begins in the entorhinal cortex, which is near the hippocampus and has direct connections to it. It then proceeds to the hippocampus, the structure that is essential to the formation of short- and long-term memories. The affected regions begin to atrophy and show a loss of synapses. These brain changes start at least 10 years before any visible signs and symptoms appear. Memory loss, the first visible sign, is the main feature of the amnestic type of mild cognitive impairment (aMCI). Many experts think aMCI is often an initial, transitional phase between normal brain aging and AD. Changes in mood (irritability, depression, anxiety) and personality (passivity) may predate cognitive symptoms by years in people with AD. This stage can last 10–30 years.

Mild Alzheimer Disease

As the disease begins to affect the cerebral cortex, memory loss continues and changes in other cognitive abilities (e.g., language, praxis) emerge. A clinical diagnosis of AD is usually made during this stage. Signs of mild AD can include memory loss, repetitive statements, taking longer to accomplish normal daily tasks, trouble handling money and paying bills, poor judgment leading to bad decisions, loss of spontaneity and a sense of initiative, confusion about the location of familiar places (getting lost begins to occur), mood and personality changes, and increased anxiety. With mild AD, one's physical abilities do not decline. Thus the individual seems healthy, but is having more and more trouble making sense of the world.

At a casual glance, these early symptoms can be confused with changes that accompany normal aging. With systematic inquiry, the clinician can reliably diagnose early AD. Mild AD does not usually result in a need for LTC unless the person has a serious disability due to other medical conditions, such as a stroke or end-organ failure. Agitation is seen in 20–45 percent of people at this stage, especially in the latter half of its time range. Major depression may be present in up to 20 percent of those with mild AD, and a depressed mood and sadness may be seen in 50–60 percent. Symptoms of anxiety are also common. This stage can last two to 10 years.

Moderate Alzheimer Disease

By the moderate stage, AD-induced cell death has spread to the areas of the cerebral cortex that control language, reasoning, sensory processing, and conscious thought. More intensive supervision and care become necessary, and many people are admitted to an LTC facility in the latter part of this stage. The symptoms of moderate AD include increasing memory loss and confusion; a shortened attention span; problems recognizing distant friends and family members; difficulty with language; problems with reading, writing, and working with numbers; difficulty organizing thoughts and thinking logically; an inability to learn new things or to cope with new or unexpected situations; occasional muscle twitches; loss of impulse control (e.g., sloppy table manners, undressing at inappropriate times or places, or vulgar language); and perceptual-motor problems (e.g., difficulty rising from a chair or setting the table). Stored long-term memories may be more-or-less spared early in this stage, prompting family members' comments such as "She remembers what happened a long time ago better than I do."

Behavioral and psychological symptoms of dementia are often the most disturbing aspect of moderate AD. Individuals evince more severe behavioral and psychological symptoms of dementia at the moderate stage than at the mild stage (Cummings 2005). The dominant behavioral and psychiatric symptoms are delusions, depression, anxiety, irritability, and agitation (restlessness, pacing, wandering). Delusions and hallucinations are much more likely in this stage than in the mild or terminal stages. At this stage, the incidence of delusions is reported at 37 percent, and of hallucinations, as high as 24 percent (Lyketsos et al. 2000). Paranoid delusions are the most usual type of false belief; commonly occurring delusions include "Someone is stealing my belongings" and "My spouse is having an affair." Psychotic symptoms frequently contribute to agitation and aggression (Gilley et al. 1997). Depression is also seen in this stage and may contribute to physical aggression (Lyketsos et al. 1999a). Major depression occurs in 10 percent of those with moderate AD, whereas the prevalence of a depressed mood and sadness is 58 percent. In moderate AD, depression often coexists with prominent anxiety symptoms. The leading features of depression in the later part of this stage may be an inversion of day and night, agitation, and aggression (Cummings 2005). Aggression occurs in 20 to 30 percent of the individuals at this stage and appears to vary with severity, correlating with frontal lobe dysfunction, a decline in ADLs, and greater cognitive impairment. The frequency of agitation is 40–55 percent and increases from the early part of this stage to the later part. Agitation is associated with shouting, pacing, restlessness, and wandering. Shouting is also associated with the later part of this stage, as shouting, although inappropriate, is a means for those with moderate AD to communicate their emotions and discomfort.

Problems of gait and movement at this stage contribute significantly to functional decline (Feldman and Woodward 2005). Some 30 to 60 percent of individuals with moderate AD may develop mild extrapyramidal symptoms (EPS) such as amimia, bradykinesia, gait impairment, parkinsonism, and paratonic rigidity (Mitchell 1999). Gait apraxia, ascribed to impaired frontal lobe function, occurs with increasing frequency. It includes a constellation of impaired trunk and leg movements as well as impaired postural reflexes, disequilibrium, dyskinetic movements, and problems with locomotion (Della, Spinnler, and Venneri 2004). Falls are associated with the severity of AD; more than one-third of residents with moderate AD experience this problem

(Camicioli and Licis 2004). The ability to move themselves and other objects about is impaired in those with moderate to severe AD. For example, a person with AD kneels on a chair instead of sitting or does not sit all the way down (i.e., lowering him- or herself part way and then getting back up). Breaking down the task into small steps by giving verbal and tactile clues (guiding the person with one's hands) helps address this problem. This stage can last one to eight years.

Severe Alzheimer Disease

The hallmark of severe AD is profound cognitive impairment. At this stage, the person may not even know his or her own name or recognize a spouse or children. Verbal ability is restricted to answering yes or no to simple questions. Even with advanced dementia, many people still have some fleeting memory of loved ones, which can surprise family and staff members. A resident who has not spoken for months may suddenly respond to his spouse's voice, and someone who has not responded to her spouse's presence may suddenly pick up the spouse's hand, kiss it, and say "love you." These moments of explicit residual continuity with the past may be most evident in the morning, after the resident has had a good night's rest. Such moments are extremely meaningful to the family. One of the authors distinctly remembers a resident who had never spoken to him or a staff member for six months suddenly blurting out "You know, I have Alzheimer's" during his visit with her. Both urinary and fecal incontinence frequently develop in those with severe AD. Incontinence is a major factor associated with the decision of caregivers to seek to admit the person to LTC (P. Thomas et al. 2004). This stage can last one to four years.

Terminal-Stage Alzheimer Disease

In the last stage of AD, plaques and tangles are widespread throughout the brain and large areas of the brain have atrophied further. Persons at this stage of dementia have lost all ability to communicate and are completely dependent on others for care. All sense of self seems to vanish. Other symptoms can include weight loss; seizures; skin infections; difficulty swallowing; groaning, moaning, or grunting; increased sleep; and a lack of bladder and bowel control. At the end, individuals may be in bed much or all of the time. As their bedridden status develops, contractures commonly occur. Myoclonus, either focal or multifocal, transient or recurrent, may also occur. Even here, some people with dementia may have emotional moments of relational recollection. But by now all of these individuals are extremely feeble, have limited mobility, and will begin to die of such things as sepsis related to incontinence or aspiration pneumonia or skin ulcers; cardiac arrest; or secondary to minimal oral intake and inanition. At this stage, in effect they are dying, and it may be appropriate to refer them to a hospice, especially after a superimposed new medical problem or sudden decline occurs. This stage can last from two months to up to two years.

Lewy Body Disease

Between 15 and 20 percent of all cases of dementia in autopsied elderly people are due to Lewy body disease, making it the most common type of dementia after AD (Barker et al. 2002; McKeith et al. 2003; Stewart 2006). Lewy bodies are round collections of proteins in the brain that are considered to be the pathological hallmark of DLB. Lewy bodies are never found in healthy normal brains. In DLB, Lewy bodies are found in the cortex as well as in an area of the brain stem called the *substantia nigra*.

The cognitive disorder in DLB is characterized by prominent anterograde amnesia and may be indistinguishable from AD. However, the most common patterns of cognitive deficits in DLB are distinct from those in AD. In AD, the first loss in thinking skills is in memory; in DLB, the earliest loss appears to be in attention and visual perception. Hence DLB has also been described as *visual-perceptual dementia* and *attentional-executive dementia* (Collerton et al. 2003). Individuals with DLB may have slightly better confrontational naming and verbal memory functions than individuals with AD, but the former have worse executive and visuospatial functions. DLB symptoms vary a great deal more from one day to the next than do symptoms of AD. In addition, up to 81 percent of individuals with DLB have unexplained periods of markedly increased confusion that lasts from days to weeks and closely mimics delirium. Individuals with DLB are typically more apathetic than those with AD.

The diagnosis and treatment of DLB are often complicated by a lack of information about the disease. The clinician should consider DLB if he or she sees spontaneous features of parkinsonism, fully formed visual hallucinations, and fluctuating cognition with pronounced variation in attention and alertness early in the course of dementia. When fluctuating cognition occurs, family or caregivers often describe the resident as "zoned out" or "not with us." Such fluctuation is often mistaken for delirium superimposed on AD. Table 3.2 lists other symptoms that may help differentiate DLB from AD, including daytime drowsiness and lethargy despite getting enough sleep the

TABLE 3.2

Differentiating Alzheimer disease, frontotemporal dementia, and dementia with Lewy bodies

Function	Alzheimer Disease	Frontotemporal Dementia	Dementia with Lewy Bodies
Short-term memory	Impaired early on	Intact in mild stage	Impaired early on
Executive dysfunction	Mild	Prominent early on	Mild to moderate
Dramatic fluctuation in cognition	Rare	Rare	Common
Recurrent falls	Seen in later stages	Seen in later stages	Seen early on
Parkinsonism	Minimal in mild stage	Minimal in mild stage	Clinically evident early on
Visual hallucinations	Rare in mild stage	Rare	Frequent early on
REM sleep behavior disorder	Rare	Rare	Seen in up to 50 percent
Social misconduct	Rare in mild stage	Present early on	Rare in mild stage
Disinhibition	Rare in mild stage	Present early on	Rare in mild stage
Capacity for empathy	Intact early on	Impaired early on	Intact early on
Extreme sensitivity to high-potency antipsychotics	Absent or mild	Mild to moderate	Severe
Response to cholinesterase inhibitors	Modest	Absent	Better than for Alzheimer disease

night before; falling asleep for two or more hours during the day; staring into space for long periods; episodes of disorganized speech; REM sleep behavior disorder (RBD); recurrent falls; and a change in personality (especially passivity) early in the course of dementia (Ferman and Boeve 2007). RBD is often a precursor of DLB and is present in about half of the individuals with DLB.

Cholinergic deficits in DLB occur early and are more widespread than in AD (Tiraboschi et al. 2002). This may explain some of the clinical differences and the somewhat better response of those with DLB to cholinesterase inhibitors (ChEIs). Individuals with DLB are more functionally impaired (due to extrapyramidal motor symptoms) and have more neuropsychiatric difficulties (e.g., visual hallucinations seen in 80 percent of the people with DLB) than those with AD who have similar cognitive scores. Also, individuals with DLB are extremely sensitive to high-potency antipsychotic medications (e.g., haloperidol, fluphenazine, risperidone). Thus the clinician should avoid prescribing these medications, due to the increased risk of morbidity and mortality.

CLINICAL CASE Mrs. H, a 79-year-old woman residing in a nursing home, was referred for a psychiatric evaluation of suspected depression. She had a history of memory problems, disorientation at times, recurrent falls, and sleep disturbances that began two to three years previously and had been progressively growing worse. The most recent fall, a week before the evaluation, caused her to have a bruise on her face but no fractures. Over the previous two weeks, Mrs. H became increasingly withdrawn, staying in her room with a mild loss of appetite. On evaluation, she complained of fatigue. Her past medical history was positive for hypertension, peripheral vascular disease, osteoarthritis of the knees, and carpal tunnel syndrome. A review of her systems revealed dysuria. She presented mentally slowed, with a flat affect, and partially oriented. Her score on the MMSE was 12. A physical examination revealed a low-frequency tremor in her arms and legs. Laboratory results were within the normal range and urinalysis revealed a bladder infection, which was treated with antibiotics. Mrs. H was taking amlodipine, acetaminophen, and lorazepam 0.5 mg three times a day. To rule out a chronic subdural hematoma, the psychiatrist recommended an emergency CT scan of her head, which showed old diffuse ischemic white matter changes and mild cortical atrophy.

The lorazepam was gradually tapered down over two weeks and then discontinued. She was started on a rivastigmine patch 4.6 mg/24 hours daily. The psychiatrist counseled her family to encourage her to walk regularly, as she had always enjoyed walking. After one month, Mrs. H was sleeping better and her dysuria had cleared up, but she still complained of fatigue. She had tolerated rivastigmine well thus far without developing any nausea or vomiting. Her tremor was no worse. The rivastigmine was increased to a 9.5 mg/24 hours daily patch. Watercolor painting was added to her activity schedule, as she had shown an interest in this activity when she was in an adult day program. After another month, Mrs. H appeared to be doing much better. She still complained of fatigue, but less often. Her family felt she was more alert and interactive. Her repeat MMSE was 15. The psychiatrist gave a final diagnosis of possible DLB.

TEACHING POINTS. The adverse effects of benzodiazepines, such as fatigue, may take several weeks to improve after the drug is discontinued. Also, a UTI may manifest as fatigue, depression, and/or increased confusion. There are often multiple causes of symptoms and disability, with untreated dementia being one. In this case, treatment of the UTI, discontinuation of lorazepam, institution of ChEI therapy, and aggressive use of psychosocial interventions helped improve the resident's quality of life.

Cerebrovascular Disease

Dementia due to cerebrovascular disease, or vascular dementia, is the third most common type of irreversible dementia. With VaD, cognitive impairment is typically abrupt in its onset and has stepwise deterioration. Cognitive impairment typically has its onset or a dramatic worsening in association with a stroke or with clear neuroimaging evidence of infarctions (Strub 2003). A physical examination reveals neurological signs typical of a stroke (focal neurological deficits, motor and reflex asymmetry). Some stroke-related syndromes include the clinical phenotype of anterograde amnesia that is identical to that of AD. A slowing of mental processing (bradyphrenia) and movement may be an early sign that helps differentiate VaD from AD. Other exhibited changes in mental status are problems with decision making, poor organizational ability, difficulty adjusting to change (due to impaired executive functions), difficulty sustaining one's attention, and an apathetic appearance. Memory function, while impaired in VaD, is not the principal and devastating feature that it is with AD. Impaired judgment, personality changes, frank aphasia, or visuospatial disturbances may predominate, either alone or in combination. Many people who have VaD also demonstrate parkinsonian symptoms (retropulsion, shuffling gait, loss of postural reflexes) and early urinary incontinence. Depression is more common in VaD than in AD.

As many as 30 percent of stroke survivors may have dementia six months after the stroke, and the risk of dementia for those suffering multiple strokes increases ninefold over that of individuals of the same age and sex who have not had a new stroke. There is a remarkably high rate of silent infarcts on imaging, perhaps as high as 20 percent, and silent infarcts increase the risk of subsequent dementia by 2.26 (Knopman et al. 2003). Besides stroke, VaD is also caused by small-vessel cerebrovascular disease, resulting from either arteriolosclerosis or amyloid angiopathy. People who have this type of VaD often have a subcortical pattern of dementia with psychomotor slowing and relative preservation of naming and other language skills. An MRI scan of the brain shows obvious evidence of severe cerebrovascular disease.

White matter hyperintensities (leukoariosis), if severe, are associated with three times the risk of subsequent dementia. White matter hyperintensities are an independent predictor of cognitive decline, even more powerful than the presence of lacunar infarcts. Infarcts may involve the hippocampus directly, and subcortical ischemic vascular disease can also affect hippocampal volume. Although the presence of hippocampal atrophy is highly indicative of AD, it cannot be taken as proof that AD, and not VaD, is the cause of a dementia. therefore, differentiating VaD from AD through neuropsychological testing or neuroimaging is not as useful as determining the burden of cerebrovascular disease in all individuals with AD. Pure VaD in people older than 70 with dementia is rare. In younger people, the possibility of pure VaD is more likely.

Parkinson Disease

The typical case of dementia due to Parkinson disease (PD)—known as Parkinson disease dementia (PDD)—occurs in a person who has well-established PD (8.5 years on average, but by definition symptoms of PD should be present for at least one year before the onset of dementia) and then develops a progressive cognitive impairment (Emre et al. 2004). The cognitive deficits of PDD are similar to those of DLB. A neurological examination may find rest tremors, hypokinesia (slowed movement), masked facial expressions, a soft voice (hypophonia), tiny handwriting (micrographia), cogwheel rigidity of the limbs, and gait problems, including an asymmetrical or decreased arm swing and abnormal postural reflexes. Approximately 1.5 million Americans have PD, and up to 80 percent eventually develop dementia (Poewe 2006).

The pathological hallmark of PD is the collection of Lewy bodies in the substantia nigra. Relatively rare syndromes of progressive supranuclear palsy (in 1 in 50,000 persons in the general population) and corticobasal ganglionic degeneration (in 1 in 100,000 persons) are both Parkinson disease-plus syndromes, in which people typically have cognitive abnormalities and rigidity without tremor (Barrett 2005). Variants of both of these syndromes, in which only cognitive abnormalities were seen in the first several years of the disease, have been reported. The cognitive deficits of progressive supranuclear palsy or corticobasal ganglionic degeneration are usually milder than those of AD or DLB and are similar to those of FTD (Knopman et al. 2003). The clinician should consider using the MMSE and the Cambridge Cognitive Examination to screen for dementia in an individual who has PD but not dementia (Miyasaki et al. 2006).

Frontotemporal Lobar Degeneration

Dementia due to frontotemporal lobar degeneration, or frontotemporal dementia, is the fourth most common type of progressive irreversible dementia, ranking behind only AD, DLB, and VaD (Boxer and Miller 2005), although the incidence of FTD is probably higher, due to problems in its recognition and diagnosis. Symptoms of FTD typically appear between the ages of 40 and 65, with a mean age of onset at approximately 52 and 58 years. In young-onset dementia (before age 60), FTD may be at least as common as—if not more common than—AD (Ratnavalli et al. 2002). Up to 25 percent of FTD cases have onset after the age of 65. Up to 40 percent of FTD cases have a positive family history of the disease, and approximately 10 percent of the cases have an autosomal dominant pattern of inheritance (Goldman et al. 2007/2008). Three clinical groups of FTD have been described: the frontal lobe variant of FTD (FTDfv), also known as the *behavioral variant* or the *social/ executive disorder variant*; and two speech and language conditions, termed *progressive nonfluent aphasia* and *semantic dementia*. FTDfv is characterized by the insidious onset of behavioral and personality changes and, typically, its initial presentation lacks clear neurological signs or symptoms.

Core diagnostic criteria for FTDfv include personality changes such as emotional blunting and a lack of insight. The clinical manifestations of FTDfv are variable, but may include poor judgment (neglecting normal responsibilities), disinhibition (impolite behavior), a loss of empathy and sympathy for others, compulsive or socially inappropriate behaviors, excessive eating and weight gain, apathy, substance abuse, and aggression early in the course of this dementia. Social misconduct, in the form of theft or offensive language, may occur in nearly half of the people with FTDfv. Behavioral symptoms such as rigidity, stubbornness, self-centeredness, and the adoption of compulsive rituals typically occur with the progression of the disease.

Individuals with FTDfv may exhibit dramatic alterations in their self, as defined by changes in their political, social, or religious values. Stereotypical behaviors, such as compulsive cleaning, pacing, and collecting, are also common. In its later stages, hyperorality, repetitive movements, and mutism may occur. Memory loss is not prominent until later in the disease. Individuals with FTD may initially be misdiagnosed as having a psychiatric disorder (e.g., major depression, bipolar disorder, personality disorder) and may have been under the care of a psychiatrist for years. Only when symptoms advance to the point of obvious cognitive (loss of speech, memory deficits) and physical deficits (stiffness and balance problems) is the correct diagnosis made. Up to one-third of the people who have FTDfv exhibit euphoria, which can take the form of an elevated mood, inappropriate jocularity, and an exaggerated self-esteem that can be indistinguishable from hypomania or mania. Gluttonous overeating and an exaggerated craving for carbohydrates are also common.

Cognitive dysfunction (specifically executive deficits) may precede dementia by decades in FTDfv. Another key clinical element of FTDfv is the relative preservation of verbal and visual memory (unlike AD). Also, individuals with FTDfv typically preserve their visuospatial functions (unlike those who have DLB). On formal testing of delayed recall, people who have FTDfv may score in the normal range. Individuals in the earlier stages of FTDfv, as compared with those with AD, often achieve higher scores on the MMSE at baseline (Mendez et al. 1996). Thus bedside cognitive testing (e.g., MMSE) is often insensitive to the early and isolated executive and/or language deficits of residents with FTDfv. Individuals with FTDfv often display echopraxia (repeating whatever the other person says), perseveration, and motor impersistence.

By the time a diagnosis is made, most people with FTDfv perform poorly on psychometric tests of executive function. People with FTDfv make more concrete, literal interpretations and have severe impairments in their social cognition (the ability to interpret social situations and ascribe mental states to others). Neuropsychological testing is highly valuable when the clinician is considering FTDfv, because bedside executive function testing is inadequate. A normal performance on neuropsychological testing does not rule out FTDfv, especially early in its course. Some individuals with FTDfv who present with predominantly behavioral and personality manifestations may have only equivocal deficits on neuropsychological tests of executive function.

Behavioral symptoms usually emerge later, in the two language subgroups. People with progressive nonfluent aphasia demonstrate expressive aphasia with a prominent difficulty in finding words, a diminished ability to produce speech, and progressive difficulty with writing and reading. Mutism eventually occurs. Progressive nonfluent aphasia typically starts in one's 40s or 50s. Individuals who have this disease remain more functionally intact than those with other subtypes, as behavioral and personality changes do not occur until the later stages (after several years). Many people with progressive nonfluent aphasia are independent in their IADLs, despite profound aphasia. People with semantic dementia exhibit a loss of knowledge in the meaning of words and objects. They have fluent dysphasia, with severe difficulty in naming and understanding words, and difficulty in stating or demonstrating the function of tools or utensils (Grossberg and Desai 2006).

Survival is typically shorter for those in the FTD subgroups, with the possible exception of semantic dementia, for which the duration of the illness is similar to that of AD. Despite their higher cognitive scores, people with FTD demonstrate profound deficits in their ability to manage daily activities. These functional losses are secondary to judgment problems and behavioral symptoms, in contrast to the memory deficits of AD. Most people with FTD, especially those with behavioral symptoms, have difficulty engaging in occupational or family pursuits. There may also be financial problems, due to the affected person's job loss, bad investments, or overspending.

FTD has a strong genetic component, with up to 20 percent of the cases showing a highly penetrant, autosomal dominant pattern of disease transmission. Progranulin mutations linked to chromosome 17q21 account for 10 percent of all cases of FTD and approximately 20 percent of the cases with a family history of the disease. However, there is great clinical variability, even within families sharing the same progranulin mutation. The motor difficulties experienced by those who have FTD with progranulin mutations frequently take the form of mild parkinsonism. In some cases, familial FTD is linked to a mutation in the tau gene, also found in chromosome 17. This disorder, called frontotemporal dementia with parkinsonism linked to chromosome 17 (FTDP-17), is like the other types of FTD, but it often includes psychiatric symptoms, such as delusions and hallucinations. FTDP-17 is relatively uncommon, even in familial forms of FTD.

FTD describes a group of diseases characterized by neuronal degeneration, primarily involving the frontal and temporal lobes. The neuropathology consists of an accumulation of abnormal proteins (tau or ubiquitin) that are thought to cause neuronal death and a loss of synapses. People with FTD are approximately evenly divided between those with tau inclusions and those with ubiquitin ones, and there are no reliable clinical differences between FTD with tau and FTD with ubiquitin inclusions. Up to 15 percent of the people with FTD have clinical and electromyographic findings consistent with amyotrophic lateral sclerosis. Table 3.2 helps differentiate AD, DLB, and FTD (Ross and Bowen 2002; Barrett 2005; Hallam et al. 2007).

The FDA has not approved any medications for the management of FTDs. Because of the well-described serotonergic deficits in FTD, selective serotonin reuptake inhibitors (SSRIs) are common first-line agents (Huey, Putnam, and Grafman 2006). SSRIs are usually prescribed to treat anxiety, depression, and/or agitation in individuals with FTD (Caselli and Yaari 2007/2008). People with FTD are particularly prone to developing extrapyramidal side effects with the use of antipsychotic drugs, because of dopaminergic deficits seen in the brain. Thus the clinician should restrict the use of antipsychotic drugs in treating behavioral emergencies and severe persistent aggression. Atypical antipsychotic drugs such as quetiapine and aripiprazole, which are least likely to be associated with parkinsonism side effects, are preferred over high-potency antipsychotic medications such as risperidone. The cholinergic system in FTD appears to be relatively intact. Thus we do not recommend the use of ChEIs for residents with FTD. The clinician may consider prescribing memantine for some residents with FTD after explaining to the family that the FDA has not approved memantine to treat FTD, but that preliminary data suggest that glutamate may play a role in FTD and memantine may produce modest benefits (Swanberg 2007).

> **CLINICAL CASE** Mr. C, a 55-year-old male, became socially withdrawn and developed poor decision-making ability and a significant weight gain over two years. He was admitted to an LTC facility for rehabilitation after surgery to repair a hip fracture. Mr. C seemed not to be bothered by his hip fracture and needed encouragement during physical therapy. He was diagnosed with depression and tried taking various antidepressants, without success. He was referred to a psychiatrist for a trial of electro-convulsive therapy (ECT). The psychiatrist ordered an MRI brain scan to rule out any neurological cause of depression, because Mr. C had no past history of depression prior to this two year period, no family history of depression, and a vague history of a possible transient ischemic attack (TIA). The MRI scan revealed right temporal, frontal, and parietal atrophy. The psychiatrist referred Mr. C to a geriatric psychiatrist at a local memory disorder clinic at an academic institution.
>
> Mr. C underwent a comprehensive evaluation, including neuropsycho-logical testing, and was diagnosed with probable FTD (frontal lobe vari-ant). Mr. C's socially withdrawn behavior was thought to reflect apathy more than depression. All antidepressants were discontinued without any worsening of his clinical symptoms. The family and staff at the LTC facility were educated about the diagnosis. Mr. C died six years after the diagnosis, due to complications of advanced dementia. A brain autopsy was performed and resulted in a pathological diagnosis of FTD (ubiquitin positive).
>
> **TEACHING POINTS** The initial presentation of FTD is often mistaken for depression. Thus an accurate diagnosis requires a high index of suspicion. A history of an insidious onset of apathy and a lack of concern for self should raise the possibility of FTD. We strongly recommend referral of such cases to a local memory disorder clinic, if available (or to a geriatric psychiatrist, geriatrician, or neurologist).

Mixed Neuropathological States

Dementia due to two or more neuropathologies (mixed dementia [coexisting AD and VaD, AD and DLB, AD and PDD, and VaD and DLB]) is common, and the clinician should consider it in a differential diagnosis. Mixed pathology is also common: concomitant AD is present in 66 percent of the people with DLB and 77 percent with VaD (Grossberg and Desai 2006). Most people with clinical VaD have coexisting low to moderate AD. Even elderly people who have a high burden of cerebrovascular disease may also have AD. More clinical evidence of cerebrovascular disease implies a greater likelihood of VaD as the dominant etiologic factor in people with dementia. Yet AD can never be ruled out on clinical or imaging grounds. When autopsied, people with PDD frequently have pathologic findings of AD as well.

HIV

The clinician should consider dementia due to HIV, or HIV-associated dementia (HAD), for any resident who is HIV positive or at high risk of being HIV positive. HAD is more frequently the first presenting sign of HIV infection in older adults than in younger adults (Skapik and Treisman 2007). HAD is associated with psychomotor slowing, abnormal gait, and hypertonia. We recommend referral to an infectious disease specialist for all residents with suspected HAD (except those in the terminal stage) to rule out reversible causes of cognitive decline (e.g., opportunistic infections related to HIV/AIDS, such as neurosyphilis).

Huntington Disease

Huntington disease (HD) is a hereditary disorder (autosomal dominant with 100% penetrance). The children of people with this disorder have a 50 percent chance of inheriting it. The disease causes degeneration in many regions of the brain and the spinal cord. Symptoms of HD usually begin when people are in their 30s or 40s. Neuropsychiatric symptoms of HD typically begin with mild personality changes, such as irritability, anxiety, and depression, and progress to severe dementia. HD causes chorea—involuntary jerky, arrhythmic movements of the body—as well as muscle weakness, clumsiness, and gait disturbance. There is no cure. The clinician may consider prescribing high-potency atypical antipsychotic medications (e.g., risperidone) to treat chorea. It may be appropriate to treat the symptoms of anxiety and depression with psychosocial (e.g., counseling) and pharmacological interventions (e.g., antidepressants).

Creutzfeldt-Jakob Disease

Sporadic Creutzfeldt-Jakob disease (CJD) is a rare type of dementia in middle-aged and elderly persons, and typical cases are clinically fairly distinct from the more common forms of neurodegenerative dementia (Knight 2006). The clinician should suspect CJD with all individuals with rapidly progressive dementia. Most people with CJD die within one year. Although the cognitive profile of CJD is not distinct from those of other dementias, people with CJD typically initially experience problems with muscular coordination, personality changes, and impaired vision. Other symptoms may include insomnia and depression. As the illness progresses, mental impairment becomes severe. People with CJD often develop myoclonus and may go blind. Eventually they lose their ability to move and speak and go into a coma. Pneumonia and other infections often occur and can lead to death. A triphasic wave pattern in an EEG in the context of a rapidly progressive dementia is strongly suggestive of CJD. There is no specific treatment or cure. Drugs such as clonazepam may help myoclonus.

Potentially Reversible Causes of Dementia

Some common reversible causes of dementia are listed in table 3.1. Some of these conditions are more often comorbid with degenerative dementias or vascular dementia, but they may cause dementia on their own (H. Wang et al. 2001; Barrett 2005). In the latter case, with treatment of the cause the dementia may be partially or completely reversible. Vitamin B_{12} deficiency is estimated to affect 10 to 15 percent of elderly people (Baik and Russell 1999). Hematologic abnormalities may not occur with a vitamin B_{12} deficiency, particularly if the nervous system is involved. Vitamin B_{12} injections to treat B_{12} deficiency should improve cognition and prevent any disability associated with progressive myelopathy and peripheral neuropathy. Vitamin B_{12} levels that are close to the lower limit of the normal range may also be treated with oral B_{12} at 1,000 mcg daily. Acute thiamine (vitamin B_1) deficiency causes Wernicke encephalopathy (characterized by delirium, ophthalmoplegia, and ataxia), and chronic thiamine deficiency causes Korsakoff syndrome (severe short-term memory impairment with confabulation) (Pepersack et al. 1999). Elderly people who are alcoholic and have poor nutrition may develop a thiamine deficiency. Individuals with diabetes mellitus may lose up to 15 times more thiamine than those who do not have diabetes. Thiamine also seems to protect those with diabetes from developing diabetic nephropathy. The treatment involves thiamine oral supplementation (100 mg thiamine daily).

The clinician may consider other vitamin deficiencies, such as a folate deficiency and pellagra (a niacin deficiency), for elderly people who are severely malnourished. Thyroid disease, especially hypothyroidism, is common in elderly persons (Diez 2002). However, apathetic hyperthyroidism (i.e., a paradoxical presentation of hyperthyroidism with fatigue, psychomotor retardation, and weight gain) also occurs in this population. A history of hypothyroidism (loss of appetite and weight gain, decreased tolerance of cold) or hyperthyroidism (increased appetite with weight loss, decreased tolerance of heat), a physical examination to look for signs of hypothyroidism (e.g., bradycardia, skin cold to the touch, the presence of goiter, dry skin) or hyperthyroidism (e.g., tachycardia, exophthalmos), and testing for thyrotropin and free thyroxine levels are indicated to evaluate this cause of reversible dementia. New-onset epilepsy in LTC residents often presents as complex partial seizures that can resemble sudden-onset dementia. The clinician should also consider trauma and anoxic encephalopathy in acute-onset dementia with no obvious evidence of a stroke. In residents who have a head injury or anoxic encephalopathy, their cognitive impairment and functional loss may not progressively worsen after the initial insult and may even improve to some extent over time.

For residents with cognitive decline and unexplained focal findings, the clinician should consider atypical presentations, including incontinence, seizures, or severe headaches early in the course of dementia, and surgically treatable causes—normal pressure hydrocephalus (NPH), a subdural hematoma, and a brain tumor—but these typically do not present as isolated dementia (Larson 2000). NPH manifests initially with gait apraxia (leading to falls), followed by urinary incontinence and, eventually, dementia. Neuroimaging shows dilated ventricles, and a diagnosis of this illness can be confirmed by demonstrating improvement in gait after the removal of some amount of cerebrospinal fluid (CSF) through lumbar puncture. The treatment involves the insertion of a ventriculoperitoneal shunt. A subdural hematoma may produce headaches and dementialike symptoms (cognitive deficits, changes in mood and/or personality for subacute onsets) because of a mass effect or the induction of nonconvulsive seizures. This treatment involves neurosurgical intervention (a burr hole and removal of the blood clot).

Tumors involving the parietal cortex may mimic AD (Barrett 2005). The parietal cortex is not directly connected to motor output systems, and paralysis and abnormal reflexes may be absent despite a significant mass effect. Although other abnormalities (i.e., sensory, complex behavioral, and visual-focal deficits) may occur, residents who have a tumor involving the parietal lobe are usually unaware of these deficits (anosognosia), and the problem may be missed on a cursory examination. Residents with dementia due to a brain tumor usually are younger (less than 70 years old) than the typical age group of residents with AD (more than 70). Neuroimaging (especially an MRI scan with and without contrast) confirms a diagnosis of a brain tumor. Primary gastrointestinal disorders, such as Whipple disease and celiac disease, may involve the central nervous system without prominent gastrointestinal symptoms (Barrett 2005). Central nervous system symptoms in Whipple disease may manifest as Parkinson disease-plus syndrome, which resembles progressive supranuclear palsy.

Amnesia and changes in mood or personality, delirium, or seizures can indicate paraneoplastic limbic encephalitis, a rare and remote effect of cancer associated primarily with non-small-cell lung cancer but also with thymoma, Hodgkin disease, and cancers of the breast, colon, bladder, and testicle (Barrett 2005). Most individuals with limbic encephalitis are not known to have cancer until their mental status changes. Most commonly, limbic encephalitis occurs rapidly, over days to weeks, and may be accompanied by other neurologic symptoms (e.g., ataxia, visual changes, neuropathy). Treatment of the primary tumor may produce substantial cognitive improvement.

For residents with a past history of a sexually transmitted disease and/ or an HIV infection, the clinician should consider paretic neurosyphilis, although it is rare in the general population. The clinical presentation is that of disinhibited frontotemporal dementia. If the clinical picture strongly suggests paretic neurosyphilis, we recommend the fluorescent treponemal antibody absorption (FTA-ABS) test. Antibiotics (e.g., penicillin) are used to treat paretic neurosyphilis. The clinician should screen all residents with dementia for the risk factors for HIV infection.

In all residents with dementia, the clinician needs to look for other potentially reversible causes of dementia (e.g., drug-induced cognitive impairment [especially benzodiazepines or anticholinergic drugs], OSA). Many people with potentially reversible dementia may not fully recover their premorbid cognitive abilities after starting appropriate therapy; however, their symptoms may stabilize for long periods and they may be protected from other significant consequences of the disorder.

Differential Diagnosis of Dementia

The clinician should differentiate dementia from age-associated memory impairment, mild cognitive impairment, delirium, depression, and schizophrenia (Ross and Bowen 2002).

Age-Associated Memory Impairment

A hallmark of normal cognitive aging is a slowed processing speed. Particularly after age 70, but most marked in the population over 85, there is a tendency to have increasing difficulty in accessing the names of people and objects; to have difficulty processing information rapidly; and to need additional time to learn things or skills (e.g., using technology), grasp new ideas (particularly complicated skills or ideas), and think through problems (Grossberg and Desai 2006). Age-associated memory impairment (also called *benign forgetfulness*) involves forgetting the name of someone, particularly someone whom one has not seen for a while; finding it difficult to recall the right word to express oneself; or even not remembering the name of an object, event, or some other thing, particularly something that is not familiar (G. Small 2002). None of these problems are sufficient to cause impairment in daily activities or in one's ability to live independently.

Memory function, as measured by a delayed recall of newly learned material, is not substantially decreased in older adults. People experiencing age-associated memory impairment complain of memory loss, but they often have normal scores on psychometric testing for their age group. The results of office-based memory testing are usually in the normal range. Although most people who have subjective memory complaints do not have a significant decline in their memory or functioning over time (months to years), subjective memory difficulties may be the earliest symptom of future dementia in highly educated people (Kawas 2003). The cognitive impairments associated with normal aging may impede one's quality of life, but a cognitive decline with aging is not inevitable, and many older adults appear to avoid cognitive decline even into the eleventh decade of life.

Mild Cognitive Impairment

Mild cognitive impairment is a syndrome characterized by impairment in a single cognitive domain, usually memory (amnestic MCI), or by moderate impairment in several cognitive domains, but individuals who have MCI do not have significant impairment in their abilities to perform ADLs and do not meet the criteria for dementia (Petersen et al. 1999). The prevalence of MCI among LTC residents varies from 5 to 10 percent in many nursing homes to up to 30 percent in some assisted living facilities. The most frequently encountered form of MCI is the amnestic type. Less-common variants of MCI present with a localized impairment of other cognitive domains (e.g., executive dysfunction in FTD) (Knopman, Boeve, and Petersen 2003). Individuals with amnestic MCI commonly progress to AD, converting from one diagnosis to the other at a rate of approximately 10–15 percent per year on average. For many people, MCI is the earliest manifestation of AD, but not all of those with MCI will convert to AD or another dementia. Although most who convert from MCI to dementia have AD, many others may convert to VaD, FTD, DLB, or other less-common dementias (Caselli et al. 2006). Depression is common in people with MCI, and its presence increases one's chances of converting to dementia in the next few years.

Although recollection is impaired in MCI, familiarity-based recognition is intact, compared with impaired familiarity-based recognition in AD (Westerberg et al. 2006). Neuropsychological testing is needed to accurately diagnose MCI and differentiate it from age-associated memory impairment and mild dementia. For residents with amnestic MCI, the clinician should discuss the potential risks and benefits of treatment with a ChEI with the resident and the family, particularly if there is a family history of AD, if the person is young (less than 70 years old), has comorbid mild depression or a subtle change in personality (passivity), has a history suggestive of RBD (indicating that he or she may develop DLB in the future), has a history of falls or a weight loss accompanying memory deficits, has family members who mention the resident's mild impairment in complex activities (not sufficient to be diagnosed with dementia), has memory deficits that have an insidious onset and are progressive, has no history of a stroke, or has an MRI scan that shows hippocampal atrophy but mild or minimal cerebrovascular disease.

Delirium

Cognitive impairment due to delirium may be confused with dementia in LTC residents. Delirium typically has an acute, dateable onset, a fluctuant level of alertness where the resident may appear drowsy, hyperalert, or alternate between them, and difficulties with attention and concentration. In addition, any and all causes of delirium may be accompanied by behavior changes (e.g., agitation) or psychotic symptoms (e.g., visual hallucinations). The clinician may also see the quiet or apathetic subtype of delirium, which is often missed. Depending on the cause, in some cases the onset of delirium may be subacute. This is in contrast to the typical insidious onset of degenerative dementia. Four key clinical features of delirium that help differentiate it from dementia (except in individuals with DLB) are acute onset, impairment in awareness (hyperalert, drowsy, stuporous), inattention, and a dramatic diurnal fluctuation in symptoms (especially cognition, but also behavior). Orientation is usually impaired, and memory deficits are also seen. Thinking is disorganized. The clinician should always assume that delirium is treatable or reversible until proven otherwise. If the clinician identifies and removes the cause, the resident should return to his or her premorbid cognitive and functional baselines (McCarty and Drebing 2001).

Depression

Major depressive disorder (henceforth simply called *depression* in this chapter) in elderly people may be associated with complaints of memory impairment, difficulty thinking and concentrating, difficulty in finding words, and an overall reduction in intellectual abilities. This condition used to be called *depressive pseudodementia*, but it is more properly termed the *dementia syndrome of depression*. This recognizes that older adults who are clinically depressed may look like and even believe that they have AD, because their depression can impair cognition. However, if depression is causing cognitive changes, once it is effectively treated the individual should return to his or her premorbid cognitive baseline. Unfortunately, depression may be an early marker, as well as a risk factor, for AD. Also, depression can coexist with AD in 30–50 percent of the people with AD. In those with dementia who exhibit acute cognitive or behavioral decline, the clinician should suspect comorbid depression (as well as delirium) and aggressively treat it.

Some residents are unaware of their mood state (alexithymia) and deny sadness, guilt, or the other usual symptoms of depression. Changes in self-attitude (e.g., helplessness, hopelessness, worthlessness, guilt), frequent crying spells, or the presence of suicidal ideas usually indicate the presence of clinical depression, especially if these symptoms persist for two or more weeks. If there is a past history of a depressive episode (single or recurrent), the clinician should treat symptoms of less than two weeks' duration as a recurrence of depression. Although apathy (lack of motivation), psychomotor retardation, weight loss, and/or impaired concentration may be present with depression and AD, it is possible to reliably differentiate depression from AD in most clinical situations (Herrmann et al. 1998; McNeil 1999; Purandare et al. 2001; H. Lee and Lyketsos 2004; also see table 3.3).

Many individuals with AD also have comorbid depression. A history of gradual cognitive decline predating the depressive symptoms may help the clinician diagnose AD with depression. To clarify the diagnosis, it is sometimes helpful to use an assessment tool, such as the GDS or the CSDD. The latter is most useful as a depression assessment tool for people with advanced dementia. In difficult cases, a close follow-up after an aggressive and successful treatment of depression clarifies the diagnosis by eliciting a continued cognitive decline in the absence of any significant depressive symptoms. Residents with late-life depression (depression after age 65 with no past history of depression) and cognitive impairment may experience improvement in specific domains following antidepressant treatment, but they may not necessarily reach normal levels of performance, particularly in memory and in executive function. This subgroup of residents with late-life depression is likely at high risk of developing progressive dementia, so the clinician should assess them every three to six months to detect the earliest signs of dementia (Butters et al. 2000).

Depression in MCI and in early dementia must also be distinguished from late-onset depression and the cognitive impairment that may accompany mood disorders. In the latter group of residents, cognitive impairment is often partially or even fully resolved with a successful treatment of the depression. However, because as many as one-half of such persons may develop dementia within five years, the clinician should closely follow them to diagnose any dementia as early as possible. Neuropsychological testing is one of the best ways to reliably differentiate cognitive deficits related to depression from MCI, MCI with depression, mild dementia, and mild dementia with depression. Neuropsychological testing may show executive dysfunction, but the typical neuropsychological profile of AD is absent in residents with depression but no dementia.

Schizophrenia
Cognitive impairment is a core feature of schizophrenia (O'Donnell 2007). Often residents with schizophrenia have a long history of psychotic symptoms and psychiatric treatment, extending back to age 20 or 30, with one or more psychiatric hospitalizations. Cognitive deficits usually involve problems with attention and executive dysfunction and are not progressive. However,

TABLE 3.3
Differentiating depression from Alzheimer disease

Clinical Symptom	Depression	Alzheimer Disease
Onset	Over weeks (subacute)	Over years (insidious)
Temporal sequence	Depressive symptoms start before cognitive symptoms	Cognitive symptoms start before depressive symptoms
Diurnal mood variations	Often present	Usually absent
Family history	Of depression (may be present)	Of Alzheimer disease (may be present)
Persistent tearfulness	Often present	Usually absent
Insomnia	Generally persistent	Usually transient
Early morning awakening	Often present	Uncommon
Decreased appetite	Frequently present	Less frequently present
Weight loss	Frequently pronounced	Mild, if present
Cognitive impairment	Attentional and motivational problems	Impaired recall of recent events
Patient complains of significant memory loss	Frequently present	Infrequently present
Memory complaints	Exceed those found during testing	Correlate with those found during testing
Patient seeks help for a memory loss complaint	Frequently	Infrequently
Language impairment	Absent	Often present
Apraxia	Absent	Often present
Clock-drawing test	Normal	Often abnormal
Agnosia	Absent	Present in the later stages
Inability to copy a drawing	Absent	Often present
Left/right disorientation	Absent	Often present
Hopelessness	Often present	Usually absent
Helplessness	Often present	Usually absent
Worthlessness	Often present	Usually absent
Guilt feelings	Often present	Usually absent
Multiple somatic complains	Often present	Infrequent
Suicidal ideas	May be present	Usually absent
Severity of depression	Correlates with cognitive impairment	Cognitive impairment much worse than depression
Response to treatment	Significant reduction of cognitive impairment	Continued cognitive impairment

a subset of chronic, institutionalized residents with schizophrenia may show some intellectual and functional decline (O'Donnell 2007). Older adults with schizophrenia may be more susceptible to developing common irreversible dementias such as AD and VaD because of the high prevalence of vascular risk factors (e.g. hypertension, diabetes mellitus, obesity, metabolic syndrome, hyperlipidemia, OSA, a sedentary lifestyle, cigarette smoking, and substance abuse). Neuropsychological testing can help the clinician differentiate residents who have schizophrenia with cognitive deficits from those who have schizophrenia and superimposed dementia.

Tools for Diagnosing Dementia

Current tools for diagnosing dementia include the following:

- a detailed history from the patient and from family or other reliable informants
- a physical and neurological examination and laboratory tests
- neuroimaging
- standardized tests to assess cognition, function, and mood (depression)
- neuropsychological testing by a neuropsychologist when the diagnosis or etiology is not clear

Tests to Clarify the Diagnosis

To date, there are no definitive antemortem tests to definitively diagnose degenerative dementias. Blood tests, such as a CBC, a basic metabolic panel, liver function tests, and tests for calcium, vitamin B_{12} and folate levels, and TSH, can help the clinician detect treatable causes of cognitive impairment, such as severe anemia, malnutrition, hyponatremia, severe renal disease, hypercalcemia, vitamin deficiencies, and a thyroid disorder. These conditions are often comorbid with irreversible dementias, but correcting them may improve cognition and slow future cognitive declines. Neuroimaging, at least during an initial diagnosis (an MRI scan, usually without contrast, is preferred over a CT scan of the brain), can help the clinician detect vascular lesions, NPH, tumors, subdural hematomas, and the like. Neuroimaging may be omitted for residents who have clinical features of degenerative dementia and are in its advanced stages, because obtaining a brain scan may be too burdensome for these residents and the findings may not influence treatment decisions. Sleep disorders, such as OSA, are also associated with cognitive impairment, and the clinician should inquire about them, especially for residents who are obese, have excessive daytime sleepiness, and snore at night. A sleep study may be warranted to confirm a diagnosis of OSA.

The prevalence of reversible dementias has been decreasing over the last few decades (Clarfield 2003), due in part to additional initial testing. Some clinicians may routinely add plasma homocysteine and C-reactive protein level tests. In selected cases (e.g., a history of a sexually transmitted disease or of intravenous drug abuse), a rapid plasma reagin test for neurosyphilis or an HIV test for central nervous system manifestations of AIDS may be warranted. A urine analysis, an EKG, and a chest X-ray may be useful to detect a comorbid UTI or lung infection if the clinician suspects that the resident has delirium superimposed on dementia. The clinician may occasionally consider a positron emission tomography (PET) scan for a resident to help differentiate between AD and FTD. (Medicare will reimburse for the PET scan only in this scenario.) Neither a CT scan nor an MRI scan can diagnose AD, but looking for the degree of atrophy or for focal and hippocampal atrophy may be useful in differentiating between FTD and AD. Atrophy out of proportion with a person's age is also important in the diagnosis of degenerative dementias.

A simple diagnosis of dementia may be inaccurate for many LTC residents (Mansdorf et al. 2008), so the clinician may consider neuropsychological testing, if available, to diagnose dementia more accurately. Neuropsychological testing is useful to clarify the diagnosis for residents with significant depression and dementia, to differentiate between MCI and dementia, and to differentiate between AD and other neurodegenerative dementias. Neuropsychological testing is also important to diagnose AD for residents who, at baseline, had extremely high or relatively low levels of cognitive or intellectual functions (e.g., residents who have mental retardation due to Down syndrome and developed insidious onset and progress cognitive and functional decline from their baselines).

The clinician should consider referral to a neurologist for an evaluation of the cause of dementia if the resident is young, if signs of parkinsonism are present, if there is history of seizures, or when neurosurgical interventions need to be considered (such as with a brain tumor, NPH, a subdural hematoma, etc.). The clinician should refer residents who have an unusually rapid symptomatic progression of dementia and the presence of myoclonus or other atypical presentations to a neurologist for spinal fluid examination to evaluate for CJD and infectious etiologies of dementia (e.g., neurosyphilis, Herpes simplex encephalitis).

We recommend genetic testing only in cases of familial AD (AD with an autosomal dominant pattern of inheritance, typically with an onset of dementia in one's 30s or 40s), some cases of FTD that have an autosomal dominant pattern of inheritance, cases of suspected Huntington disease, and cases of suspected cerebral autosomal dominant arteriopathy with subcortical infarcts and leukoencephalopathy (CADASIL). Genetic testing is currently available for only Presenilin 1 mutations in people with familial AD. We strongly recommend genetic counseling by a professional genetic counselor or a clinical geneticist or an expert in memory disorders at an academic center before any genetic testing. We do not recommend testing for the ApoE4 genotype for use in a diagnosis.

Behavioral and Psychological Symptoms of Dementia

The point prevalence of behavioral and psychological symptoms of dementia is approximately 60 percent, and the lifetime prevalence is 90 percent (Mega et al. 1996; Desai and Grossberg 2001; Steinberg et al. 2003; Aalten et al. 2007). Among the most validated syndromes of behavioral and psychological symptoms of dementia are depression, psychosis, and sleep disturbances (Meeks, Ropacki, and Jeste 2006). Apathy syndrome is also gaining research interest. The prevalence of behavioral and psychological symptoms of dementia does not vary by setting, but the prevalence of specific symptoms does, both by setting (with a higher prevalence of aggression in LTC residents than in people who live in the community) and by stage. Apathy is the most common behavioral and psychological symptom of dementia, seen in all types of dementia and across all stages. The degree to which it is present increases with advancing cognitive impairment.

Agitation is the next most common symptom, seen more often as the dementia progresses to its moderate and severe stages. Disruptive behaviors (e.g., wandering, verbal outbursts, physical threats/violence, agitation/restlessness, and sundowning) predict a cognitive decline, a functional decline, and then admission to a facility (Scarmeas et al. 2007). The prevalence of agitation and aggression is approximately 25 percent in persons who have dementia and reside at home, and 45 percent in those residing in LTC facilities. The prevalence of clinically significant depression is approximately 32 percent in its mild stage, 23 percent in its moderate stage, and 18 percent in its severe stage. We recommend a mandatory screening for depression for all residents with dementia, because this improves treatment rates (C. Cohen, Hyland, and Kimhy 2003).

Individuals with dementia frequently manifest psychotic symptoms, such as delusions and hallucinations. Sleep disturbances and anxiety symptoms are also common in residents with dementia and often occur alongside depression, psychoses, and agitation. Behavioral and psychological symptoms of dementia, especially psychosis, agitation, and problem wandering (a safety issue), are the leading triggers for admitting a person with dementia to an LTC facility (O'Donnell et al. 1992; Gaugler et al. 2000).

Although dementia itself often causes behavioral and psychological symptoms, most of these symptoms arise from the complex interaction of biological, environmental, and psychosocial factors.

Biological Factors

Several neuroanatomic and neurochemical correlates for the behavioral and psychological symptoms of dementia have been identified. Monoamine changes are a robust finding in AD and may account for many observed symptoms of depression (Meeks, Ropacki, and Jeste 2006). The risk of psychosis in AD appears to be increased by several genes that are also implicated in schizophrenia. The circadian breakdown in the sleep-wake cycle commonly seen in AD may be due to degeneration of the suprachiasmatic nucleus (the circadian pacemaker, or body clock) (Vitiello and Borson 2001). Psychosis in DLB appears to be related to cholinergic deficits. REM sleep behavior disorder is intricately related to synucleinopathies, such as DLB and PDD. Frontal lobe damage is associated with apathy and socially inappropriate behavior. Neurochemical alterations in the cholinergic and dopaminergic systems have also been implicated as a cause of apathy in individuals with dementia. The presence of cerebrovascular disease correlates with depression in persons with dementia. Low CSF 5-hydroxyindoleacetic acid and diminished orbitofrontal and caudate metabolisms occur in depressions associated with AD and PD. In AD, depression correlates with frontal hypometabolism. Depression in VaD is most common when the ischemic injury involves the deep white matter or when there are multiple lacunae in the basal ganglia. Dysfunction in a related set of frontal-subcortical structures appears to be a common underlying feature of depression in dementia. Delusions and agitation/aggression are more common and severe among homozygous ApoE ε4 carriers than among heterozygous or ApoE ε4-negative individuals with probable AD (van der Flier et al. 2007). Untreated medical conditions, such as UTIs and pain, are also common biological factors predisposing or precipitating behavioral and psychological symptoms of dementia.

Environmental Factors

Excessive noise and stimulation, inadequate lighting, a lack of structure and routine in daily life, a lack of appropriate activities, an impatient caregiver approach, confusing surroundings, and a lack of safe areas to wander in and to be outdoors are some environmental factors that often cause behavioral and psychological symptoms of dementia. The clinician should inquire into them and see that they are corrected if present.

Psychosocial Factors

Many LTC residents experience significant periods of boredom and loneliness and are unable to address this themselves, because of their dementia. In such situations, their behaviors may be an expression of their unmet psychological needs. Dementia has a tremendous negative impact on a resident's self-esteem and feelings of security, especially if the resident has partial or full insight into his or her cognitive and functional limitations. Some behaviors that are labeled disturbing could be viewed as the resident's way of overcoming feelings of fragmentation and emptiness when his or her ability to self-soothe is diminished. In such situations, the resident needs empathic, mirroring responses from caregivers who can understand the symbolic meaning of such behaviors. Take, for example, a resident with dementia who constantly follows a family or professional caregiver (such behavior is often called shadowing) and frets when that person is out of sight. To this resident, who cannot remember the past or anticipate the future, the surrounding world can be strange and frightening. Staying close to a trusted and familiar caregiver may be the only thing that makes sense and provides security. Lower premorbid agreeableness (a personality factor) is associated with agitation and irritability symptoms in AD and predicts an agitation/apathy syndrome (Archer et al. 2007).

When caring for a person with dementia, the caregiver must try to determine whether the person's behavior is dysfunctional or is a response to a particular situation. In general, the health care provider should view behavioral disturbances as an attempt to communicate or respond to a biological need, such as hunger, thirst, sex, or comfort. For example, taking one's clothes off may seem reasonable to a person with dementia who feels hot but doesn't understand or remember that undressing in public is not acceptable. Aggressive behavior is often associated with an invasion of one's personal space (e.g., during toileting or dressing). Labeling an individual's resistance to having help with personal activities as a behavioral disturbance seems inappropriate, especially if that person does not recognize the caregiver or understand the meaning of his or her actions. In this context, the individual's anger and aggressiveness may be an appropriate response to a strange situation.

A resident who screams frequently may be trying to communicate that he or she is lonely or is experiencing some discomfort (e.g., an irritating urinary catheter, arthritis pain, an uncomfortable position while sitting or lying down). Some behaviors that are labeled disturbing (e.g., persistent yelling) may represent the resident trying to assert the right to be heard and to have his or her needs met promptly. Whenever a staff member notes violent behavior, inappropriate motor activity, demanding behavior, and the like, obtaining a more detailed account of the behavior, the context in which it occurs, and the staff's approach may indicate that the behavior was a form of communication of an unmet need rather than a medical or psychiatric problem. Spending time with the resident and addressing that person's discomfort are better interventions than labeling the resident's behavior as dysfunctional and prescribing a psychotropic medication.

Many behaviors are an attempt by residents with dementia to feel connected to their surroundings. Looking for one's parent or wanting to go home, for example, may be a way of expressing the need to feel safe and secure in a strange environment. For such residents, being with one's parents or at home had calmed them and helped them feel connected to themselves and to others, as well as to objects, events, time, and place. Looking for one's small children (when the children are adults) may be a resident's way of expressing a need to be needed, to have responsibility, to be useful, to feel like a responsible adult rather than an invalid. Blaming someone for stealing one's belongings may be a mechanism to protect one's self-esteem from the blow of knowing one is losing cognitive function. Blaming a spouse for infidelity may be a way of voicing insecurity and the fear of being abandoned by one's spouse or of being admitted to a facility. Repeatedly asking the same questions may reflect a need to be reassured that everything will be okay, and that the resident will be not left to fend for him- or herself.

Verbal disruption is common and includes shouting, screaming, yelling, calling out, cursing, or using language that creates a disturbance and requires intervention by the staff. Such disruptions may be predictable or unpredictable. The clinician should consider it to be either a form of communicating a need (discomfort due to wet pants caused by incontinence, relief from hunger or thirst, a need for toileting) or a symptom of an underlying medical (e.g., pain) or psychiatric disorder (e.g., depression).

Often, the resident's reality is different from the caregiver's. The resident and caregiver could dwell in different times and places. Residents with dementia can be seen as "displaced persons, refugees without a past, occupying the present but unconnected to it." Reminiscence work may alleviate emotional distress in such situations. A catastrophic reaction is an acute expression of overwhelming anxiety and fearfulness experienced by some residents with dementia, usually triggered by a frustrating experience (e.g., difficulty dressing oneself) or in anticipation of one. These spells are typically brief, lasting less than 30 minutes, and are self-limited.

Agitation

Agitation is a generic term that includes verbally aggressive behaviors (e.g., swearing, threats), verbally nonaggressive behaviors (e.g., repetitive vocalization, pleas for help), physically aggressive behaviors (e.g., hitting, biting, scratching, kicking, pushing), and physically nonaggressive behaviors (e.g., pacing, wandering) (Cohen-Mansfield 1986). The clinician should consider agitated behaviors to be an expression of a resident's unmet needs (e.g., food, thirst, toileting, relief from environmental stress [an impatient or angry caregiver approach, excessive noise, excessive demands], relief from discomfort [due to pain, constipation]). A reaction to medication, medical conditions (e.g., OSA, pneumonia, UTI, onychomycosis), and psychiatric disorders (e.g., depression, psychoses, delirium) may also manifest as agitated behaviors.

Wandering

Wandering is one of the most common behavioral problems found in individuals with dementia, often resulting in their being admitted to an LTC facility that has locked units or other safeguards (e.g., use of a wander-guard alarm system). Wandering manifests as aimless or purposeful motor activity that involves leaving a safe place, becoming lost, or intruding into inappropriate places or situations. Residents with dementia often wander, with facilities reporting elopement rates of 35–40 percent per year (Rolland et al. 2007b; Schonfeld et al. 2007). Residents with dementia who remain ambulatory and are in relatively good physical health have a high risk of wandering. Once a resident begins to wander, more than 70 percent engage in repeated episodes (Lantz 2007), and wandering often leads to early admission to LTC.

The management of wandering primarily involves psychosocial-environmental interventions. For example, some residents may wander due to a need for socialization or stimulation and thus may benefit from a structured individualized activity schedule (e.g., a daily walking plan). The availability of safe and esthetically pleasing areas in which to wander (e.g., therapeutic gardens with walking paths) may allow residents to roam without the risk of elopement. There are no antiwandering drugs. For residents who wander but also have untreated moderate to severe depression and/or anxiety, a trial of antidepressants may be appropriate. We do not recommend the use of antipsychotic medications to manage wandering unless the resident has clear psychotic symptoms and his or her behavior is unmanageable due to physical aggression.

Other aberrant motor behaviors, such as restlessness and pacing, are also common in residents with dementia and are challenging to manage. Residents who pace a lot may need to be monitored for weight loss due to excessive caloric expenditure and for sores on their feet. Proper footwear is critical for all residents who ambulate, especially for residents who pace or wander and for those at high risk of pressure ulcers (e.g., residents who have diabetes mellitus, peripheral vascular disease). The clinician should consider referring residents who pace and/or wander to an orthopedic surgeon and a podiatrist for an evaluation of foot, knee, or hip joint problems, necessary orthotics, and pain management. We do not recommend restraining residents from pacing or wandering.

Pain

Elderly individuals with dementia are not less sensitive to pain. However, they may fail to interpret sensations as painful, are often less able to recall pain, and may not be able to verbally communicate their pain to caregivers. Hence older adults with dementia are often undertreated for pain. A label of dementia may bias the interpretation of pain cues from residents with dementia and thus may contribute to a lower use of as-needed analgesics by residents with dementia than by residents who are not cognitively impaired (Nygaard and Jarland 2005). Residents with dementia, like those who do not have dementia, are at risk of multiple sources and types of pain, including chronic pain from conditions such as osteoarthritis and acute pain. Poorly treated acute pain is a common cause of chronic pain in residents with dementia. Untreated pain in individuals with dementia can reduce their quality of life; cause depression, agitation, or aggression; delay healing; disturb their sleep and activity patterns; reduce function; and prolong hospitalization (American Geriatrics Society Panel on Persistent Pain in Older Persons 2002).

Pain influences behavioral disturbances among residents with severe dementia more often than among those with moderate or mild dementia, and residents who have both chronic pain and severe dementia exhibit more dysfunctional behaviors than residents who have chronic pain and are at earlier stages of dementia (Cipher, Clifford, and Roper 2006). Terminal-stage AD is associated with pressure ulcers, limb contractures, and pain that can be much more difficult to assess (Sherder et al. 2005). There is no evidence that surgery for a hip fracture improves the pain situation for people with advanced dementia (Christmas 2006). The primary reason to consider a surgical approach over a palliative care one is when a gain in function (especially ambulation) is the primary aim. We recommend palliative care (pain control, skin care, bed rest, deep-vein thrombosis prophylaxis, personal care) to treat hip fractures for residents with severe or terminal dementia because of their limited life expectancy and inability to participate in postoperative physical therapy (necessary to achieve a gain in function). We do not recommend the use of as-needed pain medications to manage pain for residents with cognitive impairment, because they will not ask for these medications. Regular (scheduled) administration of acetaminophen to residents with moderate to severe dementia raises their levels of general activity, social interaction, and engagement with television or magazines (Chibnall and Tait 2001).

Abrupt Decline

Over the protracted course of degenerative dementia, many residents may suddenly become more confused, with slurred speech, somnolence, agitation, tremulousness, unsteadiness, falls, or worsened incontinence. This is often due to a superimposed delirium caused by infection (e.g., UTI), a stroke, or the side effects of medication (e.g., antipsychotic drugs). Many older adults develop cognitive decline for the first time after major surgery. Several perioperative factors (e.g., hypoxia, hypocapnia, and anesthetics) can cause postoperative cognitive decline, in some cases by triggering AD neuropathogenesis. At first glance, many patients who have postoperative cognitive decline may present with delirium that seems to develop into dementia, but on further detailed inquiry, a history of subtle cognitive and functional decline for months to years before surgery indicates that the process of dementia had started before the surgery.

Treatment of Dementia

The treatment of dementia is a treatment of its cause. Thus to treat reversible dementia, treat the cause (removing offending medication, correcting vitamin and nutritional deficiencies, etc.). Table 3.4 lists goals for the treatment of irreversible dementias (G. Small et al. 1997; Doody et al. 2001; Grossberg and Desai 2003b; Snowden, Sato, and Roy-Byrne 2003). Early and aggressive management of irreversible dementias can delay the progression of symptoms and help maintain both the patient's and the caregiver's quality of life (Work Group on Alzheimer's Disease and Other Dementias 2007). Individualized and multimodal treatment plans are required to address the broad

TABLE 3.4
Goals for the treatment of dementia

Goals for the individual with dementia
  Slow his or her cognitive decline
  Slow his or her functional decline
  Improve his or her quality of life
  Prevent behavioral and psychological symptoms of dementia
  Diagnose early and promptly treat behavioral and psychological symptoms of dementia
  Treat medical comorbidity and excess disability
  Preserve his or her strengths for as long as is possible
  Achieve a timely, peaceful, and dignified death
  Achieve aging in place
  Maintain his or her dignity
  Avoid futile or unnecessary medical care
Goals for the family of the individual with dementia
  Prevent and treat the caregiver's depression
  Address the caregiver's grief
  Reduce the caregiver's stress and burden
  Improve the caregiver's confidence and comfort level in managing behavioral and psychological
    symptoms of dementia
  Improve the caregiver's confidence and comfort level in making palliative care and other difficult
    health care decisions
  Minimize the impact of the individual's dementia on the caregiver's physical health

range of cognitive, behavioral, and psychological symptoms associated with all dementias. Specialized dementia care units may offer more optimal care for residents with advanced dementia. The clinician should take into account both the resident's current level of functioning and the potential impacts on the quality of that person's life when making any treatment decisions for a resident with dementia.

Treatment for Cognitive and Functional Deficits

At present, no therapy has been shown to prevent, cure, or arrest the progression of AD, DLB, PDD, or FTD. Antidementia drugs that are currently available include ChEIs and the N-methyl-D-aspartate (NMDA) receptor antagonist memantine. The clinician should consider prescribing a trial of one of the ChEIs (e.g., donepezil, rivastigmine, or galantamine) for people with mild, moderate, or severe AD, DLB, or PDD and a trial of memantine with or without the concomitant use of a ChEI for those with moderate or severe AD. Adding memantine for a resident who is already taking a ChEI may provide benefits for some people with AD. The clinician may also consider prescribing memantine for residents with mild AD, although it is not approved by the FDA as a treatment for mild AD. LTC residents with dementia may be more at risk of adverse effects from antidementia drugs than are community-dwelling people with dementia, because of the higher prevalence of frailty, medical comorbidity, and polypharmacy in LTC residents. Thus the clinician should use extra caution in prescribing antidementia drugs for LTC populations, and we strongly recommend close monitoring for adverse effects and optimal staff education about the adverse effects of antidementia drugs. At the same time, the clinician should not routinely deny LTC residents with dementia a trial of antidementia drugs just because they are frail and have multiple medical comorbidities.

Whenever the clinician prescribes an antidementia drug, he or she should apprise residents and their families of the modest potential benefits as well as the potential adverse effects and added costs of these medications. Expectations from memantine and ChEIs are similar in that approximately 30–40 percent of the residents taking these medications show some benefit, involving a modest slowing of their cognitive and functional declines. Antidementia drugs may also reduce the risk of behavioral and psychological symptoms of dementia in the future and may reduce the need for future psychotropic medications for some residents with dementia. A few patients with dementia may show a more than modest response, but we do not currently have any reliable way of identifying such patients. Staging AD through the application of cognitive scales such as the MMSE inherently limits the applied benefit of antidementia drugs just to the drugs' cognitive effects, to the exclusion of their behavioral and functional benefits. Thus the clinician should consider not only the potential cognitive benefits, but also the potential functional and behavioral benefits of antidementia drugs.

Common adverse effects of ChEIs are nausea, vomiting, and diarrhea. These tend to be mild to moderate in their severity, but for frail residents with dementia, even mild adverse effects can significantly impair their quality of life. These effects often wane within two to four days, so if residents can tolerate such unpleasantness in the early days of treatment, they may be more comfortable later. For residents with PDD, ChEIs may worsen their tremor. Other uncommon adverse effects of ChEIs include muscle cramps, bradycardia (which can be dangerous for residents with cardiac conduction problems), syncope (and falls related to syncope), a decrease in appetite, and weight loss. ChEIs increase the production of gastric acid, a particular concern for those with a history of peptic ulcers. Preexisting bradycardia, sick sinus syndrome, or conduction defects, undiagnosed nausea, vomiting and diarrhea, gastritis, and ulcerative disease are contraindications for ChEIs (American Psychiatric Association 2007). Finally, ChEIs may induce or exacerbate urinary obstruction, worsen asthma and chronic obstructive pulmonary disease, cause seizures, induce or worsen sleep disturbances, and exaggerate the effects of some muscle relaxants during anesthesia. Thus the clinician should use extra caution in prescribing ChEIs for residents with cerebrovascular disease, seizures, or chronic obstructive pulmonary disease.

Table 3.5 shows the dosing and dosages of ChEIs. ChEIs should be given in the morning on a full stomach. If the resident tolerates the starting dose, the clinician can increase the dose after a minimum of four weeks. For frail residents and those who are sensitive to the adverse effects of the medication, their ChEI starting dose can be half the standard starting dose (e.g., 2.5 mg of donepezil should be the starting dose and may be increased by 2.5 mg increments, galantamine can be given as 4 mg once a day and then increased by 4 mg increments, rivastigmine can be given as 1.5 mg once a day with food and then increased by 1.5 mg increments). Memantine is started at 5 mg given at bedtime and increased by 5 mg a week to the therapeutic dose of 10 mg in the morning and 10 mg at bedtime. For residents with severe kidney disease, frail residents, and residents who cannot tolerate 20 mg/day, we recommend a maximum dose of 10 mg a day, given at bedtime. Adverse effects of memantine include constipation, dizziness, agitation, and hallucinations. Memantine may interact with other NMDA receptor antagonists, such as dextromethorphan (often used as a cough suppressant in LTC populations and, in combination with quinidine, occasionally used to treat pseudobulbar affect). The clinician should avoid prescribing such combinations. Memantine has 5HT3 blocking effects and may protect against some gastrointestinal side effects of ChEIs.

A relatively high proportion of LTC residents taking antidementia drugs may not be benefiting enough from these medications to warrant their continuation (J. Lee et al. 2007). To avoid a withdrawal effect, the clinician should taper antidementia drugs gradually rather than withdraw them abruptly. Gradual tapering should not result in adverse clinical outcomes or sudden

TABLE 3.5
Dosing and dosages of cholinesterase inhibitors

Drug	Starting Dose per Day	Minimal Effective Dose per Day	Therapeutic Dose Range per Day	Dosing Schedule
Donepezil	2.5–5 mg	5 mg	5–10 mg	Once daily
Rivastigmine	1.5–3 mg	6 mg	6–12 mg	In two divided doses with meals
Rivastigmine	4.6 mg/24 hr	9.5 mg/24 hr	9.5 mg/24 hr	Once-daily transdermal patch
Galantamine	8 mg	16 mg	16–24 mg	Once-daily extended release Formulation

deterioration for most patients with severe dementia. When a resident with dementia reaches the terminal stage, where no specific function is being preserved (ability to recognize family, ability to answer simple questions, ability to eat with assistance), we recommend discontinuing antidementia drugs as well as other medications that are not necessary to maintain that person's comfort (e.g., statins, vitamins, medications for osteoporosis, etc.). Ginkgo biloba may have a modest beneficial effect on cognition for residents with dementia, and the clinician may consider prescribing it for residents who cannot take antidementia drugs (Desai and Grossberg 2003b).

The clinician should recognize the potential of cognitive rehabilitation for motivated residents with mild dementia. Psychosocial-environmental interventions such as regular physical exercise (aerobics, balance and strength training), healthy nutrition (fruits, vegetables, whole grains, food rich in omega-3 and monounsaturated fatty acids, turmeric), cognitively stimulating and meaningful activities (helping other residents, reading aloud, doing puzzles, playing card or board games), yoga, meditation, and stress-management strategies (relaxation exercises, mindfulness training); pharmacological interventions (antidementia drugs); and aggressive control of cardiovascular risk factors may help highly motivated residents with mild dementia achieve their highest levels of cognitive function and slow their cognitive and functional decline. Many individuals with MCI or mild dementia may benefit from cognitive training.

Psychosocial-Environmental Interventions

Psychosocial-environmental interventions are the primary mode of intervention for all behavioral and psychological symptoms of dementia, including severe symptoms that may require the addition of pharmacological interventions. Commonly employed psychosocial-environmental interventions include the education and training of caregivers, structured and unstructured activities, exercise, music, dance, reminiscence, massage therapy, aromatherapy, pet therapy (animal-assisted therapy), therapeutic gardens, simulated presence therapy (e.g., hearing family members' taped recordings), painting, other activities that allow creative expression, and spirituality. Daily exercises (e.g., walking, resistance training, flexion and stretch exercises) improve functional fitness and are critical for maintaining muscle mass and slowing cognitive and functional decline (Struck and Ross 2006).

There is a growing consensus that spirituality is of great importance, not only for those with dementia, but also for their caregivers (Sperry 2006). Often the spiritual experiences of individuals with dementia are the most profound at the disease's later stages (and even in its terminal stage). The loss of cognitive capacity does not reflect a loss of spiritual capacity, and those with advanced dementia remain capable of high levels of spiritual well-being. Helping a resident with dementia continue to observe his or her faith can be beneficial and rewarding for both the resident and family caregivers. Songs and prayers from childhood often stay firmly rooted in memory long after dementia takes its toll. Bright light has a modest benefit in improving some cognitive and noncognitive (e.g., mood, sleep) symptoms of dementia (Riemersma-van der Lek et al. 2008).

We recommend the STAR approach for the assessment and treatment of behavioral and psychological symptoms of dementia:

- S = Safety. The clinician should assess the safety and security of the resident and others and address it first. This includes a discussion of the need for inpatient psychiatric treatment for behavioral emergencies.
- T = Team approach. We recommend a team approach to identify triggers and modifiable causes of behavioral and psychological symptoms of dementia.
- A = Action plan. The clinician should devise and implement an action plan (an individualized treatment plan with psychosocial-environmental interventions and, when appropriate, pharmacological interventions).
- R = Response to treatment. If the response to treatment is inadequate, the clinician should reassess it and modify the treatment plan appropriately.

Ensuring safety and security is crucial, as behavioral and psychological symptoms may often be severe and can even be life-threatening to the resident having the behaviors (e.g., suicide attempts) or other residents (e.g., pushing another resident and causing a fatal head injury), as well as dangerous for the staff. Also, agitation in residents with dementia may put them or others at risk of serious injury (e.g., falls, fractures). If safety cannot be ensured, alternative placement of the resident (e.g., an acute inpatient psychiatric unit for a resident who made a serious suicide attempt) may be necessary. Residents who wander may be particularly at risk of exposure to dangerous weather conditions, dehydration, being struck by another resident (because the wandering resident invades the other resident's personal space), and medical problems due to missed doses of medication. Identifying triggers is important, as modifying the triggers often ameliorates the behavioral disturbances. Medical disorders (e.g., untreated pain, UTI) and psychiatric disorders (major depression, generalized anxiety disorder) are common causes of agitation in residents with dementia and are eminently treatable. A typical psychosocial-environmental intervention can involve a therapeutic caregiver interaction and continuous activity programming tailored to each resident's unique needs, strengths, and interests, both of which can prevent and abort many agitated behaviors in residents with dementia.

> • CLINICAL CASE Mrs. L had probable dementia of the Alzheimer type at a moderate stage, and over the previous several weeks she had been growing agitated in the afternoon and evening, attempting to leave and becoming physically aggressive when prevented from leaving. Mrs. L was taking citalopram 40 mg daily, donepezil 10 mg daily in the morning, and memantine 10 mg twice daily for her dementia and anxiety symptoms. These medications helped decrease Mrs. L's agitation to some extent, but she continued to have at least one incident of physical aggression toward the staff per week. Mrs. L was referred to the consulting psychiatrist for more medication to "control her aggression."
>
> The consulting psychiatrist first ruled out easily correctable causes (anticholinergic medication, medical conditions, etc.). The psychiatrist then met with the team members (Mrs. L's family, a CNA, an LPN, and a social worker) and discussed psychosocial interventions that could be tried. Mrs. L's daughter mentioned that her mother had always loved to work in the house rather than watch television or play games. Mrs. L had never had pets and did not like them, and she had not regularly listened to music. The team decided to give Mrs. L simple tasks such as setting the table, folding napkins, and putting letters in envelopes; they did not select other psychosocial interventions, such as pets or a music group. After two weeks of implementing these interventions, Mrs. L had become significantly less agitated and more easily redirected.
>
> TEACHING POINTS Knowing the resident well (including his or her role in life before moving into an LTC facility, daily interests, and what activity gave him or her meaning in life) is key to significantly improving the success rate of psychosocial-environmental interventions. If the team had not tried to address Mrs. L's underlying need to feel useful and engage in activities that gave meaning to her life, her agitation and aggression could

have continued and she may even have been prescribed antipsychotic medications, putting her at risk of accelerated cognitive and functional decline. Agitation is best managed with psychosocial-environmental interventions, such as changing the caregiver's approach through education and training, or figuring out and meeting the resident's unmet needs (Ballard et al. 2002; Overshott, Byrne, and Burns 2004). Pharmacological interventions are not particularly effective for managing agitation in residents with dementia (Sink, Holden, and Yaffe 2005).

Palliative Care for People with Advanced Dementia

The clinician should discuss an individual's wishes regarding life-prolonging treatment during advanced dementia (moderate, severe, and terminal stages) when that person is in the disease's mild stage (preferably the first half of the mild stage), because then the individual retains the capacity to make medical decisions for him- or herself, can fully participate in the discussion, and express wishes to the family. As the dementia progresses, the burdens of life-prolonging treatment, such as hospitalization for pneumonia, often increase dramatically and the potential benefits (e.g., increased duration of survival) decrease considerably. Families of most residents in the terminal stage of dementia opt for comfort only care (indicating no life-prolonging treatment, such as the treatment of pneumonia, but a desire for any treatment interventions that improve comfort and reduce pain and discomfort). Some families of residents in dementia's severe stage may also opt for comfort only care; other families may want life-prolonging treatment. The family may choose life-prolonging treatment for persons with severe dementia for several reasons: because they are not sure what their loved one would have wanted and are erring on the side of caution; because they are not ready to "let go" or they feel that not providing life-prolonging treatment means they are giving up, instead of understanding it as letting go; or because they think that this is what their loved one would have wanted. The clinician should assure the family that there is no right or wrong answer, help the family understand what the person with dementia would have wanted, and then help them keep their promise and respect that person's wishes. The clinician should also understand the tremendous grief (and sometimes guilt) the family may be dealing with at this time, which can influence their decisions. Addressing these complex feelings can also help the family make a decision regarding life-prolonging treatment that is in keeping with the resident's wishes and values.

In addition, the clinician should discuss other aspects of palliative care—

such as when to forgo cardiopulmonary resuscitation (CPR) or hospitalization, the degree of pain control versus the adverse effects of pain medication (e.g., severely compromised awareness), and the risks and benefits of placement of a feeding tube as early as possible in the course of dementia—with both the resident and the family. In all discussions, it is crucial to focus more on understanding the values of the person with dementia, what gives that person meaning in life, and the importance that person places on how strictly his or her wishes are to be carried out by the surrogate decision maker (i.e., an advance care planning document is more than a document, it is a family covenant or promise).

Special Populations and Special Issues

Medical comorbidity, hospitalization for a psychiatry emergency, sex and sexuality, aging in place, the capacity to make medical decisions, and the caregivers' well-being are of particular concern if residents with dementia are to have an excellent quality of life.

Medical Comorbidity

More than 60 percent of residents with dementia have three or more comorbidities (Volicer and Hurley 1997; Doraiswamy et al. 2002), and residents with dementia have more comorbidities and need more assistance with ADLs than do those of the same age who do not have dementia. Hypertension, cardiovascular disease, arthritis, chronic kidney disease, anemia, diabetes, and diminution of vision and hearing, among other conditions, can be expected in the typical LTC resident with dementia. Residents with dementia have a higher incidence of Parkinsonism, seizures, infections, malnutrition, sensory impairment, hip fractures and other injuries, and pressure sores (Chandra, Barucha, and Schoenberg 1986). An optimal diagnosis and treatment of comorbid medical illnesses are essential components of the management of dementia, and they are key to sustaining the resident's cognition.

In treating medical comorbidities, the clinician should weigh the possible benefits for the resident against the burdens imposed by such treatment. Also, the goals of the treatment should be in keeping with the resident's overall goals of care (i.e., palliative [comfort only] versus life-prolonging treatment). For every resident with dementia, the clinician should consider discontinuing medications that have a potential for significant anticholinergic symptoms. Residents with dementia are frequently transferred to emergency rooms and hospitalized for medical conditions (e.g., pneumonia), putting them at high risk of delirium, falls, the need for restraints, and functional decline during and after hospitalization, despite successful treatment of the medical condition. Hospitalization is extremely stressful for residents with dementia (especially frail residents and residents with severe and terminal stage dementias). The clinician needs to discuss all of these hospitalization risks with the family before any decision is made to hospitalize the resident and soon after that person's admission to an LTC facility. We recommend psychiatric consultation (preferably by a geriatric psychiatrist) for the management of agitation in residents with dementia who have been hospitalized.

Hospitalization for a Psychiatric Emergency

Residents with dementia may require admission to a psychiatric unit for the treatment of a behavioral emergency (severe physical aggression, homicidal ideation, severe depression with a suicide attempt, or minimal oral intake). When the option is available, admission to a geriatric psychiatry or medical psychiatric unit is preferable to a general psychiatric unit. Many state laws prohibit such admission without the involvement of law enforcement agencies, which adds strain to residents, their loved ones, and the LTC staff. Although admission to a psychiatric unit for the evaluation and management of a behavioral emergency is necessary for some residents with dementia and severe psychiatric symptoms, in many such cases the admission could have been prevented by early recognition and aggressive treatment of their psychiatric disorders, either at the facility or by an outpatient psychiatric team. The clinician should order a transfer to a psychiatric unit from an LTC facility only after ensuring that such a treatment intervention is in keeping with the resident's goals for their care. For many residents with severe or terminal dementia who have documented comfort only measures as their goals of care, referral to a hospice and sedation with psychiatric medications may be more appropriate. If the resident is admitted to a psychiatric unit, the clinician should discuss palliative care goals with the resident and family as soon as possible after admission.

Sex and Sexuality

Sexuality in the broadest terms includes affection, romance, companionship, personal grooming, touch, and the need to feel attractive and either feminine or masculine. Thus sexual activity is any activity that portends the sensation of "feeling loved." Sexual expression is a basic human need, even among residents in LTC facilities (Hajjar and Kamel 2004a). Many LTC residents feel sexually unattractive. The major mode of sexual expression, as seen by residents, is trying to remain physically attractive. Sexual identity is closely interwoven with one's concept of self-worth. Denying a resident's sexuality can deleteriously affect not only the resident's sex life but also his or her self-image, social relationships, and mental health. To provide a nurturing environment that promotes the residents' health and well-being, LTC cannot ignore sexuality. Many residents have sexual thoughts and fantasies, as libido persists despite infirmity and admission to LTC. Sexual behavior in one's younger years is a strong predictor of later behavior. For many residents, sexual expression is limited to caressing, kissing, hugging, or mutual manual genital stimulation. However, self-stimulation (i.e., masturbation) is not rare, particularly among males. Female residents often find few potential partners, due to an increasing demographic gender disparity in LTC facilities. Also, for the current generation of residents, most male residents have living spouses, whereas most female residents are widowed.

Physicians, staff, and family should address sexual needs as part of their duty to enhance the residents' quality of life and well-being. The staff should make every reasonable effort to support the residents' privacy and sexuality. Staff and family members need to understand that residents (at any age) maintain significant degrees of sexuality and often wish to be sexually expressive. The clinician should carefully assess residents with dementia who are in a romantic or sexual relationship to determine their capacity to participate in such relationships. The clinician should anticipate implications the progression of dementia will have on the relationship and develop contingencies for these residents' evolving needs for supervision and advocacy. LTC facilities should protect residents' rights to homosexual and interracial relationships. Institutional and staff biases against the sexual expressions of residents should be addressed through education and training programs, and by clear institutional policies that support the residents' rights. The institution should make provisions for staff nonparticipation in direct patient care when the implications of the sexual activity in such care are unavoidable and are morally or religiously offensive to the staff member. At the same time, the facility should not permit staff members to refuse to provide care for a resident who is sexually active (Berger 2000).

A structured and regimented environment leaves residents in a situation in which their control over most aspects of their lives is eroding. Ensuring their privacy is of paramount importance. The staff should not discuss, document, judge, or gossip about the residents' personal activities. Many staff and family members may think that it is not necessary for residents to maintain their sexuality. The staff should not use fixed scheduling and treatment priorities as an excuse to deter intimacy among residents. Compromising the privacy of residents is not justified, even if their physical health can be enhanced thereby. Cultural diversity among the staff and residents is as important to addresses in areas of sexuality as it is in areas of food, clothing, and religion.

UNDERSTANDING SEXUALLY INAPPROPRIATE BEHAVIOR   Sexuality can be a difficult and challenging issue for professional and family caregivers to address with residents. This is particularly the case in responding to incidents of hypersexuality or inappropriate sexual expression as a result of dementia (Higgins, Barker, and Begley 2004). Inappropriate undressing in public or touching one's genitals may occur because of uncomfortable clothes, clothes that are too hot, or itching or discomfort. This should not be considered inappropriate sexual behavior. Staff and family members often see sexually inappropriate behaviors (e.g., using explicit sexual language, lewd sexual references, inappropriate sexual acts such as exposing one's genitalia for sexual gratification or inappropriately touching a staff member [groping], masturbating during personal care activities, reading or asking for pornographic material) as a problem rather than as an expression of the need for love and intimacy. Some other sexually inappropriate behaviors include attempting or having intercourse with another resident, fondling, and exposing one's genitalia to other residents or visitors. Sexually inappropriate behaviors are often seen in residents with a significant cerebrovascular disease (a stroke, VaD, mixed [AD and VaD] dementia) and when dementia involves the frontal lobes (advanced AD, FTD). The clinician should promptly address all sexually inappropriate behaviors using the STAR approach described above.

ROLE OF HEALTH CARE PROVIDERS   Health care providers should incorporate a discussion of the need for sexual expression into the routine care of residents, and they should learn as much as possible about the factors that influence sexual expression in residents. The availability of accurate educational materials for residents and their families, and the distribution of written materials in areas residents and their families frequently visit so that they can pick up and read these materials, are signs that health care providers welcome a discussion about the residents' sexual concerns and that family and staff members should consider these needs. The clinician should ask residents if they are sexually active, correct any misconceptions and answer any questions they might have about sexual activities, teach them about the physical changes of aging which may affect sexual functioning, and educate them about the importance of protection from sexually transmitted diseases, including HIV, for sexually active residents.

Clinicians should support the appropriate expression of the residents' sexuality and act as a resident advocate both with other health care providers and with residents who may express discomfort. If a resident who has lost a spouse feels that he or she is violating marriage vows by forming an intimate relationship with another resident or a nonresident, clinicians should provide counseling (or make a referral to a mental health care provider with expertise in geriatrics) to process this problem through discussion. Clinicians should also consider involving a member of the clergy the resident has a relationship with and trusts. Health care providers should always protect residents unable to make their own decisions about engaging in sexual activity. They should also protect residents from themselves when the residents are not in control of their own behavior. Health care providers should advocate for the healthy expression of sexual behavior. Helping residents feel physically attractive (e.g., by providing beauty salons and cosmetic services) can dramatically improve ways the residents can satisfy their sexual needs. Health care providers should not make assumptions about the residents' sexual preferences. Many older gay men and lesbians may be reluctant to identify themselves as such. However, as they enter LTC facilities, many find that their previously private lives are now open for scrutiny. Health care providers need to challenge their own preconceived notions, explore their own homophobic attitudes, and advocate for all residents, irrespective of sexual orientations.

INTERVENTIONS   We recommend meeting the residents' need for intimacy and affection by allowing appropriate touching, hugging, and hand-holding. Male residents exhibiting sexually inappropriate behaviors should be seated away from female residents. The clinician should request male staff members to care for male residents who exhibit sexually inappropriate behaviors during personal care. Choosing clothing that opens in the back and considering twin beds for a husband and wife if one of them engages in sexually inappropriate behavior are other examples of environmental strategies. The LTC facility should provide a private space for residents who wish to engage in sexual activity. The staff must strive to maintain the privacy of information and associations, although this is difficult within closely monitored quarters. The staff should not infantilize residents who voice an interest in sexual expression, and clinicians should routinely consider sexuality in their overall assessments of residents. The staff can address a situation in which two residents show sexually intimate behaviors in public (e.g., kissing or groping) by discretely taking the residents to their room, closing the door, and putting a Do Not Disturb sign outside the room (table 3.6).

Staff members should be flexible in their actions as advocates, and their role should evolve as conditions warrant. The staff may be obligated to disallow a physically intimate relationship if the residents' interests (however those interests are defined) are not served or the integrity of their lives is violated. The staff may need to negotiate some limited breaches of privacy with the couple (and their families) in order to assess, over time, the kind of advocacy the residents need and whether the relationship has continued to be in the residents' best interests and in keeping with their values before dementia. The greater a resident's cognitive capacity, the less paternalistically the staff should behave. Psychiatric and neuropsychological evaluations may clarify a resident's decision-making capacity.

TABLE 3.6
Strategies to meet residents' needs for intimacy and sexual expression

Educate staff members and provide sensitivity training

Obtain a detailed sexual history for each resident

Encourage staff to openly discuss their attitudes and concerns, and to pick up any cues that may indicate a resident's needs for intimacy

Promote privacy (minimize room sharing; provide a Do Not Disturb sign; before entering a resident's room, knock on the door, call the resident's name, and ask permission to enter)

Allow conjugal visits and/or home visits

Provide individualized high-touch, low-tech care

Encourage alternative forms of sexual expression, such as hugging and kissing

Provide beauty salons and cosmetic services in the long-term care facility, and attend to the personal appearance of residents

Educate residents and family members about the residents' rights and recourses to meet their sexual needs

Encourage friendships and relationships between residents, with appropriate guidance and supervision

Reassign care to another staff member if there is a conflict between the duty to address a resident's sexual needs and the staff member's personal value system

Address residents' physical limitations and poor health (e.g., manage pain better, correct hearing and vision deficits)

Offer appropriate means and encouragement to residents to help them meet their sexual needs (e.g., privacy to masturbate)

BEHAVIOR THERAPY   Redirecting behavior verbally or physically, telling the resident in a firm but kind manner that his or her behavior is inappropriate, improving the consistency of the staff's approach, ignoring unwanted behaviors and encouraging appropriate behaviors, and avoiding inadvertent reinforcement of unwanted behaviors (smiling and laughing when redirecting, or saying "You are being naughty again, stop that") are some examples of behavior therapy.

PHARMACOTHERAPY   No practice guidelines are available for the pharmacological treatment of abnormal sexual behaviors in LTC residents or in cognitively impaired elderly populations. Nor are there any large, randomized controlled trials investigating pharmacological interventions to treat sexually inappropriate behavior in LTC populations. Pharmacotherapy includes SSRIs as first-line agents for moderate to severe sexually inappropriate behaviors (Hajjar and Kamel 2004b). SSRIs may reduce impulsivity, but they may have adverse sexual effects (e.g., reduction in libido) as well as antidepressant and anxiolytic effects (depression and anxiety symptoms often are comorbid with sexually inappropriate behaviors). The clinician may consider prescribing antipsychotic medications when there is persistent sexual aggression and he or she suspects that psychotic symptoms underlie the behavior. Hormonal interventions are controversial, but the clinician may consider them if a male resident is engaging in or threatening dangerous acts involving physical contact. In such situations, sexually aggressive behavior is severe and persists despite all other interventions, and the resident cannot be managed without control of these symptoms. Among hormonal interventions, antiandrogens (medroxyprogesterone acetate or cyproterone acetate) are first-line agents (Guay 2008). The clinician may consider prescribing luteinizing hormone-releasing hormone agonists (e.g., leuprolide, triptorelin) as a first choice and estrogens (oral, transdermal) as a second choice if antiandrogens are contraindicated or ineffective. Combination therapy is reasonable if the resident fails to respond to monotherapy. We recommend thoroughly educating the surrogate decision maker about the risks and benefits of hormonal interventions before initiating these interventions.

EDUCATING AND COUNSELING THE FAMILY AND STAFF   Family and staff members need to be educated about the fact that dementia may result in an inappropriate expression of sexual needs (because of disinhibition), although these needs are still real. Residents with dementia often misinterpret staff actions; for example, they may interpret a staff member's bending over to provide care as an invitation to undo a blouse or pull down a zipper. Occasionally, dementia can cause a seemingly indefatigable desire for sexual gratification, but the resident does not comprehend the act itself or the emotions involved. The clinician should address a spouse's guilt about not wanting to be a willing partner and counsel that spouse regarding what is appropriate and acceptable for the spouse and the resident. No spouse should feel guilty about a decision to forgo gratifying a partner's sexual needs. The integrity of the resident's and the spouse's life journeys needs to be protected against the waywardness created by dementia. For example, if a resident is unable to recognize her husband, the potential emotional trauma she may feel after the sexual act may be a serious enough concern to ask the husband to forgo his wish to be sexually intimate (Post 2000).

Conflicting duties to promote residents' health and to protect them from abuse, injury, and neglect can raise ethical issues when trying to meet some residents' needs for sexual expression. Conflicts between prevailing social moral values and a resident's behavior are also a concern. Staff members may express confusion, embarrassment, anger, denial, and helplessness when they discover residents having sexual relations. The staff are often not sure when to involve the family, and they feel torn between moral norms and their duty to respect residents' rights. Clinicians should improve their own knowledge and skills to enhance the sexual expression of residents and take a leadership role in educating and training the staff to meet the need for optimal sexual expression for all residents.

> **CLINICAL CASE** Ms. H was a 78-year-old woman who had been living in a nursing home for two years. Since she was admitted, the staff had noticed that Ms. H had invited various male residents to her room and had tried to kiss them. A psychiatrist was consulted because of the staff's report that Ms. H was "sexually aggressive" toward male residents. The psychiatrist, after a detailed interview and input from various staff members, found out that the nursing assistants involved in caring for Ms. H for the first one-and-a-half years had left. The new nursing assistants had just obtained their certification and were not sure how to deal with Ms. H's sexually inappropriate behavior. One nursing assistant felt that the behavior was "cute" and "funny" and even giggled with Ms. H, while another felt that the behavior was "abhorrent" and should be stopped. In fact, this nursing assistant had told Ms. H that she was

not behaving like a "lady" and another staff member found Ms. H crying
after this exchange. The sexually aggressive behavior that precipitated
the consultation was that Ms. H was found kissing a male resident in her
room.

During the interview, Ms. H, a cheerful woman, asked the psychiatrist
to give her "just one kiss." The psychiatrist showed her his wedding ring,
but Ms. H said, "Your wife won't know." The psychiatrist told her that
he loved his wife and could not grant Ms. H her wish. The psychiatrist
was pleasant and nonjudgmental during the interview, and shook Ms.
H's hand when it was completed. The psychiatrist spent time educating
the staff caring for Ms. H that her need for sexual gratification was normal, but that it was expressed inappropriately because of her dementia;
the damage to her frontal lobe or its connections was predisposing Ms.
H to sexually disinhibited behavior. The psychiatrist also discussed the
importance of being nonjudgmental and the need for a consistent staff
approach. Over the next eight weeks, with a nonjudgmental approach and
firm and consistent redirection by all the staff, encouraging Ms. H to hug
and hold the hands of male residents who liked these gestures (and whose
families were in agreement with such contact), Ms. H's sexually inappropriate behavior became more manageable. The psychiatrist also met with
the facility's director of nursing and its administrator, and together they
decided to have a facility-wide in-service addressing this topic.

TEACHING POINTS At times, nursing assistants may have a high turnover rate. Adequate education of new nursing assistants regarding
sexually inappropriate behaviors (as well as other behaviors) and ongoing
training are key to preventing a misinterpretation of a resident's sexual expressions as something that needs to be fixed, that is, stopped or eliminated.

CLINICAL CASE Mr. S was a 58-year-old single male with chronic
paranoid schizophrenia who lived in a community nursing home. He had
been moved there several years previously from the state hospital. Mr. S
was stable on his antipsychotic drug regimen of clozapine 100 mg in the
morning and 300 mg at bedtime. He was mostly seclusive, but he did leave
his room to go to the dining room for meals. Mr. S collected pornographic
magazines and videotapes, which he would read and watch in the privacy
of his room. One day, on returning from breakfast in the dining room,
he found his dresser and other belongings in the hallway. He apparently
was not told that his room would be recarpeted. His magazines and tapes

were also moved into the hallway. He became angry, agitated, and upset, accusing the staff of messing with his personal belongings. His dormant suspiciousness became blatant, and he required hospitalization after a suicide attempt.

TEACHING POINTS Assuring privacy and respect is not only ethically necessary, but also important in maintaining the emotional well-being and dignity of all residents.

Aging in Place

Early and aggressive management of dementia and of the behavioral and psychological symptoms of dementia can increase the chances of a resident's aging in place (i.e., if the person is in an assisted living facility, he or she can delay for a few years having to move into a nursing home and can thus save money, as the cost of staying in a nursing home is much higher than the cost of staying in an assisted living facility). With the availability of hospice care and a slowly improving understanding of palliative care for people who have dementia, many residents may live the last years of their lives in an assisted living facility without having to transfer to a nursing home or hospital.

Capacity to Make Medical Decisions

Assessing a resident's capacity to make medical and financial decisions is one of the important skills that are essential for physicians working with LTC populations. Decision making requires that a person understand information, be able to communicate choices, understand the situation and its consequences, and manipulate information in a rational manner (Ganzini et al. 2004). The communication framework of Charles, Gafni, and Whelan (1999), which defines three distinct components of decision making—information exchange, deliberation about treatment options, and responsibility for the choice—may help model the physician-resident encounter.

The clinician should give the person with dementia whose capacity to make decisions is being assessed all the information about the benefits and risks of a proposed treatment or recommendation (e.g., a recommendation to stay in an LTC facility), the implications of not having this treatment, available alternatives, and the practical effects of having or not having the treatment. An individual's cognitive ability may vary from day to day, and decision making is not an all-or-nothing phenomenon. A resident may not have the decision-making capacity to make major decisions about health care, but he or she may have the capacity to decide whether to take a sleeping pill. Not having the capacity to make decisions is not always a permanent condition. For example, residents with delirium may lack decision-making capacity, but once the delirium resolves they may regain that capacity. Any physician or licensed psychologist with a doctorate can and should be able to assess a resident's decision-making capacity. Residents have a right to trust that their health care providers and legal advisors will not divulge confidential information without their express permission, even when a resident has diminished capacity.

The capacity for decision making should be differentiated from competency to make decisions for oneself. Competency to make health care and financial decisions or to delegate the right to make such decisions is a legal conclusion, requiring help from an elder-law attorney. Western civilization's concept of personal autonomy and self-determination are at the core of health care decision making, but health care providers must be aware that other cultures do not always share that value system. Sensitivity to multicultural diversity is imperative to maintain individual self-esteem and respect for both the resident and the resident's family.

We recommend five principles of care regarding the evaluation of capacity in residents with dementia:

1. Preserving patient autonomy should be the guiding principle in exercising professional judgment regarding a person with a diminished capacity. This requires upholding the values of individual choice, control, privacy, and dignity in the nursing home setting (Hayley et al. 1996).
2. The clinician should always presume that an individual with dementia is capable of making health care decisions, unless a formal evaluation of capacity by two physicians has shown the opposite.
3. The clinician should not treat an individual with dementia as being unable to make a decision unless the clinician has taken all practicable steps to help him or her do so without success.
4. For an individual with dementia to give valid consent, he or she must be capable of making decisions in his or her own best interest, be acting voluntarily, and be provided with enough information to enable decision making.
5. Whenever possible, the clinician should consider enlisting the assistance of family, friends, caregivers, and advocates who can help the

person with dementia understand the issues and make his or her own decisions.

Caregivers' Well-Being

Perhaps the greatest cost of dementia is the physical and emotional toll on the family, caregivers, and friends (Gwyther 1998). Caring for a loved one with dementia increases the risk of death for the caregiver, as dementia puts a gradually increasing burden on caregivers as the disease progresses. Caregivers commonly report poor self-rated health, increased levels of depressive symptoms, and greater use of psychoactive medications (Baumgarten et al. 1994). Caregivers often experience a profound sense of loss as the dementia slowly takes their loved one. The relationship as it once was gradually ends, and plans for the future must be radically changed. Caregivers must come to terms with "the long goodbye." Family caregivers of residents with dementia may have experienced many negative effects of caregiving (employment complications, emotional distress, fatigue and poor physical health, social isolation, family conflict, and less time for leisure, self, and other family members), but research has shown that caregiving may also have important positive effects (e.g., a new sense of purpose or meaning in life, fulfillment of a lifelong commitment to a spouse, an opportunity to give back to a parent some of what the parent has given to them, a renewal of religious faith, closer ties with people through new relationships or stronger existing relationships).

Most primary caregivers are family members. Spouses are the largest group of caregivers. Most are older, too, and many also have to deal with their own health problems. Daughters are the second largest group of primary caregivers. Many daughters are married and raising children of their own, and juggling two sets of responsibilities is often very difficult for these members of the sandwich generation. Daughters-in-law (the third largest group of family caregivers), sons, brothers, sisters, grandchildren, friends, neighbors, and fellow faith-community members constitute the remaining groups of caregivers. In general, caregivers who are male spouses, who have few breaks from caregiving responsibilities, or who have preexisting medical or psychiatric disorders are most vulnerable to the physical and emotional stresses associated with caregiving. It can be emotionally and spiritually draining to watch as dementia takes the memory and sense of self from a loved one. Caregivers should be supported in their efforts to continue to hold a spiritual perspective on life (i.e., to have spiritual beliefs that are incorporated into their philosophy of life).

LTC staff can facilitate caregiver well-being by providing peer support programs (or information on where to find one) that link caregivers with trained volunteers who have been dementia caregivers. Such programs are especially useful for the family members of residents admitted to an LTC facility for the first time and for family members with weak social support networks or who are undergoing caregiver burnout. Family caregivers must be reminded that there is no one right way to help a loved one with dementia. Even small interventions (referral to a support group, expressing support) may translate into improvements in the family caregiver's quality of life or confidence. We recommend educating family members about dementia, its effects on the individual, how best to respond to symptoms, and how to access and use available resources (e.g., involving other willing family members, contacting the local chapter of the Alzheimer's Association). We also recommend counseling and ongoing support for family members, including individual and family counseling, telephone counseling, and encouragement for caregivers to join support groups, especially caregivers who have limited social support and those experiencing depression. We recommend improving social support and reducing family conflict, both to help the caregiver withstand the hardships of caregiving and to help family members understand the primary caregiver's needs and how best to be helpful (Mittelman et al. 2004).

For community-dwelling people with AD, improving caregiver well-being delays admission to a nursing home (Mittelman et al. 2006). This may help the person entering LTC adjust to the facility better, as he or she may be less aware of being admitted to a facility because of advanced dementia and thus may make less effort to leave. Using a structured multicomponent intervention (in-home sessions and telephone sessions over several months to address the caregiver's depression, burden, self-care, and social support and the care recipient's problem behaviors) adapted to individual risk profiles can increase the quality of life for ethnically diverse caregivers (Belle et al. 2006).

Conclusion

Residents with dementia are at risk of becoming medical orphans in a long-term health care system geared toward cure and in a culture in which it is considered normal for elderly people to suffer. Residents with dementia, and their family members, have a right to receive care that is competent, compassionate, appropriate to the stage of the disease, and consistent. Appropriate care can substantially reduce the number of residents with dementia who have pain, depression, and agitation, as well as the number who receive inappropriate medical treatment (e.g., hospitalization, surgery, medication, CPR) and futile procedures (e.g., tube feeding). Although most dementias are incurable, appropriate comprehensive treatment can substantially improve the quality of life for that person, the family, and professional caregivers.

CHAPTER 4

Delirium

Delirium is a classic geriatric psychiatric syndrome that occurs commonly among elderly people who are frail or have dementia, that is, those who make up most of the residents in a long-term care facility (Inouye 2006; Eeles and Rockwood 2008). When screened, up to 15 percent of the people admitted to a postacute facility are delirious (Kiely et al. 2003). Among LTC residents older than age 85, up to 60 percent may have delirium at some point during their stay (Fann 2000). The prevalence of delirium in an LTC setting may be increasing as a result of the pressure to reduce the length of hospital stays (Lyons 2006). Delirium in elderly people is also called *acute confusion, acute confusional state,* and *cognitive/mental status change.* Central features of delirium are an acute onset and a fluctuating course, a disturbance of consciousness (hyperalert or drowsy), and inattention (a reduced ability to focus, sustain, or shift attention). Disturbances of the sleep-wake cycle, of perception, and of thinking (disorganization, incoherence) and a reduced awareness of one's environment generally accompany delirium. Although the onset of these symptoms is typically described as acute (often within hours or one to two days), a subacute onset of delirium over days to weeks is not uncommon in LTC populations. Psychosis can accompany delirium, irrespective of the latter's cause. At the cellular level, delirium is considered to be a reversible dysregulation of neuronal membrane function. This involves the selective vulnerability of certain populations of neurons (e.g., the reticular activating system) and neurotransmitter dysfunction (e.g., acetylcholine and gamma-aminobutyric acid).

There are four subtypes of delirium:

- Agitated (hyperactive) delirium is characterized by agitation, hallucinations, hyperalertness or vigilance, and inappropriate behavior. It accounts for 25–30 percent of the cases of delirium.
- Quiet (hypoactive) delirium is characterized by somnolence (the resident tends to sleep all the time), apathy, sluggishness, lethargy, and withdrawn behavior. It accounts for 50–55 percent of the cases of delirium. Quiet delirium is more likely to be overlooked or to be misdiagnosed as depression, and it may carry a higher risk of mortality than agitated or mixed delirium. Often, quiet delirium goes unrecognized until the resident becomes stuporous (difficult to arouse) or comatose (unarousable).
- Delirium with normal psychomotor activity carries the lowest risk of mortality, compared with other types of delirium.
- Mixed delirium is characterized by a pattern of fluctuating symptoms, including periods of agitation and times when the resident is quietly confused and withdrawn.

Risk Factors and Etiological Factors

In LTC populations, dehydration and infection are the two most common causes of delirium. Constipation and drug-induced delirium are also common. Table 4.1 lists risk factors for delirium in LTC populations (Flaherty and Morley 2004). Although all LTC residents have at least one risk factor for delirium, many have several, and these residents are at highest risk of delirium. Table 4.2 lists some of the common causes of delirium in LTC populations (Inouye 2000; Flaherty and Morley 2004). Although typically one or two of the common causes of delirium can be identified as precipitating, delirium is multifactorial in most residents. Thus solving one factor alone is unlikely to resolve the delirium. In high-risk residents, a relatively benign insult, such as the addition of a sleeping pill or sleep aids containing diphenhydramine (e.g., Tylenol PM), may be sufficient to precipitate delirium.

Diagnosis and Work-Up

Recognizing delirium may be difficult, but its diagnosis can be improved through a cognitive assessment and the use of simple diagnostic tools (Lyons 2006). Chapter 2 contains clinical pearls to detect delirium early and tools to identify delirium. Delirium is often noticed in an agitated or noisy resident, but it is easily missed in a quietly confused, apathetic resident or a resident

TABLE 4.1
Risk factors for delirium

Recent transfer from a hospital for a postacute rehabilitative stay in a long-term care facility
Underlying or preexisting dementia (especially advanced dementia)
Underlying or preexisting mild cognitive impairments
Advanced age (more than 85 years old)
Moderate to severe cerebrovascular disease (large and small strategic strokes, lacunar infarcts)
Loss of hearing and/or vision
Frailty
Poor nutritional status (such as protein energy malnutrition)
Polypharmacy
Heart failure
Inadequate relief of pain
Physical restraints
Indwelling urinary catheter
Certain medications (drugs with high anticholinergic activity, benzodiazepines, opiates, steroids)
Chronic end-organ failure (end-stage chronic obstructive pulmonary disease, end-stage renal disease, end-stage liver disease)
Metastases
Prolonged sleep deprivation
Social isolation
Bedfast status

Source: Adapted from Flaherty and Morley 2004.

with psychomotor retardation who is staying in his or her room. Underlying dementia, impaired vision, and being older than 80 have also been associated with the underdiagnosis of delirium (Inouye et al. 2001). For many residents, delirium may be the only manifestation of a serious medical problem (e.g., the sudden onset of a change in mental status without typical symptoms such as speech disturbances, a focal neurological deficit [in the case of a stroke] or dyspnea, tachypnea [in the case of respiratory failure], chest discomfort or pain [in the case of myocardial infarction], shortness of breath [in the case of heart failure], and a fever or leukocytosis [in the case of infection]). The clinician should have a high index of suspicion regarding occult infections in LTC populations.

Delirium is primarily diagnosed from the resident's history and mental status examination. The setting (e.g., postacute stay in an LTC facility) and the presence of several risk factors add to the acumen of the diagnosis. The clinician should consider new-onset falls in LTC residents to be the equivalent of delirium (Flaherty and Morley 2004). To establish an accurate diagnosis, the clinician should speak to various staff members who know the resident well (e.g., CNAs, LPNs, RNs, dietary staff, housekeeping) and to the resident's

TABLE 4.2
Mnemonic for common treatable causes of delirium in long-term care residents

D   Dehydration
    Deficient nutrition (such as Wernicke encephalopathy due to a thiamine deficiency in a resident
    with alcohol dependence)
E   Electrolyte imbalance (such as hyponatremia, hypercalcemia)
    Endocrine disorders (such as diabetes, thyroid disorders)
    End-organ failure (kidneys, liver, lungs, heart)
    Electrical disturbances in the brain (seizures) and heart (arrythmias)
    ETOH (alcohol)-induced (intoxication, withdrawal)
L   Lack of oxygen to the brain (hypoxia/hypoxemia) and hypercarbia (stroke, heart failure,
    myocardial infarction, acute blood loss, pulmonary embolism, exacerbation of chronic
    obstructive pulmonary disease, occult respiratory failure)
I   Injury (hip fracture, head injury after a fall or due to physical abuse [resulting in a subdural
    hematoma])
    Intestinal obstruction
    Impaction (fecal)
R   Rule out psychiatric disorders (mania, depression, psychosis, acute stress disorder, post-traumatic
    stress disorder)
I   Infection (urinary tract infection, pneumonia, cellulitis)
U   Urinary retention
    Unfamiliar environment
M   Medications (steroids, drugs with high anticholinergic activity, benzodiazepines [intoxication,
    withdrawal], opiates)
    Malignancy (includes paraneoplastic syndromes)

family regarding the onset and nature of the resident's change in mental status. The clinician should take subsyndromal delirium as seriously as delirium. In subsyndromal delirium, only one or two of the features of delirium are present (e.g., a sudden increase in confusion but no significant fluctuation in sensorium, no perceptual disturbances or disorganized thinking). In cases involving an uncooperative resident, it may not be possible to establish a diagnosis with certainty. In these instances, it is reasonable to make a tentative diagnosis of delirium and then search for reversible causes until further confirmation can be obtained.

Following a diagnosis of delirium, we recommend a work-up that includes meticulous history taking, a physical examination (including a focused neurological examination), a detailed mental status examination, and tests (e.g., blood, urine) guided by that person's history and a physical examination of the resident. If the clinician suspects a UTI, he or she should send a clean-catch urine specimen for culture and testing for sensitivity to antibiotics. The need for further laboratory testing (e.g., a stool examination, an EKG, a thyroid function test, a vitamin B_{12} level, drug levels or a toxicology screen, an ammonia level measurement, a chest radiograph, an arterial blood gas test) will be determined according to the individual's clinical picture. The goal of such a work-up is to identify all potential predisposing, precipitating, and aggravating factors. In some cases (e.g., falls or a head injury), the clinician may consider neuroimaging. A CT scan may be preferred over MRI to detect intracerebral or extracerebral bleeding in emergency settings. A CT scan is also preferred over MRI for some residents with advanced dementia, because of the increased stress and anxiety associated with the need to be still for a longer time to obtain a high-quality MRI brain scan as opposed to a CT scan. Examination of the cerebrospinal fluid is indicated for a resident with delirium if the clinician suspects meningitis (because of fever, neck rigidity) or encephalitis (fever, seizures). The clinician may consider an EEG if he or she suspects occult seizure (e.g., complex partial seizures), as well as to differentiate delirium from other psychiatric disorders.

A differential diagnosis includes the following:

Depression: Delirium (especially quiet or hypoactive delirium) is often misdiagnosed as depression (Farrell and Ganzini 1995). Residents with depression demonstrate a normal level of alertness, intact thought processes, a depressed affect, and poor motivation to participate in activities. Onset is usually gradual, over weeks to months. There may be a past history of a depressive episode.

Dementia with delirium: At least two-thirds of the cases of delirium occur in residents with underlying dementia or a cognitive impairment (Inouye 2006). There usually is a documented history of preexisting dementia or an obvious history of cognitive decline before a person develops delirium. Cognitive symptoms (e.g., disorientation, memory impairment, inattention, poor thought organization) are worse in individuals with delirium superimposed on dementia than in those with delirium alone (Voyer et al. 2006). Residents with both dementia and delirium often display significantly more physical agitation than those who have dementia without delirium.

Dementia without delirium: Residents with dementia, such as probable Alzheimer disease, have an insidious onset of cognitive decline over months to years and demonstrate a normal level of alertness. Dementia with Lewy bodies (DLB) shares clinical features with delirium (e.g., visual hallucination, fluctuating symptoms), but a resident with DLB also has signs of parkinsonism and symptoms that persist over months to years. Vascular dementia may present with an acute onset of cognitive impairment, but the characteristic features of delirium (such as fluctuating sensorium and inattention) are usually not seen. With advanced dementia, residents may be inattentive and their speech may be aphasic, which makes it challenging to differentiate advanced dementia from delirium. In advanced dementia, the person's level of alertness is not impaired and inattention and speech impairments have been progressing over several months. Disorientation and memory impairment do not help differentiate dementia from delirium, as they may be seen in both.

Bipolar disorder, manic episode: Residents in a manic state have a long history of psychiatric illness, have clinical symptoms of elated or irritable moods, talk excessively, have a diminished need for sleep, exhibit grandiosity, and have a normal level of alertness. Steroid-induced delirium may have symptoms of mania (e.g., grandiosity, excessive talking), but it usually has altered sensorium and a fluctuating course.

Acute exacerbation of a chronic psychotic disorder: Exacerbation of a preexisting chronic psychotic disorder, such as schizophrenia or schizoaffective disorder, may present with acute-onset agitation, hallucinations, and delusions, but dramatic fluctuations in consciousness, orientation, and attention are usually absent and the individual has a past history of severe and persistent mental illness.

Acute exacerbation of a chronic anxiety disorder, such as post-traumatic stress disorder (PTSD): Acute exacerbation of PTSD may manifest as agitation, inattention, and hypervigilance, but there is no alteration in consciousness and no disorganized thinking. The presence of other symptoms of PTSD (e.g., nightmares, flashbacks, a history of abuse or trauma) and a past history of similar symptoms help clarify this diagnosis.

Delirium with acute psychiatric illness: Residents who are in a manic state or who have acute psychotic symptoms or severe depression may develop delirium for a variety of reasons (e.g., noncompliance with medications [such as diabetes medications]). A high index of suspicion, a thorough history, and the time period of the symptoms help identify the nature of this dual diagnosis.

CLINICAL CASE Mr. A, an 80-year-old male with hypertension, benign prostatic hypertrophy, hyperlipidemia, and arthritis, was transferred from a hospital to a nursing home for rehabilitation after surgery to repair a hip fracture. In the hospital, Mr. A had become disoriented after surgery, insisting that he needed to go to work, trying to climb out of bed, and becoming aggressive when the staff tried to redirect him. He was given haloperidol (2 mg twice daily) and his physician recommended that he continue taking haloperidol when he was transferred to the nursing home. Mr. A developed drooling, tremors, daytime sedation, and periods of agitation. The staff requested a psychiatric consultation. The psychiatrist asked Mrs. A about Mr. A's cognitive functioning before surgery. Mrs. A insisted that Mr. A's memory was "good" but added that "he is old, you know." Mr. A's daughter reported that for the past two years, her father had been increasingly forgetful, repeating himself often, becoming irritable, and that in the last six months he began making mistakes in paying bills, got lost while driving, began avoiding social gatherings, and refused to wear a hearing aid.

During the examination, the psychiatrist found Mr. A to be somewhat drowsy, with poor attention and concentration. Mr. A did not recall having been hospitalized and had slurred speech. The psychiatrist reviewed test results done in the hospital. A CT scan of the brain showed diffuse moderate cerebral atrophy, urinalysis was negative for infection, and the results of blood tests (including a chemistry panel, a thyroid profile, and folate levels) were within normal limits. Vitamin B_{12} was at the lower limit of normal (a level of 220). The psychiatrist made a diagnosis of dementia of a probable Alzheimer type (AD) accompanied by postoperative delirium. He discontinued haloperidol due to its adverse effects, added vitamin B_{12} (1,000 mcg daily), and started donepezil (5 mg daily in the morning). The psychiatrist also met with the nursing home staff to discuss instituting various psychosocial-environmental interventions (e.g., letting him listen to his favorite music, aromatherapy with lavender lotion, one-on-one supervision at times, minimizing nighttime noise, and lowering expectations for Mr. A to remember and follow directions). The psychiatrist then had a lengthy family meeting in which he explained his diagnosis, recommended a support group for Mr. A's wife and daughter, and discussed the prognosis. Over the next several days, Mr. A gradually become less agitated and started taking part in physical therapy (although he required constant reassurance and redirection). The drooling was markedly reduced, his tremors and slurred speech decreased significantly, and his daytime sleepiness was completely resolved. After six weeks, Mr. A smiled and joked, although he still asked when he could go home.

TEACHING POINTS Mild dementia often goes unrecognized and undiagnosed. It predisposes the person with dementia to develop postoperative delirium. Therefore, for any resident with postoperative delirium, the clinician must inquire about that person's cognitive functioning before surgery. In addition, it is common for delirium to be treated with much larger doses of haloperidol in the hospital, and patients are often discharged on haloperidol or another antipsychotic medication. Haloperidol is associated with a high incidence of EPS in older adults with dementia, especially at doses of more than 1–2 mg/day (although EPS can be seen even at doses as low as 0.5 mg/day). Hence, in the management of delirium, the clinician must promptly discontinue haloperidol or any other antipsychotic as soon as possible, especially if adverse effects arise. Finally, the treatment of delirium consists primarily of treating the cause and establishing psychosocial environmental interventions, although cholinesterase inhibitors may also help residents with AD recover from delirium.

CLINICAL CASE Mrs. S was a 72-year-old woman with multiple chronic medical problems (diabetes for 30 years, hypertension, osteoarthritis, chronic liver disease due to alcoholism, peripheral neuropathy) who recently developed right-sided hemiplegia due to a stroke. After some initial anxiety and depression after moving into an assisted living facility, she had been doing well for the previous three months. Mrs. S was a frail, petite woman who had a body mass index (BMI) of 16 (normal range 18–25). She was taking 12 different medications for her many medical conditions, including amitriptyline (10 mg) for peripheral neuropathy pain and insomnia. Mrs. S had developed urinary frequency and incontinence over the past several weeks, and for the last week she was started on oxybutynin (5 mg daily) for a suspected overactive bladder. Urinalysis was negative for infection. The staff noticed that for the last five days she had become more confused and irritable, had fallen twice (no injuries), and was unable to sleep for more than two to three hours at night. The health care provider recommended discontinuing amitriptyline, but the resident and her family refused, as Mrs. S had taken amitriptyline for more than 15 years and it had helped her peripheral neuropathy pain and insomnia. The staff obtained a psychiatric consultation.

The psychiatrist, after assessing Mrs. S, recommended discontinuing oxybutynin and suggested a scheduled toileting program to treat her overactive bladder. Over the next 72 hours, Mrs. S's delirium resolved and she was back to her level of functioning before starting oxybutynin. The psychiatrist then met with Mrs. S and her family, explaining the risk of cognitive impairment with amitriptyline and the potential benefits of alternatives such as gabapentin or nortriptyline. Mrs. S agreed to try switching to gabapentin with the assurance that if it did not help, she could restart the amitriptyline. The psychiatrist checked Mrs. S's renal function before starting gabapentin. Her serum creatinine was 1.8, indicating mild chronic kidney disease. Amitriptyline was decreased to 5 mg daily at bedtime for two weeks and then discontinued. Gabapentin was added at 100 mg daily at bedtime, and over a two-week period it was increased to 300 mg at bedtime. Mrs. S had mild insomnia for a few days but no increase in her peripheral neuropathy pain. The psychiatrist recommended that, to improve her sleep, the staff encourage Mrs. S to step up her physical activity, increase her exposure to sunlight, and minimize her daytime napping. After two weeks of taking gabapentin and not amitriptyline (along with psychosocial-environmental interventions), Mrs. S felt that she was doing "quite well." The staff noticed that Mrs. S's constipation was replaced with mild diarrhea, which resolved once her medications for constipation (docusate sodium and senna) were discontinued.

TEACHING POINTS Prescribing an anticholinergic medication such as oxybutynin for a frail resident who is already taking other medications with high anticholinergic activity (amitriptyline, in this case) and had a compromised neurological status (in this case, cerebrovascular disease) puts that resident at high risk of drug-induced delirium. Drugs for an overactive bladder, such as tolterodine and oxybutynin, may precipitate delirium and should be prescribed with great caution for frail residents, residents with a history of liver disease, or residents who are taking multiple drugs metabolized through the cytochrome P450 system (Chancellor and de Miguel 2007). We recommend a rigorous trial of scheduled toileting and prompt voiding before prescribing drugs for an overactive bladder.

Each assessment for change in a resident's mental status is an opportunity to review the resident's medications and reduce the anticholinergic load. Gabapentin has no anticholinergic activity and is a better choice than amitriptyline to treat peripheral neuropathy in LTC residents. Because gabapentin is primarily excreted by the kidneys, it is important to start with a low dose for residents who have chronic kidney disease, and low doses may be sufficient for a therapeutic response. Also, for residents who have been taking psychiatric medications for a long time, discontinuing such medications is a major decision, which may be associated with significant anxiety. Hence, before instituting any change, the clinician and the resident's family should discuss the risks of continuing current psychiatric medications and the benefits of safer alternatives. Finally, anticholinergic medications are constipating, and most residents need medications to treat the constipation these drugs cause. By reducing the anticholinergic load, the clinician may also be able to decrease many residents' need for medications to treat constipation, thus reducing polypharmacy and its harmful consequences.

Complications Associated with Untreated Delirium

Untreated delirium in a hospital setting is associated with increased mortality rates, ranging from 10 to 65 percent—as high as the rates associated with acute myocardial infarction or sepsis. Older patients whose delirium was not detected by the hospital's emergency room physician or nurse had a high rate of mortality (30.8%) over six months (Kakuma et al. 2003). Delirium in LTC populations is also associated with high mortality, much greater rates of hospitalization, an increased risk of falls, wandering, injury, pneumonia, pressure ulcers, increased caregiver burden, and accelerated preexisting cognitive decline (Gleason 2003). In hospitalized elderly people, delirium may result in a longer stay in the hospital and is highly predictive of future cognitive and functional decline and subsequent admission to LTC (Inouye 2000). Delirium during hospitalization is also a risk factor for subsequent hospitalization (Bourdel-Marchasson et al. 2004). Even subsyndromal delirium carries a significant risk of morbidity and mortality (Cole et al. 2003). Delirium markedly and independently affects resident outcomes, such as functional declines and loss of the ability to live independently. Complications associated with delirium are more likely in residents with preexisting unstable medical conditions (e.g., brittle diabetes, protein energy malnutrition, advanced Parkinson disease) and those with advanced dementia.

Treatment of Delirium

The clinician should always assume that delirium is reversible until proven otherwise. The primary goal is to reverse the delirium and thereby mitigate associated morbidity and mortality. Delirium in LTC residents requires aggressive treatment because the experience is frightening to residents and their families, with an increased risk of wandering, falls, self-harm, and death. The treatment of delirium is much more than a treatment of its cause (e.g., UTI). This treatment should also address predisposing and precipitating factors for delirium, because delirium in LTC populations is typically multifactorial.

The treatment begins with a thorough evaluation of the causes and risk factors, unless the resident is at the end stage of life, in which case palliative and hospice care are more appropriate. If the offending agent is obvious (e.g., diphenhydramine), discontinuing it may be a sufficient intervention, without the need for any tests. The clinician should eliminate all nonessential drugs. Addressing safety (falls, injury due to the accidental removal of tubes, etc.), preventing complications (seizures, coma, death), removing restraints, and treating agitation should all be done at the same time as treating the cause of the delirium. Avoiding drugs with high anticholinergic activity whenever possible is a cornerstone in the management of delirium. Even after a thorough assessment and once all diagnostic tests are completed, the clinician may still not know the cause of delirium. We recommend close observation of the resident to ensure that person's safety, to see if an obscure confusion (perhaps related to a medication) may clear up, or to see if new clues to an underlying medical condition may appear.

Psychosocial-environmental interventions are the primary mode of treatment for delirium, and the clinician should institute them for all residents with delirium (Inouye et al. 1999; Cole 2004). We recommend the use of bright or blue light for circadian rhythm disturbances, massage, soothing music, aromatherapy, one-on-one monitoring (encouraging the presence of family or staff members, using sitters), and reorientation strategies (clocks, calendars, a daily schedule) as appropriate, as well as minimizing the need for physical restraints by using intramuscular injections instead of intravenous injections. The clinician can minimize sensory deprivation by encouraging the use of hearing aids and eyeglasses when appropriate. For hearing impairments, we recommend the use of hearing aids, amplifying devices, and disimpaction of ear wax. We recommend a quiet environment with appropriate lighting, and the staff should make every effort to allow an uninterrupted period for sleep at night. The staff should address sleep deprivation with interventions such as warm drinks (warm milk, herbal teas) at bedtime, relaxation tapes, and back massage. Aggravating environmental factors and others, such as sleep deprivation, immobilization, pain, sensory overload, or deprivation, can place excessive demands on the cognitively compromised resident; the clinician should identify any such problems and address them.

The clinician should reserve pharmacological interventions for residents whose severe agitation will result in an interruption of essential medical therapies or who pose a danger to themselves (e.g., vivid hallucinations causing a resident to attempt to jump out of a window) or to others (because of physical aggression). Although antipsychotic medications are considered first-line agents in the pharmacological management of severe agitation and/or physical aggression for residents who are experiencing delirium, these drugs do not carry an indication from the FDA that they can be used for the management of delirium (Seitz, Gill, and van Zyl 2007). Antipsychotic medications have just started to be rigorously studied in large, well-designed, randomized controlled studies for the management of severe agitation for individuals with delirium. We usually recommend haloperidol because of its wide therapeutic margin of safety, ease of administration by a variety of routes (oral [pills and liquid], intramuscular, and intravenous), and relative lack of cardiopulmonary and anticholinergic effects at low doses. We usually recommend oral (liquid) or intramuscular haloperidol for LTC residents and reserve the intravenous form to treat delirium in a hospital setting. The recommended doses of haloperidol to treat delirium in LTC populations are low (0.25-0.5 mg repeated every 30 minutes to achieve sedation [up to 4 mg/day]). A younger resident with a high BMI may need a higher dose. The major problems with the use of haloperidol are EPS (e.g., tremors, hypokinesia, drooling) and akathisia. EPS may be associated with discomfort, choking, falls in ambulatory residents, and increased immobility in nonambulatory residents.

The use of liquid risperidone (0.125-0.25 mg repeated every 30 minutes to achieve sedation [up to 2 mg/day]) or orally dissolvable risperidone (M-tab risperdal) in place of haloperidol may also be appropriate. The adverse effects of risperidone are similar to those of haloperidol. For agitated residents, especially those with parkinsonism, low-dose quetiapine (12.5-25 mg two to four times a day, which may be increased to up to 200 mg/day if the initial doses are tolerated]) may be useful. The use of quetiapine and, less commonly, of risperidone may be associated with orthostatic hypotension. Once initial sedation is achieved, one-half of the loading dose of the medication may be given in divided doses (two to four times a day) for one to two more days, with a tapering of the doses over the next few days. The clinician may consider prescribing intramuscular ziprasidone (10–20 mg one to four times a day) for an agitated delirious resident for whom the use of haloperidol is contraindicated (e.g., a resident with drug-induced EPS, parkinsonism, or Parkinson disease) or a resident who refuses oral atypical antipsychotic medications such as quetiapine. The use of antipsychotic medication is associated with sudden cardiac death, and Ziprasidone may prolong the QT interval.

Except for behavioral emergencies, we recommend obtaining a baseline EKG before prescribing antipsychotic medications. The clinician should avoid prescribing ziprasidone for residents with a preexisting prolonged QT interval. We do not recommend the use of olanzapine to treat behavioral emergencies for a resident with delirium because of the potential for an anticholinergic effect, although such an effect in the elderly population has not been clinically established as an issue. Considering the possible antipsychotic-agent-related adverse effects of torsades de pointes, hypotension (especially with intravenous haloperidol), and neuroleptic malignant syndrome, the clinician must evaluate the safety of these agents in the context of their potential benefits. Titrating medications to resident-specific, goal-directed target sedation levels (where the resident is awake and manageable), rather than to unresponsive resident status (where the resident is lethargic), may be helpful in reducing iatrogenically induced morbidity and mortality.

The clinician should prescribe antipsychotic medications only for short-term treatments (a few days), using the lowest effective dose appropriate for a particular resident. Lorazepam and oxazepam may be useful for residents who are experiencing withdrawal from alcohol or sedative-hypnotic agents or if the clinician suspects seizures as a cause of the person's delirium. Otherwise, the use of these drugs may be associated with a worsening of the delirium, falls, and agitation. Individuals with dementia are at increased risk of a stroke and strokelike events, as well as a higher rate of mortality, with the use of antipsychotic medications. Before instituting treatment for residents with delirium and dementia, the clinician should weigh the risks of antipsychotic medications against the risk of not treating severe agitation. Treating pain may reduce agitation in individuals with delirium who are in physical pain.

Recovery from Delirium

The goal of the treatment is a complete resolution of the delirium and the resident's return to his or her predelirium level of functioning and cognition. Residents whose delirium resolves quickly (within two weeks) without recurrence usually regain 100 percent of their predelirium level, while those for whom this is not the case regain less than 50 percent of their predelirium level. Thus a substantial number of residents do not return to their predelirium level of functioning and cognition. Delirium can be a persistent issue for a resident, lasting weeks or months. It is essential that the clinician follow up to confirm resolution of the delirium once its cause is found and treated, as persistent delirium or delirium of unknown etiology carries a high risk of morbidity and mortality.

The speed of delirium resolution for residents newly admitted to a skilled nursing facility for rehabilitation after hospitalization correlates with the ability of those residents to carry out activities of daily living and reach their prehospital functionality (Kiely et al. 2006). If, after six months, a resident has not reached his or her prehospital functionality, the prognosis for significant further recovery is poor.

Outcomes of delirium include the following:

Complete resolution over days to weeks: This is usually seen in residents with intact baseline cognition, an absence of preclinical degenerative changes in the brain, minimal cerebrovascular disease, and a good premorbid cognitive reserve.

Persistent delirium: In this form of delirium symptoms persist for weeks to months. Persistent delirium is much more common than was previously believed, and it is usually seen in residents with significant cerebrovascular disease and/or another medical comorbidity (e.g., end-organ failure of the liver, kidneys, heart, or lungs), poor cognitive reserve, and impaired predelirium cognition (e.g., the presence of dementia).

Delirium followed by neurodegenerative dementia: Here the resident usually has preexisting dementia but with subtle or mild symptoms, and further brain damage due to the factors causing the delirium results in obvious symptoms of dementia and its subsequent typical progression (Inouye and Ferrucci 2006). Anesthetic agents may have a role in accelerating neurodegenerative processes.

Delirium causing dementia: This outcome is controversial. Neuroimaging studies have documented regions of hypoperfusion in individuals with delirium, suggesting that delirium may trigger a derangement in the brain's vascular function that leads to dementia in some cases (Inouye 2006).

Accelerated cognitive decline in residents with preexisting dementia: In this instance the resident does not recover enough to reach his or her pre-delirium baseline, but instead is in the next stage of dementia. Because the resident developed delirium, the cognitive decline was accelerated over a period of days to weeks, when it would otherwise have taken several months. The clinician should suspect the existence of delirium in a resident with progressive dementia (such as AD) who begins to show an abrupt downward course.

Prevention of Delirium

Research to identify strategies to prevent delirium in LTC populations is sparse. Table 4.3 lists some strategies based on our clinical experience and on extrapolating evidence from studies on preventing delirium in hospitalized patients (Inouye 2000; Siddiqi et al. 2007). Many cases of delirium in LTC populations may be preventable through the routine use of these strategies. Instituting palliative and hospice care when appropriate (in keeping with the resident's wishes and advance directives) instead of hospitalization may prevent delirium due to aggressive medical care (tube feeding, CPR). The clinician should follow residents with urinary incontinence due to an overactive bladder who have been prescribed antispasmodic medications for the development of drug-induced delirium. Trospium is eliminated from the body as an unchanged drug and, in the context of polypharmacy or for residents with liver disease, it may be a safer treatment option for an overactive bladder than other medications (e.g., tolterodine or oxybutynin) because there is less risk of a drug-drug interaction (Chancellor and de Miguel 2007).

By changing the care processes, we can prevent delirium in many residents. Barriers to an early recognition of delirium—such as a high workload that allows less time for the staff to spend with the resident, fragmented clinical care because knowledge about the course of a resident's mental status changes is missing, and a lack of recognition that delirium is a medical emergency—need to be addressed at the administrative level to improve outcomes.

TABLE 4.3
Strategies to reduce the risk of delirium in the long-term care population

Obtain proactive geriatric consultation (with a geriatrician, geriatric psychiatrist, geriatric nurse practitioner, or pharmacist who has training in geriatric pharmacology) for residents admitted from a hospital for rehabilitation and for other high-risk groups of residents (e.g., residents with advanced dementia)

Decrease the anticholinergic load

Reduce medication errors

Reduce inappropriate medication prescriptions

Monitor for the presence of a urinary tract infection

Reduce the use of physical restraints and indwelling catheters

Diagnose and treat dementia in its early/mild stages

Institute interventions to reduce infection (e.g., pneumococcal and flu vaccines, prophylactic antibiotics for a resident with a recurrent urinary tract infection)

Reduce inactivity and immobility (walking and other exercise one to three times a day)

Treat pain and depression optimally

Institute sleep-enhancing strategies (to reduce chronic sleep deprivation)

Correct hearing and vision impairments with adaptive equipment

Improve nutritional status (to prevent dehydration, protein energy malnutrition)

Provide appropriate daily cognitive stimulation (to slow cognitive decline)

Provide regular orienting communication in written form (e.g., the day's schedule)

Provide adequate therapeutic activities and continuous activity programming (to prevent boredom, sensory deprivation)

Reduce the time the resident spends in bed, reduce noise, minimize bed-rest orders, and encourage self-care as much as possible

End-of-Life Delirium

Delirium is the most common mental disorder at the end of life, especially in LTC populations (Ganzini 2007). Delirium is one of the natural manifestations of the dying process. Among dying residents, delirium progresses to a coma preceding death. Dehydration and drug-induced delirium (particularly opiate-induced delirium) are among the most treatable causes of delirium at the end of life. We recommend atypical antipsychotic medications or low-dose haloperidol to treat agitation associated with delirium. Benzodiazepines may worsen confusion, but they may be needed in the final hours or days of life to induce calm and reduce the risk of seizures that can occur with the use of antipsychotic medications.

Conclusion

Untreated delirium carries a high rate of morbidity and mortality. A high index of suspicion, prompt recognition, a thorough diagnostic assessment, an appropriate work-up, and an evidence-based treatment of delirium are essential to reduce morbidity and mortality. Effective strategies to resolve delirium promptly and prevent its recurrence in a long-term care setting are crucial for maintaining the residents' optimal level of functional capacity and emotional well-being. For residents with end-of-life delirium, we recommend palliative and hospice care.

CHAPTER 5

Mood Disorders

Mood disorders (especially depression) are the second most common psychiatric disorder (after dementia) for residents in long-term care facilities (Mulsant and Ganguli 1999; Payne et al. 2002). Mood disorders often impede compliance with medical treatment, a response to analgesics, activities of daily living (e.g., bathing, dressing, feeding, toileting), and rehabilitation, and they are associated with increased morbidity and mortality (whether or not from suicide). Strategies to prevent mood disorders and to provide an early diagnosis and vigorous treatment are crucial to improving the quality of life for LTC residents. Mood disorders include depression, apathy, suicidality, mania, and pseudobulbar affect.

Depression

Depression is not a natural consequence of aging or of living in an LTC facility. Older adults biologically appear to be at greater risk of major depression, such as depression resulting from vascular changes, yet the frequency of depression is lower among community-dwelling elders than among younger adults (Blazer and Hybels 2005). This may be because of the protective effects of wisdom, a capacity to de-emphasize negative experiences, and a capacity to prioritize emotionally meaningful goals, all of which are thought to increase with age. The comorbidity of depression and other psychiatric disorders (e.g., substance abuse) is less frequent in late life than earlier in the life cycle (the various dementias being an exception).

Although at any one time most residents of LTC facilities are not depressed, depression is the most common mood disorder of LTC residents (Blazer 2002; Kallenbach and Rigler 2006), affecting them at rates three to five times higher than those of older adults living in the community. The prevalence of major depression ranges from 10 to 30 percent, and depressed mood is even more common (Mulsant and Ganguli 1999; Payne et al. 2002). In LTC populations, depression is most strongly associated with aggressive behavior, but it is also linked to delusions, hallucinations, and constipation (Leonard et al. 2006). The recognition and treatment of depression is an indicator of the quality of an LTC facility. Despite being eminently treatable, depression is often unrecognized in LTC populations (Thakur and Blazer 2008). Residents with physical or cognitive impairments, residents aged 85 or older, and residents from ethnic minority groups are particularly less likely to be diagnosed and treated for depression (Levin et al. 2007). Stigmas and myths about aging hinder an early diagnosis and appropriate treatment. Table 5.1 lists some common myths about depression in older adults.

Screening for depression in LTC populations is crucial. Not only is the frequency of depression high, but suicidal ideation can also be detected by screening. The standard use of screening tools, such as the GDS and the CSDD, may improve the recognition of depression in LTC populations. All residents should be screened for depression within four weeks of admission. The clinician should ask about any recent or past occurrences, or a family history of depression, or suicidal thoughts or attempts. Even when depression is recognized, less than one-quarter of those who are diagnosed receive treatment, and, when they are treated with medications, they often receive a suboptimal dose.

Depression can occur at any time during a resident's stay in an LTC facility, ranging from minor to major in its severity. Depression in LTC has been found to be associated with severe cognitive impairments, behavioral symptoms, pain, and the for-profit status of the facility. LTC residents with depression have greater functional impairment and need additional staff time for their care. Depression is associated with a reduced quality of life, higher mortality (due to suicide or another cause), increased rates of hospitalization,

TABLE 5.1
Myths about depression in long-term care residents

Trivialization ("Wouldn't you be depressed, too?")
Belittling of psychiatric treatment ("Does it really work for these people when it is too late, anyway?")
Belief that older persons do not want psychiatric treatment
Belief that depression is a normal part of aging or cannot be distinguished from normal aging
Belief that depression is a normal part of adjusting to living in a long-term care facility

longer hospital stays, and increased physical pain. Clinical depression is one of the most common causes of excess disability (i.e., dysfunction beyond an impairment caused by dementia and/or other chronic conditions alone) in LTC residents. Among individuals who have a physical dependency following a catastrophic illness (e.g., a stroke or a hip fracture), persistent depression is often associated with a delay in recovery or a failure to improve during the rehabilitation process. Depression in older adults increases their risk of myocardial infarction and adversely affects the course of medical illnesses such as diabetes and coronary artery disease. Depression accelerates the cognitive and functional declines associated with dementia, and late-onset depression may be a prodrome of Alzheimer disease (Schweitzer et al. 2002). Thus the clinician should closely follow all residents with late-onset depression and no dementia, looking for signs of mild cognitive impairment or mild Alzheimer disease. A score of less than 24 on the MMSE or a decline of more than three points from a stable baseline is thought to be clinically significant and warrant evaluation for dementia (H. Lee and Lyketsos 2004). Many residents are affected by depression before being admitted to an LTC facility, and depression in older adults is a modifiable risk factor. We thus recommend a comprehensive evaluation for and treatment of depression before admission to LTC.

Table 5.2 enumerates multiple risk factors for depression in LTC populations (Jongenelis et al. 2004; Achterberg et al. 2006; Levin et al. 2007; Llewellyn-Jones and Snowdon 2007). Various losses in old age may precipitate or exacerbate depression. Physical illness (especially chronic pain) and disability are major factors in the development and persistence of depressive disorders in LTC populations. Recognizing risk factors, such as recent losses, is often key to developing a management plan.

Diagnosis and Work-Up

Diagnosing depression in LTC populations is complex. The high prevalence of cognitive and sensory impairments and of apathy, and a lack of adequate time and training for the staff (including physicians, nurse practitioners, physician assistants) in recognizing depression in this population, makes accurate diagnosis challenging. Furthermore, the symptom profile of depression in older adults may not resemble that in younger adults. LTC residents are less inclined to express their feelings openly and are more apt to present with somatic complaints (e.g., weakness, fatigue, dizziness) or to display a loss of interest, anhedonia, a loss of appetite, sleeplessness, or pessimism. Anxiety symptoms, agitation, aggression, social withdrawal, and accelerated

TABLE 5.2
Risk factors for depression in long-term care residents

General risk factors for depression in older adults
  Past history of depression
  Past history of suicide attempts
  History of alcohol or drug abuse
  Family history of depression or suicide
  Recent loss of a family member or another negative life event (e.g., loss of the ability to drive or loss
    of one's own home)
  Sensory impairment (e.g., severe loss of hearing and/or vision)
  Chronic pain
  Alzheimer disease
  Cerebrovascular disease (includes stroke, widespread white matter hyperintensities in the brain on
    magnetic resonance imaging) and vascular dementia
  Frailty
  Parkinson disease
  Hip fracture
  Urinary incontinence
  Obstructive sleep apnea
  Chronic insomnia
  Severe functional disability (e.g., severe arthritis or end-organ failure of the heart, lungs, liver, or
    kidneys, causing functional disability)
  Some medications (e.g., interferon, benzodiazepines, opioids)
  Abuse (verbal, physical, sexual, financial, neglect)
  Premorbid personality disorder (e.g., a personality disorder before the onset of dementia or of a
    stroke)
Risk factors related to institutionalization
  Existential distress (demoralization)
  Admission to a long-term care facility for the first time
  Admission to a long-term care facility without preparing the resident for the move psychologically
  Change from one long-term care facility to another
  Change of one's room within the facility
  Change or loss of a roommate or a staff member with whom the resident has developed a close
    relationship
  Loneliness, social isolation, boredom, and too much "down time" (too much time spent alone and
    without engagement in meaningful activities)
  Countertherapeutic staff approaches and interactions (e.g., staff constantly correcting the
    resident's recall of events, excessively burdening the resident)
  Perceived inadequacy of care
  Inadequate exposure to sunlight
  Excessive noise or interruption of sleep
  Meals not in keeping with the resident's preference and/or ethnic and cultural background
  Cognitively intact residents (i.e., residents who do not have dementia) living with residents with
    advanced dementia

cognitive and functional declines may be the predominant manifestations of a depressive disorder in LTC populations.

The clinician can differentiate clinical depression from normal sadness by taking into account the intensity, duration, and number of depressive symptoms, any functional impairment due to depressive symptoms, and the context in which the depression occurs. The symptoms of clinical depression are usually moderate to severe and persistent, and they are associated with a moderate to severe impairment in functioning, suicidal ideas, and/or psychotic symptoms. Clinical depression usually occurs in the context of one or more risk factors. Statements made by residents that may indicate clinical depression as opposed to normal sadness include (but are not limited to) "I don't care anymore," "I wish I were dead," and "Help me, please help me." The DSM-IV-TR defines major depressive disorder (MDD) as the presence of five of the following symptoms nearly every day for most of the day for at least two weeks: depressed mood, lack of interest, appetite change or significant weight loss or gain, insomnia or hypersomnia, psychomotor agitation or retardation, loss of energy or fatigue, feelings of worthlessness or excessive guilt, difficulty in concentrating or in making decisions, and recurrent thoughts of death or suicide, including plans or attempts (American Psychiatric Association 2004). A diagnosis of MDD also requires that at least one of the five symptoms be a depressed mood or a lack of interest. In addition, these symptoms should cause significant impairment in the person's daily functioning.

Minor depression is defined by criteria similar to those for MDD, except that the total number of symptoms needed is three or four rather than five. A self-rated mood inventory, such as the GDS, is also useful. However, many LTC residents are unable to report these symptoms accurately. For such residents, the criteria for major depression may be met by using an observer-rated scale. We recommend that the clinician use the CSDD for residents with advanced dementia (a score of less than 15 on the MMSE) (McGivney, Mulvihill, and Taylor 1994). Table 5.3 lists common symptoms of depression in LTC residents.

An assessment of potentially depressed residents involves both clinical evaluation and, when feasible, the use of specific assessment tools. Typically, older persons are less likely to acknowledge symptoms such as a depressed mood or sadness. They may be more preoccupied with somatic complaints or may have prominent anxiety symptoms. Clinical signs and symptoms of depression may also be modified or masked by comorbidities or causative disease processes, such as severe chronic pain or advanced dementia with agitation. Bradykinesia and the flat affect of Parkinson disease may be mistaken for depression. Poor appetite, fatigue, and sleep disturbance symptoms may overlap with a wide variety of medical illnesses. Depression is usually comorbid with anxiety and agitation in LTC residents, and the comorbidity of anxiety with depression rises with an increase in the severity of the depression. Physical aggression may be associated with depression in more severe dementias. The

TABLE 5.3
Main features of depressive disorder in long-term care residents

Core symptoms
  Lack of interest in daily activities
  Depressed mood or affect
Additional symptoms
  Lack of appetite or weight loss; increased appetite or weight gain
  Insomnia or hypersomnia
  Recurrent thoughts of suicide or a wish to die or a suicide attempt
  Decreased energy or fatigue
  Hopelessness
  Helplessness
  Worthlessness
  Inappropriate or excessive guilt
  Loss of self-confidence
  Excessive time spent in bed
  Multiple somatic complaints
  Chronic pain not responding to medication
  Hypochondriasis
  Marked anxiety symptoms
  Agitation (especially in residents with advanced dementia)
  Verbal aggression or verbally abusive behaviors (especially in residents with advanced dementia)
  Physical aggression (especially in residents with advanced dementia)
  Decreased spontaneous speech
  Psychomotor retardation
  Refusal of medications
  Resistance to care
  Refusal to participate in therapy (physical, occupational, speech)
  Sudden decline in cognition
  Subjective memory complaints
  Failure or lack of progress in rehabilitation (e.g., after a hip fracture)

clinician should suspect depression if a resident has been staying in his or her room more or if a resident takes to bed.

Depression in LTC residents is frequently present in the context of physical problems that complicate a diagnosis and impede the management of the illness. If depression and physical illness coexist, the clinician may assume that the depression is a result of a general medical condition or that the concomitant illness contraindicates antidepressant therapy, and he or she may therefore withhold antidepressants. Although the core symptoms of depression are similar to those found in younger populations, additional symptoms are considerably different and varied in LTC residents. Core depressive symptoms are also similar across cultures, but cultural factors may modify the presentation of a depressive disorder (Mackinnon et al. 1998). For example, older depressed people from Southeast Asia often present with physical complaints (e.g., weakness, dizziness) without a depressed mood. African Americans may complain of irritability or hostility, or have vague somatic complaints.

Latinos may complain of having problems with "nerves" or having "heart-aches."

The diagnostic work-up of depression in LTC residents involves a thorough history, pertinent physical and neurological examinations, and laboratory studies (e.g., TSH level, vitamin B_{12} level). For a resident suspected of having vascular depression, the clinician should consider reviewing the most recent MRI brain scan (if one was already done) or ordering an MRI scan to look for evidence of significant cerebrovascular disease (e.g., the presence of periventricular white matter hyperintensities). A low BMI, a history of recent weight loss, low albumin, and low cholesterol levels are markers of poor nutritional status and thus are critical for the clinician to assess, given the risk of frailty and failure to thrive in depressed residents, especially those who are very old (more than 85 years old). Depression and malnutrition are a dangerous combination, because the resident's immune functioning may also be affected. This is a psychiatric/medical emergency, and clinicians need to act quickly to provide nutritional supplementation and an aggressive treatment of depression secondary to a high risk of mortality.

The clinician should assess the general health perceptions as well as the functional status of all residents suspected of having depression. An assessment of social functioning, medications, mobility and balance, sitting and standing blood pressure, and (if indicated) a urine analysis, a metabolic panel (e.g., electrolyte and renal function abnormalities may signal dehydration), a CBC to rule out anemia, and an EKG (if tricyclic antidepressants or stimulants are being considered) round out a diagnostic work-up. The clinician should differentiate clinical depression from bereavement-related depression, apathy, and dementia (see chapter 3 for differentiating depression from dementia).

Bereavement-Related Depression

Although bereavement is not a disease and most people adjust without professional psychological intervention, it is associated with an excess risk of mortality, particularly in the early weeks and months after a loss (Stroebe, Schut, and Stroebe 2007). Bereaved individuals report diverse psychological reactions. The resident may be sad and tearful in response to a recent loss (or losses), such as the death of a spouse. After a lifetime together, often with increasing interdependence during retirement and dependence due to dementia, the loss of a spouse may result in a chronic or inhibited bereaved state (Stadeford 1984). A recent loss can also reactivate grief from a previous bereavement (especially if those feelings were not acknowledged and expressed).

In the early stages, a bereaved person may have symptoms similar to those of someone with major depression (Zisook and Kendler 2007). Hence differentiating grief and bereavement from depression can be difficult. The DSM-IV-TR excludes a diagnosis of MDD in the first two months of a bereavement-related depression. Symptoms of bereavement usually do not last beyond two years, although some widows and widowers experience symptoms beyond that period (Turvey et al. 1999). The most severe symptoms usually improve within six months. The circumstances surrounding the death of the loved one, intrapersonal and interpersonal variables, and ways of coping are some of the common determinants of severe bereavement-related depression.

Symptoms that indicate complicated grief include having trouble accepting the death, being unable to trust others since the death, being excessively bitter regarding the death, feeling uneasy about moving on, being detached from formerly close individuals, feeling that life is meaningless without the deceased, feeling that the future holds no prospect for fulfillment without the deceased, and feeling agitated since the death (Zhang, El-Jawahri, and Prigerson 2006). We recommend psychotherapy and psychosocial interventions to treat complicated grief. For cognitively intact residents, the clinician may consider encouraging the bereaved resident to share the details of the loved one's death and have an imaginary conversation with the deceased, and helping that person confront avoided situations. For residents with cognitive impairment, complicated grief may manifest as agitation, aggression, somatic symptoms, and an accelerated cognitive and functional decline.

Severe depressive symptoms persisting beyond two months, the presence of suicidal thoughts at any time during bereavement, an intense wish to join the deceased, early-morning awakening, severe anxiety symptoms, feelings of excessive guilt, psychomotor retardation, mummification (maintaining grief by keeping everything unchanged), and overwhelming pessimism about others all point toward the need for antidepressant treatment. Interventions should be targeted at high-risk residents. Potential therapies for bereavement-related depression include pharmacologic agents, psychotherapy, and psychosocial/spiritual support. Often a combination of these treatments is optimal. We also recommend that religious residents continue with their spiritual observances.

Types of Clinical Depression

DEMENTIA WITH DEPRESSION   Dementia with depression is probably the most common diagnosis in LTC residents with depressive disorder.

This is because of the high prevalence of dementia in LTC populations and the high prevalence of depression in people with dementia (Lyketsos et al. 2002; Blazer and Hybels 2005). The presence of depression in residents with dementia is associated with an accelerated cognitive and functional decline, higher rates of mortality, and an impaired quality of life. Depression occurs in approximately 20–40 percent of the people with Alzheimer disease, 30–40 percent of those with Parkinson disease dementia, 35–50 percent of those with vascular dementia, and 50–60 percent of those with dementia with Lewy bodies (Ballard et al. 1996; Brodaty and Luscombe 1996; Zubenko et al. 2003; Borroni, Agosti, and Padovani 2008). MDD can be reliably diagnosed in residents with mild to moderate dementia (I. Katz 1998). Depressive symptoms in residents with dementia often fluctuate over time (crying spells in the evening but a bright affect in the morning) and include a reduction in one's positive affect or pleasure (e.g., a resident who rarely or never smiles), irritability, verbal and physical aggression, social withdrawal, and isolation.

The key sign of depression in people with dementia is depressed affect. A resident with depression and dementia appears sad, is often tearful, has sleep and appetite disturbances, is easily discouraged, may withdraw socially, and may voice multiple vague somatic complains (e.g., loss of energy, headache). Feelings or expressions of worthlessness ("I am stupid" or "I am useless"), hopelessness ("Why bother?" or "Nothing is going to help me"), helplessness ("Help me, help me"), and guilt ("I am a burden to my family"), a wish to die ("I wish I were dead"), and suicidal plans may be present, indicating severe depression. The clinician should inquire about these symptoms even if the resident has dementia and thus may not comprehend some of the questions. Diagnostic errors are common when attempting to distinguish between depression and dementia. Marked forgetfulness often accompanies depression; memory loss due to depression may be misinterpreted as dementia. Residents with dementia can appear apathetic and withdrawn. This can be especially true once their executive function is impaired. Many residents with dementia say "No" when asked if they feel depressed and say "Yes" to feeling lonely, bored, or useless. In advanced dementia, depression may manifest as irritability, anger, verbal and physical aggression, an absence of smiles, agitation, persistent moaning, yelling, and a wish to go home. Comorbid delusions are often seen in residents with dementia and depression.

The DSM-IV-TR criteria for major depression and minor depression identify clinically relevant syndromes of depression in Alzheimer disease. Mild levels of depression can produce a significant functional impairment, and the severity of psychopathological and neurological impairments increases with the growing severity of the depression (Starkstein et al. 2005). In a resident with dementia who has been stable but either deteriorates rapidly or develops an acute behavioral disorder, depression, in addition to the many causes of delirium, may also be the culprit. Differentiating MDD with cognitive impairment (and subjective memory complains) from mild cognitive impairment plus depressive symptoms and from mild Alzheimer disease with depressive symptoms is difficult. A gradual cognitive decline over several years, accompanied by a recent onset of depression, a lack of insight about one's own obvious decline in a depressed resident, and continued cognitive decline despite an improvement in depressive symptoms are all likely indicators of mild cognitive impairment or mild Alzheimer disease with depression (H. Lee and Lyketsos 2004).

Depression in residents with dementia is eminently treatable (Lavretsky 2003). The clinician should avoid prescribing antidepressants that have significant anticholinergic properties (e.g., tricyclic antidepressants, paroxetine) because of the risks of direct cognitive toxicity and blunting the potential benefits of ChEIs. The treatment of depression in residents with dementia may also reduce other behavioral and psychological symptoms associated with depression (e.g., aggression, anxiety, agitation, insomnia, apathy), and even mild psychotic symptoms may improve.

POSTSTROKE DEPRESSION AND VASCULAR DEPRESSION   The prevalence of depression after a stroke ranges from 30 to 60 percent and depends on the location and size of the stroke (dominant-hemisphere frontal strokes have the highest association with depression), physical disabilities after the stroke, the presence of cognitive impairment with the stroke, whether the person had to move from his or her home to an LTC facility after the stroke, and the extent of that person's social support (Blazer and Hybels 2005). The course of depression after a stroke varies widely. For many people, their depression remits approximately one to two years after a stroke. However, as many as 14 percent may have continued symptoms of MDD and 18 percent may have symptoms of dysthymia (chronic minor depression) two years after a stroke. Depression occurring within a few days after a stroke is more likely to be associated with spontaneous remission than the onset of depression several weeks after a stroke. The course of depression after a stroke increases one's disabilities, adversely affects rehabilitation outcomes, impairs recovery from illness, and contributes to an increased rate of mortality.

The term *vascular depression* is used to describe a subtype of late-onset depression associated with cerebrovascular risk factors (e.g., diabetes, hypertension, hyperlipidemia, obesity), an accompanying executive dysfunction, evidence on brain imaging of significant cerebrovascular disease (especially periventricular white matter hyperintensities in an MRI scan), and an increased risk of being refractory to treatment with antidepressant medication monotherapy. Vascular depression may account for 5–20 percent of late-onset depression. Residents with vascular depression usually have a later age of onset and may exhibit symptoms of motor retardation, apathy, poor insight, and impaired executive function (Alexopoulos et al. 1997). They may not have a high score in traditional scales to assess depression, such as the GDS (H. Lee and Lyketsos 2004). There is usually no family history of depression in older adults with vascular depression.

DEPRESSION IN RESIDENTS WITH PARKINSON DISEASE   Depression is common in people with Parkinson disease, but symptoms of Parkinson disease, such as a flat affect and hypokinesia, may be mistaken for depression. The clinician may consider using the Beck Depression Inventory-I, the Hamilton Depression Rating Scale, or the Montgomery Asberg Depression Rating Scale to screen for depression in Parkinson disease (Miyasaki et al. 2006). The clinician should consider recommending psychosocial interventions (e.g., counseling) and regular exercise (e.g., strength training using Pilates), especially for cognitively intact residents with Parkinson disease. For this latter category of residents, the clinician may also consider prescribing low-dose tricyclic antidepressants (e.g., 5–25 mg of nortriptyline) to treat depression. Tricyclic antidepressants may also help reduce drooling, inhibit an overactive bladder, and treat insomnia. For residents with Parkinson disease dementia, the use of selective SSRIs (e.g., sertraline, citalopram, escitalopram), bupropion, venlafaxine, duloxetine, or mirtazapine is preferred, as they carry less risk of anticolinergic toxicity than tricyclic antidepressants. In addition to treating depression, mirtazapine may improve tremor and levodopa (L-dopa)-induced dyskinesias in people with Parkinson disease (Pact and Giduz 1999). SSRIs may worsen parkinsonian symptoms such as tremors, and they may also worsen REM sleep behavior disorder. Thus the use of SSRIs for residents with Parkinson disease requires close monitoring for these adverse effects. Because of its dopaminergic activity, bupropion may precipitate psychosis in residents with Parkinson disease.

The antiparkinsonian medication selegiline is now available in patch form as an antidepressant and may be considered the drug of first choice for residents with Parkinson disease and depression, although it has not been well studied in LTC populations. Other antiparkinsonian drugs, such as pergolide and pramipexole, are reported to have antidepressant effects, and the clinician may consider prescribing them to treat depression accompanied by Parkinson disease (Rektorova et al. 2003). We recommend ECT for residents with medication-refractory or life-threatening depression and for depressed residents with Parkinson disease who cannot tolerate antidepressants. ECT may also improve motor function. Psychotherapy may be helpful for residents with Parkinson disease (and no dementia) who have mild depression, and it may also be used to augment the response to pharmacotherapy.

DEPRESSION DUE TO GENERAL MEDICAL CONDITIONS   Medical disorders such as chronic pain, hypothyroidism, hyperthyroidism, anemia, adrenal insufficiency (Addison disease), Cushing syndrome (excessive corticosteroids), hypercalcemia, pancreatic cancer, neurological conditions (e.g., brain tumors, multiple sclerosis, central nervous system infections), autoimmune disorders (e.g., systemic lupus erythematosus), paraneoplastic syndromes, and end-organ failure of the kidneys, liver, lungs, and heart all have the potential to cause depressive symptoms. Depression frequently results from and complicates the recovery of older patients who experience myocardial infarction and other heart conditions, diabetes, and hip fractures (Blazer and Hybels 2005). Treatment of the medical condition thought to cause depression is usually sufficient to resolve depressive symptoms. Dispensing eyeglasses to treat uncorrected refraction errors, other interventions to correct impaired vision or hearing, and the aggressive treatment of pain can also lead to decreased symptoms of depression. For some residents with depression due to medical conditions (e.g., multiple sclerosis), antidepressants may be necessary to improve their depressive symptoms.

MEDICATION-INDUCED DEPRESSION   To identify medication-induced depression, the clinician should review the prescribed and over-the-counter medications, as well as the herbs and supplements, being taken by residents with depression. Common medications that often induce depression include interferon alpha, benzodiazepines, antipsychotics, opioids, some antihypertensives (e.g., propranolol, clonidine), and steroids (Desai 2004). Discontinuation of the offending drug usually suffices. More often, the resident has depression due to multiple causes (e.g., dementia, medications, psychosocial stressors/losses), so discontinuation of the offending drug is not sufficient to resolve the depressive symptoms, although it is necessary if other treatment options are to be effective.

Primary Depressive Disorders

Primary depressive disorders include MDD (single episode and recurrent), dysthymia, adjustment disorder with depressed mood, depression occurring in the context of bipolar disorder (types I and II), cyclothymia, schizoaffective disorder, schizophrenia, delusional disorder, and personality disorder (especially borderline personality disorder).

MAJOR DEPRESSIVE DISORDER   Major depressive disorder usually lasts two or more weeks (typically from weeks to a few months), has symptoms that do not fluctuate in residents with depression and no dementia, and has symptoms that occur on most days for most of the time. Core symptoms include a depressed mood, a lack of interest or pleasure in normal activities, decreased energy, a change in one's appetite and sleep patterns, impaired concentration, psychomotor agitation or slowness, suicidal ideation, guilt feelings (being a burden), and feelings of hopelessness, helplessness, or worthlessness. There may be complaints of memory problems and a lack of effort in answering memory questions, with "I don't know" answers being common. Usually there is high medical comorbidity, and depressive symptoms precede memory problems. Depressive symptoms may occur with or without accompanying psychotic symptoms. Late-onset depression is defined as a first episode of depression occurring after age 60 and is characterized by a greater degree of apathy, cognitive dysfunction, and temporal lobe abnormalities (Krishnan et al. 1995).

DYSTHYMIA   Individuals with dysthymia have depressive symptoms for two or more years that do not meet the criteria for MDD. Some LTC residents are admitted to the facility already having dysthymia, and the loss of autonomy, a decline in functional competence, and other circumstances related to life in an LTC facility provide a climate for the persistence and worsening of preexisting depression. The clinical profile of late-life dysthymia may be different from that of dysthymia in younger adults. Late-life dysthymia is often associated with medical illness, admission to a facility, progression to major depression, and an inadequate response to antidepressant treatment. Health care providers often overlook or discount symptoms such as blunted affect, anhedonia, a lack of energy, and other somatic complaints, erroneously assuming that these are a normal part of aging, particularly in the context of medical illness and residence in an LTC facility (Devanand et al. 1994).

ADJUSTMENT DISORDER WITH DEPRESSED MOOD   Individuals with adjustment disorder may have depressive symptoms in response to an identifiable stressor (other than bereavement), and their symptoms do not meet the criteria for MDD. After moving from their home to an LTC facility, new residents commonly experience adjustment disorder with depressed mood or with mixed anxiety and depressive symptoms. Other common situations in which residents may experience adjustment disorders include a change in their room or their roommate, transfer to another LTC facility, a sudden decrease in visits from close family/friends (e.g., due to the hospitalization of a spouse), and the absence of a staff member the resident has become attached to. Symptoms include tearfulness, insomnia, anxiety, restlessness, irritability, attempts to leave, and (sometimes) aggression. Typically, these symptoms gradually decrease in intensity over a one to two month period. Such symptoms are best managed by psychosocial-environmental interventions (e.g., empathic support from family and staff), provision of an outlet for the resident to express distress (e.g., therapeutic listening), the use of reminiscence, engagement in activities preferred by the residents, and counseling for family members regarding strategies to ease their loved one's transition to an LTC facility. On occasion, the clinician may consider prescribing the short-term use of hypnotic drugs (e.g., zolpidem) to treat severe insomnia or benzodiazepines (e.g., lorazepam or oxazepam) to treat severe anxiety symptoms. For some residents, these symptoms may progress to a more severe depression. In such situations, the clinician may need to add antidepressants to psychosocial-environmental interventions.

PSYCHOTIC DEPRESSION (UNIPOLAR OR BIPOLAR)   Individuals with psychotic depression often are rigid in their thinking, have more severe depression, and exhibit delusions that are usually congruent to mood, including delusions of poverty, somatic illness (e.g., preoccupation with having a terminal illness such as cancer), and paranoia. Hallucinations, which occur less commonly than delusions in these residents, are more likely to be auditory than visual or somatic. Residents with psychotic depression are much more likely to display agitation (the classic pacing and wringing of hands) and greater cognitive disturbance and have a family history of MDD or bipolar disorder. A past history of delusions in a depressive episode or profound anxiety in a depressed resident are major clues to possible psychotic depression.

Psychotic depression carries a high risk of suicide and does not respond to antidepressants alone. Hence it is important to diagnose this entity as early as possible. Additional antipsychotic medications are usually prescribed along with antidepressants. The clinician should consider hospitalization and ECT early in the course of treatment, especially for life-threatening cases of psychotic depression. ECT can be used safely with this population and may be life saving in severe cases of psychotic depression (e.g., with inanition or catatonia).

MIXED MOOD DISORDERS   The most common co-occurring mood disorders are major depression and apathy in residents with dementia, and other common co-occurring ones are medication-induced mood disorders in residents with MDD or dementia with depression, mood disorders due to alcohol use in combination with MDD, and dementia with depression. MDD co-occurring in residents with dysthymic disorder is also common, and it typically presents with the resident or the family reporting that the resident has been depressed "all her life," with an exacerbation of this depression (i.e., the development of MDD) during past stressful events/losses or admission to the LTC facility.

DEPRESSION AND FRAILTY   Depression often contributes to the etiology of frailty. Residents with depression often lose weight, become less active, can therefore lose muscle mass, strength, and exercise tolerance, and may be more prone to acute illness. On the other hand, frailty may contribute to the etiology of depression. Residents who are frail due to other factors—such as anemia, immune system dysfunction, malnutrition (e.g., being underweight, having sarcopenic obesity), advanced age, or high medical comorbidity—may lose muscle mass, strength, and exercise tolerance, which can result in decreased participation in pleasurable activities and subsequent depression. For some residents, strength training may increase their muscle strength, break the cycle of frailty by stimulating increased activity, and thus prevent depression (Espinoza and Fried 2007).

Treatment of Depression in Long-Term Care Residents

Although the treatment of depression is not as rigorously studied in the LTC setting as it is in the young adult population, it is important to recognize that depression in LTC residents does respond to treatment. A recent consensus statement specific to LTC is available to guide depression screening, evaluation, and treatment in nursing facilities (American Geriatrics Society and American Association for Geriatric Psychiatry 2003b). It can also be extended to residents in assisted living.

An accurate diagnosis and the identification of potential causes of depressive disorders (e.g., medications, medical illness) are key to successful outcomes. We recommend implementing the American Medical Director's Association's *Clinical Practice Guidelines* for the treatment of depression in LTC residents (www.amda.com/tools/guidelines.cfm). The clinician should discontinue medications that may be causing or exacerbating depression and treat pain and other partially or completely reversible physical symptoms or problems (e.g., a UTI, a vision or hearing impairment, a vitamin B_{12} deficiency, a vitamin D deficiency, undercorrected or overcorrected hypothyroid disorder, constipation, dehydration) before or along with initiating specific antidepressant treatment. The choice of treatment options for depressive symptoms (psychosocial intervention, pharmacological interventions, ECT) depends on the severity of the depressive symptoms, the person's past response to treatment interventions, and resident and family preferences. In general, if a resident has no past history of major depression, depressive symptoms that meet the criteria for minor depression or mild major depression can be successfully managed with psychosocial-environmental interventions. We recommend a combination of antidepressants and psychosocial-environmental interventions for some residents with mild MDD (especially if there is a past history of MDD) and those with dysthymic disorder. For residents with moderate to severe MDD (primary or secondary to dementia or a stroke), psychotic depression, or depression due to bipolar disorder, treatment with medications and/or ECT is of prime importance.

Initiating antidepressant therapy for LTC residents is a complex decision. The choice of an antidepressant should be informed by individual medication and resident factors: the adverse effects profile of the medication, the tolerability of the treatment (including the potential for interactions with other current medications), the person's response to prior treatment, and resident or family preferences. We do not recommend tricyclic antidepressants for LTC populations because of the risk of an added cognitive impairment (due to the drugs' anticholinergic properties) and cardiac toxicity associated with their use. SSRIs, venlafaxine, bupropion, mirtazapine, and duloxetine are all appropriate first-line antidepressants for LTC populations. Among SS-

RIs, we prefer sertraline, citalopram, and escitalopram over fluoxetine and paroxetine. Fluoxetine has a long half-life, and paroxetine has some anticholinergic properties. In addition, both fluoxetine and paroxetine are associated with a greater risk of drug-drug interaction than are sertraline, citalopram, and escitalopram. A resident who has depression, is doing well on an antidepressant, and is tolerating it well should continue taking the same antidepressant. The earlier the antidepressant starts to work, the better the chance of a good outcome, as research data support the correlation between a person's earlier clinical improvement and a more robust recovery. The key to successful pharmacotherapy for depression is giving an adequate dose of antidepressants for a long enough period. If the resident is not responding to treatment after six to eight weeks, treatment options include switching to another agent, augmenting or combining antidepressants, and having a geriatric psychiatry consultation.

Residents with depression present three key challenges to treatment: comorbid medical conditions that may complicate the treatment for depression; comorbid medications that may contribute to depression; and a slow metabolic rate (Hybels, Blazer, and Steffens 2006). The presence of neurovegetative symptoms (e.g., severe appetite and weight loss), suicidal ideation, and psychotic symptoms may indicate a need for more vigorous and aggressive therapies (e.g., higher medication dosages, multiple trials of medications, or ECT). Referral to a mental health specialist with geriatric expertise is appropriate when the diagnosis of depression is unclear, the syndrome is severe, a risk of suicide is present, residents do not respond to treatment, or other complicating factors exist that may affect the choice of treatment. ECT and/ or hospitalization to an inpatient psychiatric unit (preferably a geriatric psychiatry unit) may be necessary for the treatment of life-threatening or refractory depression, even for residents with dementia (Rao and Lyketsos 2000).

• **CLINICAL CASE** Mr. B was an 82-year-old nursing home resident with severe obesity. He was experiencing a lack of interest in activities, decreased appetite, decreased energy, and agitation during personal care, and he was making statements such as "I don't care" for the previous two to three months. This started a few weeks after he was moved from an assisted living facility to the nursing home wing of the facility, due to advancing dementia and recurrent falls. He also had a recent history of gastrointestinal bleeding, due to his peptic ulcers. When clinically examined, he had a depressed affect and made poor eye contact. A diagnosis of dementia of probable Alzheimer type with major depression was made. SSRIs were considered but not prescribed, due to his recent history of gastrointestinal bleeding. Mirtazapine was considered but not prescribed, due to obesity. Bupropion was started at 75 mg daily in the morning and after 7 days was increased to 75 mg in the morning and at 5 p.m. His family was encouraged to bring the grandchildren to visit Mr. B, as they cheered him up. The psychiatrist recommended that the staff bring Mr. B's former roommate to visit Mr. B, as they had become close friends over the two years that they lived together in the assisted living facility. Over the next four weeks, Mr. B gradually started talking more and eating more. The bupropion was changed to bupropion sustained release preparation, given as 150 mg once daily in the morning. After eight weeks, he was attending activities and eating better, and his agitation during personal care was dramatically reduced.

TEACHING POINTS The selection of antidepressants needs to take into account the resident's medical problems as well as what side effects of the various antidepressants one wants to have or to avoid. There is no compelling evidence that one antidepressant works better than any of the others for this population. Antidepressants, when used appropriately and in combination with individualized psychosocial-environmental interventions, can dramatically improve depressive symptoms and a depressed resident's quality of life.

Starting and Ending Antidepressants

It is crucial to educate residents, families, and staff about what to expect in the course of antidepressant therapy. Difficulties can develop at any time, but they seem to cluster at the beginning, during any increase in dosage, and during discontinuation of the drug. Although it usually takes weeks for a therapeutic response to occur, most adverse effects (e.g., nausea, diarrhea, constipation, sedation, lethargy, headache, anxiety, insomnia, and agitation) appear shortly after the first dose and after any increase in the dosage. Thus it is vital to educate the resident and his or her caregivers that adverse effects, when they occur, usually precede therapeutic effects. In general, if the dose is started low and increased slowly, early adverse effects are mild, self-limiting, and remit within one to two weeks. For residents who are particularly prone to developing adverse effects (especially anxiety and insomnia), the risk of these adverse effects can be minimized by reducing the antidepressant dose to an even smaller starting dose, increasing it even more slowly, and using lower final doses. For residents who develop significant anxiety, restlessness, or insomnia after starting an antidepressant, the clinician may consider a brief course of a low-dose benzodiazepine or low-dose hypnotics (e.g., zolpidem, eszopiclone).

When some of the commonly used antidepressants are abruptly discontinued after several weeks or more, discontinuation syndrome is common. Discontinuation syndrome involves manifestations of dizziness, paresthesias (typically electric-shock-like sensations), muscle jerks and twitches, and agitation. Drugs such as paroxetine and venlafaxine carry the highest risk of discontinuation syndrome, due to their short half-life. Discontinuation syndrome is milder with intermediate-acting antidepressants (e.g., citalopram, sertraline, and escitalopram). Typically, discontinuation syndrome remits within one to two weeks. The treatment may involve reinstating the antidepressant and tapering it off more slowly. Serotonin syndrome is a serious and potentially fatal condition that may develop with the use of high doses of SSRIs or of SSRIs in combination with other medications that also increase serotonin neurotransmission (e.g., lithium, trazodone). The clinical manifestation of serotonin syndrome includes hyperreflexia, agitation, insomnia, myoclonic jerks, autonomic instability, fever, and delirium. The treatment involves discontinuing the offending drugs and hospitalizing residents with severe symptoms.

CLINICAL CASE Mr. G, a 79-year-old resident who had had a stroke causing left hemiparesis four months previously, was referred for psychiatric consultation because of frequent episodes of irritation and actions such as hollering at staff members almost daily, making sexually inappropriate comments, and attempting to touch them inappropriately during personal care. These symptoms were present for three months. Mr. G's wife (who was also Mr. G's legal surrogate decision maker) had refused antidepressant treatment for Mr. G from his primary care physician because Mr. G had become "wild" after the initiation of an antidepressant (paroxetine) five year previously, after his first stroke. On a mental status examination, Mr. G showed evidence of executive dysfunction and depressed mood, but his affect was broad. He enjoyed socialization and his conversation with the psychiatrist and seemed to crave social interaction and personal attention. A diagnosis of poststroke depression and impulse control disorder due to frontal lobe dysfunction was made.

The psychiatrist reviewed previous records, which indicated that Mr.

G was treated with 20 mg of paroxetine for depression five years previously. The psychiatrist and Mrs. G reviewed the possible adverse effects and benefits of a second trial with an antidepressant at a low dose. The psychiatrist assured Mrs. G that Mr. G would be closely monitored for any adverse effects and that the antidepressant would be promptly discontinued if its adverse effects were moderate to severe. Mrs. G agreed to this plan. A decision was made to start Mr. G on sertraline 12.5 mg daily in the morning, to be increased to 25 mg daily in the morning after seven days. Mr. G developed transient mild nausea and anxiety for three days, which resolved spontaneously. After treatment for four weeks, the staff noticed that Mr. G was less irritable, but his sexually inappropriate behaviors and occasional episodes of hollering (at least once a week) continued. After four weeks, his dose was increased to 37.5 mg daily for seven days and then to 50 mg daily. Mr. G once again developed transient mild nausea and anxiety, which cleared up spontaneously over a one week period. After six more weeks of treatment, the staff reported that Mr. G's sexually inappropriate behavior had decreased considerably and his episodes of hollering now occurred less than once a week.

TEACHING POINTS Some individuals may have an overly sensitive subtype of serotonin receptor and respond to small final doses of SSRIs, but they are prone to develop adverse effects (e.g., severe anxiety) if the starting dose is not very low. SSRIs (except paroxetine and fluoxetine) are good first-choice antidepressants for people with cardiovascular or cerebrovascular disease because of their negligible cardiac toxicity and anticholinergic properties. Paroxetine carries a small but significant anticholinergic effect and thus is not the SSRI of first choice for people with cognitive impairments. SSRIs are also good first-choice antidepressants for people whose depression coexists with sexually inappropriate behavior, as serotonin dysfunction has been associated with impulse control disorders. Also, sexual adverse effects associated with the use of SSRIs (e.g., decreased libido) may be therapeutic in this situation. Education of the family and staff in the management of adverse effects is also key to a successful outcome.

Augmentation Strategies

A partial response to antidepressant monotherapy for severe MDD in older adults is common and may be seen in as many as 60 percent of the cases. This often requires augmentation strategies for further improvement, although increasing the dose of the antidepressant the resident is already taking still further may also be appropriate. Residual symptoms are strong predictors of relapse that may place the resident at a higher risk of suicide. Older adults whose mobility is limited or who present with underlying signs of chronic depression may be most at risk of a partial response (Hybels, Blazer, and Steffens 2006). The most common augmentation strategy is to add another antidepressant that acts on different receptors and neurotransmitters. For example, if the resident's depression improves partially with citalopram (or another SSRI), adding mirtazapine or bupropion is reasonable. We do not recommend combining SSRIs with venlafaxine. Combining venlafaxine or duloxetine with mirtazapine is also a good augmentation strategy, because mirtazapine targets different combinations of neurotransmitters (e.g., norepinephrine, histamine) from venlafaxine or duloxetine (e.g., serotonin, norepinephrine). Other strategies for augmentation include adding a psychostimulant (e.g., methylphenidate), buspirone, or tri-iodothyronine, as well as ECT and psychotherapy (for cognitively intact residents). We do not recommend augmentation with lithium for most LTC residents because of the high risk of toxicity. Augmentation with aripiprazole may be an appropriate strategy for the treatment of resistant depression. For residents with severe agitated depression, the clinician may consider adding low-dose atypical antipsychotics (e.g., quetiapine) to an antidepressant.

Treatment of Medical Comorbidity to Improve the Response to Treatment

Aggressively treating medical comorbidity (e.g., anemia, pain, under- or overcorrected hypothyroidism, and vitamin deficiencies [e.g., vitamin B_{12}, folate, vitamin D]) may improve not only the resident's functional status, but also his or her mood and response to the treatment of depression with antidepressants and/or psychosocial-environmental interventions.

Treatment-Resistant Depression

Some 25–35 percent of patients show only minimal improvement in their depressive symptoms when treated. Many patients do not improve because antidepressants are not given a long enough time to work, and psychosocial-environmental interventions are not individualized and are used aggressively. The clinician should inform family and professional caregivers that these medications take six to eight weeks to begin to show results. Also, what could seem to be resistance to treatment might be depression that is being treated inadequately with too low a dosage, too short a treatment period, or premature discontinuation due to side effects or cost. Unaddressed underlying triggers (e.g., pain, thyroid problems, anemia, malignancy) also might prevent an adequate response to antidepressant therapy. Other barriers to a treatment response include an incorrect diagnosis and use of the wrong drug. Recent data suggest that, after an initial benefit, elderly people may benefit further from prolonged courses (two years) (Reynolds et al. 2006).

Vascular depression is of particular concern, as it is more difficult to treat. If the first trial of an antidepressant at an adequate dose and duration fails, the clinician should initiate a second trial with another class of antidepressant. If the second trial also fails, then the clinician should try a secondary tricyclic amine (e.g., nortriptyline) if there are no contraindications (e.g., severe heart disease). The FDA recently approved aripiprazole as an adjuvant to antidepressant therapy for the treatment of resistant depression, and the clinician should consider its use in LTC populations. The clinician should also consider ECT if the tricyclic antidepressant fails. For residents with a past history of a good response to ECT, the clinician should consider ECT early in the course of their treatment. A selegiline transdermal patch has not been studied in LTC populations, but the clinician may consider it for refractory cases, especially for residents with Parkinson disease, as selegiline increases dopaminergic neurotransmission in the brain. If two trials of antidepressant monotherapy fail, the clinician should seek a psychiatric consultation. An assessment of suicide risk at every step is critical, as elderly people have the highest rate of suicide. This suicide risk exists even for LTC residents with depression.

Supplements and Herbal Remedies

We rarely recommend the use of supplements such as S-adenosyl methionine (SAM-e) or St. John's wort to treat depression in LTC populations, as such supplements are not well studied in these populations and may have a clinically significant drug-drug interaction with conventional antidepressants and other medications. One exception to this recommendation is for residents with depression who strongly believe in these supplements and refuse to take conventional antidepressants.

Electroconvulsive Therapy

Electroconvulsive therapy is a safe and rapidly effective option for the treatment of depression and mania in older adults (van der Wurff et al. 2003).

The clinician should consider ECT for any resident with severe depression, as it is life-saving for many of them. For a resident with severe depression and cachexia, for whom we don't have the luxury of time for medications to work, or for residents who are actively suicidal or psychotically depressed, we strongly recommend ECT. Residents with depression and dementia can be given ECT with good effect, but post-ECT delirium is a greater risk (Rao and Lyketsos 2000).

Psychotherapy and Psychosocial-Environmental Interventions
Psychotherapy and psychosocial-environmental interventions are important in all types of depression and may prove more effective than the use of antidepressants for milder disorders (Llewellyn-Jones and Snowdon 2007). Many residents feel that initiating action in an environment that cannot be changed is futile (learned helplessness). Also, many residents may have expectations that are not realistic, may overgeneralize or overreact to adverse events, and may personalize events (cognitive distortions). Perceived negative interpersonal events are also associated with depression, particularly in residents who demonstrate a high need for approval and reassurance in the context of interpersonal relationships. Other psychosocial factors, such as a mutual social and affective withdrawal between residents and their social environment (family, friends), inadequate compensation for lost interests, failure to optimize abilities, and the poor quality of social supports (e.g., significant family conflicts), may also need to be addressed to achieve a successful outcome. For ongoing loss-related depression, including sadness about one's loss of health, the clinician can help the resident ventilate feelings and either reacquire what is lost (e.g., use physical therapy to reacquire the ability to ambulate after a stroke) or grieve and then adapt to the new situation.

Some cognitively intact residents may prefer psychotherapy instead of, or in addition to, medication. Moreover, psychotherapy may be indicated for residents who are relatively intact cognitively but cannot tolerate medication, or who are dealing with grief or other stressful situations or interpersonal problems. Social factors and perceptions of health and well-being may be important predictors of the outcome in older adults with MDD, and these can be addressed during psychotherapy. Several types of psychotherapy have been found to reduce the symptoms of depression, including cognitive-behavioral therapy, interpersonal therapy, problem-solving therapy, family therapy, and brief psychodynamic therapy. The clinician may also consider life review or reminiscence psychotherapy, group therapy, music therapy, and meaning-centered therapy (logotherapy). Psychosocial interventions, including psychoeducation, family counseling, and the provision of counseling for spouses, may also be helpful.

The clinician may consult mental health care providers with expertise in geriatrics (social workers, psychologists, psychiatrists, and geriatric psychiatrists) to provide psychotherapy for residents with depression who are relatively intact cognitively. Residents with a preexisting personality disorder, a long-standing history of poor coping skills, or difficulty with interpersonal relationships may benefit from long-term psychotherapy in which the social worker or psychologist sees the resident every one to four weeks for months to years. A significant barrier to this arrangement is lack of access to professionals able to provide psychotherapy for LTC populations. In many instances, the resident may need to go to an outpatient clinic that provides such treatment. In an increasing number of LTC facilities, a social worker or psychologist with expertise in providing psychotherapy for LTC residents visits the facility to provide therapy to residents that the consulting psychiatrist identified as potentially benefiting from psychotherapy. However, most of the social workers in LTC facilities do not have the time or the training to provide formal psychotherapy for the residents.

Complementary and Alternative Treatments

The clinician may consider interventions such as daily exercise programs, tai chi, yoga, exposure to sunlight, bright light therapy (with high-lux light built into the environment), music therapy, aromatherapy, a daily schedule of pleasant activities, activities promoting spirituality and creative expression, mindfulness and breathing exercises, massage therapy, Reiki, gratitude journaling, pet therapy, intergenerational activities, and an omega-3-rich diet (or omega-3 fatty acid supplements) in addition to conventional interventions (antidepressants, psychotherapy) to treat depression in LTC populations (Lyketsos et al. 1999b; Williams and Tappen 2007). For residents with better cognitive functioning, the clinician should routinely inquire about the resident's and family's preferences for such interventions. Family members may also express a wish to add these interventions to conventional treatments. One advantage of including such interventions is that the staff and family can be actively engaged in helping the resident recover from depression, thus indirectly addressing their own stress and increasing their feelings of usefulness.

CLINICAL CASE Mrs. U, a 90-year-old woman with a history of dementia, had been experiencing severe depressive symptoms for the previous four months. She was also experiencing severe anxiety, insomnia, a lack of appetite, and irritability. Her primary care physician referred her to a psychiatrist when her depression did not respond to two trials of antidepressants.

The psychiatrist found that Mrs. U had tried taking citalopram 20 mg daily for four weeks and then tried sertraline 50 mg for four weeks before the referral. Her primary care physician was reluctant to use higher doses of antidepressants because of Mrs. U's advanced age and dementia. In the week before evaluation by the psychiatrist, Mrs. U had developed abdominal pain, was found to have a UTI, and was given antibiotics. The psychiatrist found Mrs. U to be severely depressed. She was tearful throughout the interview, expressing hopelessness and a wish that she were dead. She was also distraught because she had developed mild antibiotic-induced diarrhea. Her score on the MMSE was 13. Mrs. U's liver function and kidney function tests were within normal limits. The psychiatrist considered prescribing one of the SSRIs again, but because of the risk of worsening the antibiotic-induced diarrhea, he decided to avoid SSRIs and prescribe mirtazapine instead. Mrs. U started taking 7.5 mg of mirtazapine daily at bedtime, and the dose was increased after seven days to 15 mg daily at bedtime. She began sleeping better after two weeks of treatment, her diarrhea resolved when the course of antibiotics was over, her UTI cleared up, and her abdominal pain improved. However, her tearfulness, daytime agitation, and hopelessness persisted, so the dose of mirtazapine was further increased to 22.5 mg daily at bedtime for seven days. Mrs. U was able to tolerate this dose without sedation or other adverse effects. The family and staff were counseled to try to walk with her daily, and the family hired a massage therapist to come twice a week. After eight weeks, her mood had improved significantly, her anxiety decreased, her appetite had returned to near normal, and her feelings of hopelessness had resolved.

TEACHING POINTS Some oldest old residents (over age 85) may tolerate antidepressants at final doses similar to those taken by younger residents to treat severe depression. As long as the dose of antidepressant is increased slowly and the resident is being monitored closely for adverse effects, there is no reason not to prescribe adequate doses of antidepressants for a sufficient time before abandoning the trial and trying other antidepressants. It is possible that higher doses of citalopram (up to 40 mg) or sertraline (up to 100 mg) for a longer period (six to eight weeks) would have improved Mrs. U's depression. Complementary and alternative treatment interventions (in this case, massage therapy) may also have contributed to the successful treatment outcome.

Apathy

Apathy is the most ignored and underdiagnosed behavioral and psychological symptom of dementia, despite being the most common one, occurring in up to 92 percent of residents with dementia (Overshott et al. 2004). The Greek word *pathos* refers to passions. Apathy is characterized by indifference, often in situations that would normally arouse strong feelings or reactions. Residents with apathy lose initiative and drive for their usual activities. They may complain of an inability to finish tasks. Family members and staff usually report that the resident is showing a lack of concern for daily events or even for personal care. Despite these issues, the resident appears emotionally absent or unconcerned (Orr 2004). Apathy often includes a lack of motivation, a lack of interest and emotion, periods of sitting and staring blankly, and, in severe cases, self-neglect (not bathing or changing clothes for days or even weeks). It manifests in behaviors such as poor persistence, diminished initiation, low social interaction, indifference, and blunted emotional response.

Apathy is distinct from depression, although its symptoms are often mislabeled, and it can be reliably identified in residents with dementia (Landes et al. 2001). Residents who exhibit apathy lack the dysphoria (tearfulness, expressions of sadness, irritability), suicidality, loss of appetite, agitation, anxiety, restlessness, insomnia, verbalization of hopelessness, worthlessness, and guilt seen in residents with depression. Apathy increases in severity as the dementia progresses, in contrast to a decrease in the prevalence of depression with the progression of dementia. Apathy is also commonly seen in residents who do not have dementia, especially those with delirium (particularly quiet delirium) or who have had a stroke involving the frontal lobe or its connections. Apathy also often accompanies end-organ failure of the kidneys, liver, heart, or lungs. Apathy and depression are often comorbid in residents with dementia. Table 5.4 lists common causes of apathy (Aalten et al. 2007; Borroni, Agosti, and Padovani 2008). All of these causes involve damage to or impairment of the frontal lobe or connections to the frontal lobe. Most residents with apathy also exhibit executive dysfunction.

By its very nature, apathy prevents residents from bringing up such issues with health care providers. Family and/or staff are the first to raise concerns.

TABLE 5.4
Common causes of apathy in the long-term care population

Apathy secondary to physical illnesses or conditions
  Alzheimer disease
  Other dementias (vascular dementia, dementia with Lewy bodies, Parkinson disease dementia, frontotemporal dementia)
  Delirium
  End-organ failure of the kidneys, liver, heart, lungs
  Pain
  Medications (e.g., selective serotonin reuptake inhibitors, antipsychotics, interferon)
  Infections (e.g., urinary tract infection, pneumonia, "flu")
  Brain tumors involving the frontal lobe or its connections
  Strokes involving the frontal lobe or its connections
  Head injuries with damage to the frontal lobe or its connections
  Medical conditions (e.g., dehydration, hyponatremia, hypothyroidism)
Apathy accompanying primary psychiatric disorders
  Major depression and vascular depression
  Schizophrenia
  Schizoid personality disorder
  Schizotypal personality disorder

The treatment of apathy is a treatment of its cause. For most residents, apathy is due to dementia or a stroke, in which case the treatment consists primarily of psychosocial-environmental interventions. (See table 5.5 for interventions to treat apathy.) Apathy is stressful to both the family and the staff. Educating them about apathy, its neurological basis, and its difference from depression is useful in alleviating family and staff stress. Whenever possible, the clinician should discontinue or lower the dosage of medications that may cause or exacerbate apathy. Occasionally, apathy in residents with Alzheimer disease, dementia with Lewy bodies, or Parkinson disease dementia improves to a modest extent with the use of ChEIs. In severe cases, the clinician may consider prescribing a trial of psychostimulants (e.g., methylphenidate) or dopaminergic agents (e.g., amantadine) (Marin et al. 1995). Apathy typically does not improve with antidepressant treatment. In fact, certain antidepressants, such as SSRIs, may exacerbate apathy. Apathy is often comorbid with depression, in which case the clinician may consider prescribing a trial of non-SSRI antidepressants (e.g., bupropion, duloxetine, or stimulants). For residents who have severe apathy and mild parkinsonism, the clinician may consider prescribing dopamine agonists.

CLINICAL CASE Mr. L was an 80-year-old married man who moved to an assisted living facility after experiencing difficulties managing his daily activities and an inability to take care of his home. He was also forgetting to

TABLE 5.5
Interventions for the treatment of apathy

Psychosocial-environmental interventions
  Education of the family and staff regarding the differences between clinical depression and apathy,
    the neurological basis of apathy, and the need to lower the expectations of residents with apathy
  Music (e.g., listening to preferred music, live music, group singing)
  Exercise
  Reminiscence
  Intergenerational interventions
  Animal-assisted therapy
  Nature (e.g., gardening, sunshine)
  Spirituality (e.g., going to church, listening to bible readings, singing or listening to religious songs)
Medications to consider for the treatment of severe apathy*
  Stimulants (e.g., methylphenidate)
  Modafinil, Armodafinil
  Bupropion
  Dopamine agonists (e.g., selegiline, amantadine)
  Cholinesterase inhibitors (e.g., rivastigmine, donepezil, galantamine)

*The U.S. Food and Drug Administration has not approved any drug for the treatment of apathy.

take his medications. His wife of 48 years moved with him, as Mr. L would not move otherwise and his wife was undergoing severe stress from caregiving and could not continue to care for Mr. L at home. Mrs. L also had health problems, including severe rheumatoid arthritis. Over the previous six months, Mrs. L had noticed that Mr. L had stopped initiating conversations, avoided going to any social gatherings, and became irritated when she would insist that they attend at least some of the family functions that they had been going to for more than four decades. Mr. L would spend the major part of the day watching television. Mrs. L also noticed that Mr. L avoided changing clothes and would take baths only when she became adamant that he do so. Mrs. L was concerned that her husband was depressed and requested a psychiatric consultation. Mrs. L told the psychiatrist that her husband had always enjoyed company, had many interests that he shared with friends and family (e.g., golf, hunting), and had always looked forward to family events. She stated that Mr. L had bypass surgery one year previously and had recovered slowly. Some of the symptoms of his lack of motivation may have started a month or two after the surgery, but Mrs. L noticed that in the last six months, Mr. L was "not himself."

Mr. L did not mind being interviewed by the psychiatrist, although he felt he was "fine" and did not understand his wife's concerns. Mr. L had no past history of depression and no family history of depression. He answered all of the psychiatrist's questions in short sentences and did not initiate conversation. Mr. L denied feeling down, reported that he was content with his life, denied any sleep or appetite problems, and denied feeling pessimistic or hopeless or that he was a burden to others. He denied feeling that life was not worth living. He said that he had several interests but that he was "too old" for golf and hunting and enjoyed watching television. His score on the MMSE was 23. A CT scan showed several lacunae in the right basal ganglia and pons. All other laboratory tests were normal.

The psychiatrist diagnosed Mr. L with apathy in the context of mild vascular dementia. Neuropsychological testing confirmed a significant frontal lobe dysfunction (as indicated by severe executive dysfunction). Mr. L's wife was educated about apathy and how it was different from depression. The psychiatrist also explained various treatment options. Mrs. L preferred psychosocial-environmental interventions over experimental medication trials. Mr. L had always loved music and agreed to see a music therapist once a week on an individual basis. Mr. L also agreed to help his great-grandson with the latter's life-history project, which would involve reminiscing about Mr. L's successful professional career. The psychiatrist counseled Mrs. L not to insist that Mr. L attend various social and family events and to be content with Mr. L's bathing twice a week. The psychiatrist also recommended that Mrs. L see a social worker for individual counseling to address the stress of caregiving and the grief of losing parts of her husband's original personality. After 12 weeks, Mrs. L's depression had decreased significantly and Mr. L showed a mild interest in music therapy and in the life-history project. He was agreeable to continuing these activities.

TEACHING POINTS Apathy can be reliably differentiated from depression. The occasional irritability in Mr. L could be considered mild depression, but because it was short lived and usually in the context of when his wife was trying to motivate him for social events, rather than a pervasive change in mood, it was more likely a part of apathy.

Suicidality

Suicidality is one of the most serious clinical concerns in LTC residents. Manifestations of suicidality range from passive suicidal ideation to completed suicide. Older adults (> 65 years old) are at a higher risk of suicide than any other age group. Suicidality in older adults is a complex phenomenon with multiple risk correlates. Its prevalence increases in late life and reaches a rate of 17.6/100,000 for the population aged 75–84. Among all adults, elderly people are most likely to die as a result of their suicide attempts, with the ratio of completed to attempted suicides increasing from 1:200 in young adult women to 1:4 in elderly persons. These statistics are primarily for community-dwelling elderly people, as suicidality has not been rigorously studied in residents of LTC facilities. Besides demographic factors (older age, male gender, white race), the presence of mood disorders (most notably depression), physical health factors (perception of poor health status, poor sleep quality, smoking, high medical comorbidity), and psychosocial factors (stressful life events such as the loss of spouse, the loss of a job, marital discord, low social interaction, a lack of social support, financial stress, lack of a purpose to live) increase the risk of suicidality. Depression, a family history of suicide, pervasive feelings of hopelessness, feelings of being a burden, social isolation, and a past history of suicide attempts are the most important risk factors for future suicidality. Most residents who completed suicide had depression, although most did not have a prior lifetime history of psychiatric treatment (Suominen et al. 2003). Most victims of completed suicide are male, and firearms and hanging are the two most common methods used. In contrast, self-harmful behaviors among LTC residents are more strongly associated with dementia and may not necessarily reflect depression or a wish to die (Draper et al. 2002).

Self-harming behaviors associated with depression may take the form of a refusal to eat, to take medications, or to undergo life-extending or life-saving interventions. Increased risk is also associated with resolved plans for suicide, a sense of courage or competence regarding suicide, and access to a means of suicide (e.g., pills, a gun). Residents with severe and persistent mental illness may attempt suicide by throwing themselves down a flight of stairs or out a window. Most studies have not associated dementia with suicidality (Conwell et al. 2002). We recommend assessing all new residents for suicide risk. If the clinician suspects that a resident is suicidal, the staff may need to search the resident's belongings for drugs on which he or she could overdose. It is also important to check for medication hoarding. Among community-dwelling elderly people, the most common means of committing suicide is the use of a firearm. The clinician should screen residents who are suicidal and are requesting a visit home for the presence of a firearm at home and then implement the necessary interventions to limit that resident's access to firearms. Involving the family (with the consent of the resident whenever possible) to help reduce suicide risk is crucial.

About 10 to 15 percent of those with bipolar disorder commit suicide, and 25 percent attempt suicide during their lifetimes. For older adults who attempt suicide, the presence of bipolar disorder may be associated with a higher risk of suicide than from any other psychiatric or medical disorders. The presence of other severe and persistent mental illnesses (e.g., schizophrenia and schizoaffective disorder) is also associated with a high risk of suicide. Although frail or confused LTC residents may have greater difficulty physically carrying out suicidal acts, the clinician should take any suicidal ideation seriously.

We recommend a referral to a psychiatrist if the clinician suspects a resident is at high risk of suicide (see table 5.6). When in doubt, the clinician should still initiate a referral to a psychiatrist. For residents at imminent risk—those who have made a serious suicide attempt (evidence of high lethality [a violent, near-lethal, premeditated attempt; precautions to avoid rescue]) or are voicing suicidal ideas with a plan or intent, and those who have severe depression with suicidal ideas, psychotic depression with suicidal ideas, poor judgment, or medical complications and are refusing treatment— we recommend hospitalization in a psychiatric inpatient unit (preferably a geriatric psychiatry unit).

A suicide prevention program may involve the following five principles:

1. A focus on new admissions, inquiring about any past histories of depressive episodes (e.g., a history of outpatient treatment for depression, a history of severe depression or a "nervous breakdown" requiring inpatient treatment), suicide attempts, suicidal thoughts (or a family history of suicide), alcohol abuse, and other substance abuse.
2. The early involvement of a mental health professional (preferably with expertise in geriatrics) in managing residents with suicidal ideas, psychotic depression, bipolar depression, schizophrenia and related disorders.
3. Staff education to closely monitor suicidal thoughts when they are present.
4. A routine assessment of suicide risk factors in residents with clinical depression.

TABLE 5.6
Situations in which residents are considered at high risk for suicide

The resident made a suicide attempt in the recent past
The resident is voicing suicidal ideas and has a past history of a suicide attempt
The resident has severe depression and is feeling hopeless
The resident has depression and suicidal ideas
The resident has depression and a family history of suicide
The resident expresses a wish to die and has a plan

5. The implementation of an interdisciplinary care plan to reduce the risk of suicide in residents with risk factors.

Mania

Mania involves a distinct period of abnormally and a persistently elevated mood or an irritable mood (lasting at least one week), along with other symptoms (excessive talking, pressure of speech [the inability to interrupt speech], grandiosity, distractibility, increased goal-directed activity [or psychomotor agitation], no need for sleep). Classic mania is not hard to recognize. Mania in older adults often is characterized by grandiose delusions, irritability, dysphoria, and sexually inappropriate behaviors that are not characteristic of the individual and often surprise those closest to him or her. Hypomania is a milder form of mania, and it is often hard to elicit a past history of a hypomanic episode.

The differential diagnosis of mania includes the following:

- primary mania or hypomania (Bipolar I and Bipolar II disorders, cyclothymia, schizoaffective disorder-bipolar type)
- secondary mania or hypomania (e.g., mania or hypomania due to medications, a stroke)
- mixed (primary and secondary causes) (e.g., bipolar disorder and steroid-induced mania)

Bipolar Disorders

Bipolar disorder is a life-long illness and confers a susceptibility to recurrent episodes of depression and mania or hypomania. Most people with bipolar disorder spent a large part of their lives experiencing depressive symptoms. Depression during bipolar disorder in older adults is often melancholic in nature and includes disturbances in sleep and appetite as well as a cognitive impairment that mimics dementia. As a result of population aging, the number of older persons with bipolar disorder (and other severe psychiatric disorders) will increase two- to threefold over the next several decades. Some 50 percent of patients in a Veterans Administration bipolar disorder registry are over age 50, and the proportion of those with bipolar disorder over age 65 increased fivefold between 1980 and 1998 (Almeida and Fenner 2002; Sajatovic et al. 2004). The majority of older adults with bipolar disorder experience its onset before age 30 and have simply gotten older (early-onset bipolar disorder). About 10 to 15 percent of people with bipolar disorder experience the onset of this illness after age 50 (late-onset bipolar disorder).

The psychopathology of bipolar disorder among older adults can be severe. Neurological comorbidity/signs (e.g., white matter hyperintensities in an MRI brain scan indicating cerebrovascular disease) appear to be more prevalent in the late-onset form of the disease, similar to what has been found in late-onset depression. Medical comorbidity (especially diabetes, obesity, hyperlipidemia, heart disease, hypertension, metabolic syndrome, and pulmonary disorders) is common in older adults with bipolar disorder, but comorbid substance abuse is uncommon in this population. However, the baby boom generation has had greater exposure to street drugs or other substances, and thus the next wave of older adults with bipolar disorder will be more likely than the current generation to have substance use disorders. A variety of cognitive deficits in people with bipolar disorder persist between episodes of depression and mania. Almost 50 percent of the people with bipolar disorder who are older than 60 showed impairment on cognitive screening tests (Gildengers et al. 2004), and functional limitations are also common in older adults with this disorder.

Older adults can and do experience the full range of manic, mixed, and depressive symptoms that characterizes bipolar disorders. In persons with bipolar disorder, normally the first episode, and most other episodes, are depressive. A depressive episode meets the criteria for MDD. For individuals with recurrent MDD, the clinician should always keep a diagnosis of bipolar disorder in mind, as the first manic or hypomanic episode may not occur for years to decades after the first episode of depression, and it may occur after many more episodes of depression. Differentiating bipolar depression from MDD is critical to successful treatment outcomes, because not only are the treatments of the two disorders different, but antidepressants may also worsen the symptoms and course of bipolar disorder. A past history of hypomania or mania, a family history of bipolar disorder, an early age of onset for MDD, a higher number of prior depressive episodes, and symptoms related to anxiety indicate bipolar depression rather than MDD (Perlis et al. 2006). A mixed episode involves symptoms that meet the criteria for MDD and mania lasting for at least seven days.

Treatment of Bipolar Disorders

The symptoms of bipolar disorder can be severe among elderly people. The treatment of bipolar disorder in elderly adults is similar to its treatment in younger adults, although the incidence and severity of adverse effects are greater among older people. Older people are also more likely to be taking several medications that may interact with one another, are more likely to have comorbid physical conditions, and tend to adhere poorly to treatment. Resistance to treatment is common, recurrences are frequent, and there is a high incidence of mortality. Hence bipolar disorder in LTC populations is best managed by a psychiatrist.

Treatment strategies for controlling bipolar disorder consist of pharmacotherapy and psychosocial interventions. Pharmacotherapy involves mood stabilizers (e.g., lithium, valproate, carbamazepine, lamotrigine) and atypical antipsychotics. The use of antidepressants for residents with bipolar disorder type I is controversial, because of the potential for antidepressants to worsen the course of bipolar disorder (e.g., an increased risk of rapid cycling) and their potential for switching a resident with depression to mania. This risk is particularly higher with antidepressants that have serotonin and norepinephrine reuptake inhibition properties, such as tricyclic antidepressants, venlafaxine, and possibly duloxetine. If the clinician prescribes antidepressants, one of the SSRIs or bupropion is preferred, and the clinician should closely monitor the resident for a switch to mania and rapid cycling. Antidepressants should only be used for a short period and should be accompanied by a mood stabilizer or an atypical antipsychotic medication. The use of antidepressants may carry less risk with bipolar disorder type II than with type I. Rapid cycling (four or more episodes of mania or hypomania or MDD or mixed episodes in one year) is associated with a higher prevalence of hypothyroidism. Hence all residents with rapid cycling should have their TSH levels checked. Even for residents with rapid cycling and a normal TSH level, augmenting with tri-iodothyronine may help control bipolar symptoms (especially depression).

Although lithium is the gold standard of treatment for bipolar disorder (especially bipolar disorder with classic euphoric mania), LTC residents usually develop toxicity even with low doses of lithium, due in part to lower renal clearance of the drug and in part to its interactions with diuretics. The most common symptoms of lithium toxicity in this population include neurocognitive adverse effects (e.g., disorientation, memory impairment), diarrhea, falls, and tremors. LTC residents are also at higher risk of serious lithium toxicity (e.g., delirium, myoclonic jerks, severe diarrhea, a coma, cardiovascular collapse, and seizures) than are older adults in the community, who, in turn, are at higher risk than middle-aged and younger adults. Hence we recommend avoiding lithium for treating bipolar disorder in LTC residents unless they are already taking lithium, are tolerating it well, and have benefited from it. Also, for patients with mixed episodes and those with rapid cycling, lithium is not as effective as valproate, carbamazepine, or atypical antipsychotics.

Valproate is much better tolerated than lithium by LTC residents with bipolar disorder, and it is one of the first-line agents for the treatment of bipolar mania, hypomania, and mixed episodes; other first-line agents include atypical antipsychotics. Carbamazepine is a third-line agent because of its substantial risk of drug-drug interactions and adverse effects. Atypical antipsychotics are preferred over mood stabilizers for treating bipolar symptoms associated with psychotic symptoms. Risperidone, olanzapine, quetiapine, aripiprazole, and paliperidone are preferred over ziprasidone, which has not been well studied in elderly patients. Although olanzapine has lost its place as a drug of first choice in young adults with bipolar disorder, primarily due to its risks of metabolic complications (weight gain, diabetes, hyperlipidemia, metabolic syndrome), it remains one of the first-line agents for older adults with bipolar disorder, because the risk of metabolic complication is probably lower in older adults and weight gain may be beneficial for residents who are underweight. The clinician should avoid prescribing typical antipsychotics (e.g., haloperidol, fluphenazine, and thioridazine) for LTC residents with bipolar disorder, due to the much higher risk of adverse effects (e.g., parkinsonism, falls, cognitive dysfunction, tardive dyskinesias) with these drugs than with atypical antipsychotics. To prevent future episodes, we recommend lamotrigine for the treatment of bipolar depression. We recommend quetiapine monotherapy or a combination of an SSRI (e.g., citalopram, sertraline, escitalopram) with olanzapine for the treatment of a depressive episode of bipolar disorder.

Many residents with bipolar disorder may need complex medication regimens, including more than one mood stabilizer and antipsychotic. Bipolar disorder is often comorbid with other psychiatric disorders, such as anxiety disorders (generalized anxiety disorder, panic disorder) and substance abuse. The clinician should inquire about the presence of these comorbid disorders and, if present, appropriately treat them. The clinician may consider prescribing the short-term use of low doses of a benzodiazepine (e.g., clonazepam or lorazepam) to control symptoms of severe agitation and/or severe anxiety.

Residents with bipolar disorder have a high risk of suicide, so the resident, the staff, and the resident's family need to be educated regarding this risk. We strongly recommend close monitoring for suicidality during an acute episode of depression or of mania and a mixed episode. The clinician must take all statements of suicide, hopelessness, and a wish to die seriously, as people with bipolar disorder are at high risk of suicide. Besides treating bipolar symptoms, the clinician should take appropriate suicide precautions for residents who express suicidal ideas or hopelessness. The clinician should consider hospitalization in a psychiatric unit (preferably a geriatric psychiatry unit or a med-psych unit) for residents who have made suicidal attempts or have suicidal ideas, severe symptoms, psychotic symptoms, and symptoms that are not responding to treatment. ECT is one of the first-line treatment options for rapid control of manic, mixed, and depressive symptoms.

Psychosocial interventions include psychoeducation for the resident, the family, and the staff. Residents, family members, and staff members can be trained to recognize early signs of symptom exacerbations and adverse events as they occur. Families of residents with bipolar disorder may have been under considerable strain for decades before the person's move to LTC. Thus their well-being also needs to be addressed.

CLINICAL CASE Mrs. F, an 85-year-old woman, had recently been admitted to a nursing home for rehabilitation after surgery for a hip fracture. She had a long history of bipolar disorder type I, with multiple suicide attempts and hospitalizations, but she had been stable for the previous 10 years by taking olanzapine 5 mg at bedtime, lamotrigine 100 mg daily in the morning, and valproate extended release 500 mg daily at bedtime. The olanzapine was discontinued in the nursing home, due to her experiencing "lethargy" and not participating in physical therapy. Her daughter strongly opposed this intervention, and after Mrs. F started showing a recurrence of symptoms of bipolar depression (frequent tearfulness, loss of appetite), her daughter insisted that olanzapine be restarted. The staff decided to ask for input from the consulting psychiatrist. The psychiatrist obtained feedback from Mrs. F's daughter, who was her primary caregiver and had helped Mrs. F through previous bouts when her bipolar illness was exacerbated. The psychiatrist felt the daughter was knowledgeable about both bipolar disorder and her mother's treatment history. The daughter was concerned about the discontinuation of olanzapine, due to her mother's past history of severe depression and serious suicide attempts. Mrs. F's valproate levels were 45. On reviewing Mrs. F's medications, the psychiatrist noted that she was taking hydrocodone as needed for pain three to four times daily. The psychiatrist recommended trying up to 4 grams/day of acetaminophen, restarting olanzapine 5 mg at bedtime, and using hydrocodone only if acetaminophen was not helping. Over the next four weeks, the as-needed hydrocodone use decreased to once a day, Mrs. F's lethargy cleared up, her depressed mood lifted, her appetite and sleep improved, and she started taking part in physical therapy.

TEACHING POINTS People whose bipolar disorder is well controlled with psychiatric drugs should keep taking these drugs as much as possible, because the symptoms of bipolar disorder (especially depression) are difficult to treat. The management of bipolar disorder is complex, and the clinician should consult a psychiatrist before changing any psychiatric medication.

Secondary Mania

Secondary mania is mania due to a general medical condition or to medications (Brooks and Hoblyn 2005). Manic symptoms can be caused by a variety of general medical conditions, such as neurological conditions affecting the inferomedial frontal lobes (e.g., infarcts, frontotemporal dementia, a brain tumor, a head injury), epilepsy, Huntington disease, multiple sclerosis, Cushing syndrome, neurosyphilis, and medication-induced effects (e.g., due to corticosteroids, stimulants). Older people with new-onset mania are more than twice as likely to have a comorbid neurological disorder, including silent cerebral infarcts (65 percent in new-onset versus 25 percent in chronic illness) (Fujikawa, Yamawaki, and Touhouda 1995). The clinician should consider that all residents who have a first episode of mania also have secondary mania, at least until proven otherwise. Residents with secondary mania require a comprehensive assessment (including a detailed neurological exam) and testing (blood and neuroimaging) to identify the cause. The treatment of secondary mania involves a treatment of its cause. Some residents with secondary mania (e.g., due to frontotemporal dementia) may need medications (e.g., atypical antipsychotics, valproate) to treat manic symptoms.

CLINICAL CASE Mr. L, a 62-year-old realtor, had been transferred to a nursing home after being treated in a hospital for severe pneumonia. In the hospital, he had been diagnosed with bipolar disorder and treated with haloperidol and lorazepam for his aggressive behavior there. Mr. L was having falls and being belligerent with the staff at the nursing home, so he was referred to the consulting psychiatrist for an urgent psychiatric evaluation. Mr. L had been experiencing mood swings and aggressive verbal and physical behaviors that had progressively worsened over one-and-a-half to two years. Mr. L had also been irritable, and over the past year he had engaged in several failed schemes to make money by buying and selling real estate in impoverished areas. Mr. L had assaulted his friend at his friend's home and then had decided to walk for two miles in bitter cold to go home. As a result, he developed pneumonia. He refused antibiotics and had to be hospitalized for high-grade fever, severe cough, and fatigue. Mr. L also had a history of making lewd comments during social situations and becoming verbally abusive toward the people he was working with. Mr. L had been a congenial and easygoing person all his life and had no past history of psychiatric problems. He had a brother who was diagnosed at age 59 with frontotemporal dementia. On a mental status examination, Mr. L reported feeling "fine" and believed that his friend "deserved" to be hit because the friend had declined Mr. L's offer to make money for his friend by buying some real estate on the friend's behalf. Mr. L's MMSE score was 28. On a neurological exam, Mr. L had mild extrapyramidal signs (tremors, stiffness, and hypokinesia).

After a thorough assessment, including neuropsychological testing that showed significant executive dysfunction and an MRI brain scan that revealed moderate asymmetric atrophy of both the frontal lobes and the insula, a diagnosis of frontotemporal dementia with secondary mania was made. Mr. L was prescribed valproate and quetiapine, haloperidol was discontinued, and lorazepam was switched from scheduled dosing to as-needed dosing. Over the next four weeks, Mr. L became much less aggressive and more manageable by the staff.

TEACHING POINTS The clinician should consider a change in personality in a middle-aged person with mood symptoms as a secondary mood disorder until proven otherwise. The long duration of manic symptoms and a family history of frontotemporal dementia in this resident's brother strongly suggested secondary mania rather than bipolar disorder. For patients with secondary mania (as for all older adults), the clinician should avoid prescribing haloperidol to treat manic symptoms, due to the higher risk of EPS (which probably led to Mr. L's falls). The clinician should also avoid prescribing lithium for patients with secondary mania, due to the higher risk of lithium-induced adverse effects (especially delirium). Valproate and/or atypical antipsychotics with a low risk of EPS (e.g., quetiapine, aripiprazole) are the drugs of choice to treat manic symptoms in residents with secondary mania.

Pseudobulbar Affect

Pseudobulbar affect is a dramatic disorder of emotional expression and regulation characterized by a syndrome of uncontrollable laughter or crying that is unrelated or out of proportion to the eliciting stimulus (H. Rosen and Cummings 2007). Pseudobulbar affect is also known as *involuntary emotional expression disorder, pathological laughing or crying,* and *emotional incontinence.* Pseudobulbar affect may relate to the release of the brain stem's emotional control centers from regulation by the frontal lobes. LTC residents with pseudobulbar affect tend to become emotional over trivial matters and usually cannot understand or explain these episodes. Typically, pseudobulbar affect is not associated with an underlying depressed or happy mood and is not amenable to voluntary control. Alzheimer disease is the most common cause of pseudobulbar affect in LTC residents. Other common causes include strokes, Parkinson disease, traumatic brain injuries, amyotrophic lateral sclerosis, and multiple sclerosis.

Pseudobulbar affect can lead to significant stress or embarrassment for the resident and the family and, in severe cases, it can be disruptive to the milieu. Pseudobulbar affect can also lead to social isolation, the obstruction of normal relationships with family and friends, and, rarely, choking if it occurs when the resident is eating or drinking. In most cases, education of the resident and of the family and staff caring for the resident, as well as other psychosocial-environmental interventions (distraction, reassurance, activities), are sufficient for treatment. Although the FDA has not approved any antidepressants for the treatment of pseudobulbar affect, in moderate to severe cases the clinician may consider prescribing a trial of an antidepressant (e.g., SSRIs or tricyclic antidepressants). For residents with amyotrophic lateral sclerosis or multiple sclerosis with pseudobulbar affect, the clinician may consider prescribing a combination of dextromethorphan and quinidine (H. Rosen and Cummings 2007). The most common side effects of dextromethorphan and quinidine include dizziness and nausea, and the clinician should also consider potential drug interactions with quinidine (especially with memantine, as both are NMDA receptor antagonists).

Conclusion

Mood disorders, especially depression and apathy, are prevalent in long-term care populations. We recommend periodic screenings for depression for all residents, and in particular recently admitted residents, to increase the identification of depression in LTC populations. We also recommend a screening for suicide for all new residents, as suicide and self-harmful behaviors are more prevalent in LTC than previously thought. Mania, although uncommon in LTC populations, is associated with high morbidity and mortality. Residents with depression that is not responding to treatment and residents who have made suicide attempts and/or have persistent suicidal ideation, psychotic depression, or mania are best managed by a mental health clinician (psychiatrist, psychiatric nurse practitioner, psychiatric physician assistant) with expertise in geriatrics. Comprehensive assessment and aggressive treatment strategies for all mood disorders and suicidality can dramatically improve the quality of life, and may even be life saving, for all residents with mood disorders.

CHAPTER 6

Psychotic Disorders

Psychotic disorders are serious psychiatric conditions because of their clinical significance and social impact. Delusions and hallucinations are the hallmarks of psychotic disorders, although catatonic and bizarre behaviors may also be evidence of impaired reality testing. Delusions are false, unshakeable beliefs that are not in keeping with the person's cultural beliefs. Hallucinations are perceptions (in any sensory modality) in the absence of any stimuli. In older adults who experience hallucinations, visual hallucinations are the most common, followed by auditory hallucinations, and then by others (gustatory, tactile, and olfactory). A lack of insight, emotional suffering, and impairment in daily functioning are required for symptoms such as hallucinations and delusions to be considered part of a clinically significant psychotic disorder.

Elderly people have a higher incidence of psychotic disorders than younger adults. The prevalence of psychotic disorders in elderly people ranges from 0.2 to 5.7 percent in community-based samples to 10 percent in a nursing home population (Grossberg and Desai 2003a). Among community-dwelling elderly people who do not have dementia, the lifetime prevalence of psychotic symptoms may be even higher, up to 10% (Ostling and Skoog 2002). The prevalence of psychotic symptoms in people with dementia ranges from 50 percent for those with Alzheimer disease to 80 percent for those with dementia with Lewy bodies. Late-onset psychoses account for about 10 percent of the psychiatric admissions for older adults (Webster and Grossberg 1998). Thus as the population ages, the absolute number of elderly individuals who develop psychotic symptoms will rise dramatically. Risk factors for psychotic symptoms in elderly people include cognitive impairments, sensory deficits (e.g., hearing deficits), female gender, social isolation, certain premorbid personality traits (e.g., cold and querulous, schizotypal, paranoid), bedridden conditions, polypharmacy, and substance abuse (Grossberg and Manepalli 1995; Ostling and Skoog 2002). Most of these risk factors are more prevalent in long-term care populations than in community-dwelling elderly people.

Psychotic symptoms in LTC populations are common and independently predict functional decline. Psychotic symptoms due to delirium and dementia are the two most common categories of psychotic disorders in LTC populations. In people with dementia, psychotic symptoms are associated with a greater risk of admission to a facility and with mortality. Screening for and appropriately managing delusions and hallucinations in LTC residents may substantially improve their quality of life and functional status.

Assessment of Psychotic Symptoms in Long-Term Care Populations

Psychotic disorders in LTC populations are predominantly due to toxic (e.g., drugs), metabolic (e.g., thyroid dysfunction), infective (e.g., UTI), vascular (e.g., stroke), or neurodegenerative (e.g., AD, DLB) etiological factors. The primary goal of an assessment is to identify one or more of these factors. A comprehensive assessment of psychotic symptoms in LTC populations includes a thorough history, a detailed mental status examination, pertinent physical and neurological examinations, and laboratory tests (e.g., blood, urine, EKG, neuroimaging) as necessary. The clinician should assess residents who show verbal or physical aggression for the presence of psychotic symptoms (Leonard et al. 2006). In some cultures, visual or auditory hallucinations with a religious content may be a normal part of a religious experience (e.g., seeing the Virgin Mary, hearing God's voice). Language barriers, sensory impairment, and cultural issues may impede an accurate diagnosis of psychotic symptoms, especially for residents with dementia. We recommend using interpreters and soliciting input from the family to clarify cultural issues. Residents who confabulate (typically individuals with Korsakoff syndrome, due to a thiamine deficiency, but also occasionally those with dementia) and residents who have incoherent speech (e.g., residents with Wernicke aphasia [receptive aphasia]) may be mistakenly diagnosed as having a psychotic disorder. Careful assessment of a person's language and memory during the mental status examination will usually identify these patients. We recommend assessing hearing and vision for all residents with psychotic symptoms.

Differential Diagnosis

Table 6.1 lists common causes of psychotic disorders in LTC populations (Grossberg and Desai 2003a; Khouzam and Emes 2007).

Primary Psychotic Disorders

Primary psychotic disorders include affective psychoses (psychotic symptoms associated with depression or mania), schizophrenia, schizoaffective disorder, delusional disorder, and brief psychotic disorder. These are serious disorders associated with high morbidity, a risk of suicide, and increased mortality (due to suicide or another cause). Approximately 2 percent of the population over age 54—about 1 million people—have severe mental illnesses (including schizophrenia, bipolar disorder, schizoaffective disorder) (Grossberg and Desai 2003a). Older persons with schizophrenia make up the majority of these patients, and the number and proportion of older adults with schizophrenia are expected to double in the next three decades. As the availability of beds in psychiatric hospitals declines, increasing numbers of persons with severe mental illnesses are housed in nursing homes (Mechanic and McAlpine 2000). In response to this trend, the Omnibus Budget Reconciliation Act of 1987 (OBRA-87) was passed. It was intended to improve nursing home care for persons with mental illnesses and to prevent inappropriate admissions.

TABLE 6.1
Common psychotic disorders in the long-term care population

Primary psychotic disorders
    Affective psychoses (major depression with psychotic symptoms, bipolar disorder with psychotic symptoms)
    Schizophrenia
    Schizoaffective disorder: unipolar type, bipolar type
    Brief psychotic disorder
    Delusional disorder
    Hallucinations during grief
Secondary psychotic disorders
    Dementia with psychotic symptoms
    Delirium with psychotic symptoms
    Medication-induced psychotic symptoms
    Psychosis associated with Parkinson disease
    General medical conditions causing psychotic symptoms
    Street drugs and/or alcohol-use-related psychotic symptoms
Mixed psychotic disorders
    Dementia with psychotic symptoms and delirium with psychotic symptoms
    Schizophrenia and medical conditions causing psychotic symptoms
    Other combinations of primary psychotic disorders and secondary psychotic disorders or two
        secondary psychotic disorders

OBRA-87 mandated preadmission screening (to ensure that only persons in need of nursing care were admitted) and annual reviews of residents to screen them for mental health problems and service needs.

Primary psychotic disorders are best managed by a mental health team. Such a team would consist of the resident, the family, a social worker, a certified nursing assistant familiar with the resident, a licensed practical nurse or a registered nurse, and a geriatric psychiatrist (or other mental health provider with expertise in geriatrics). Residents with these disorders who are experiencing severe symptoms may need prompt hospitalization in an inpatient psychiatric unit (preferably a geriatric psychiatry unit) to prevent complications such as suicide, physical aggression and/or agitation leading to serious injury to oneself or to others, and severe malnutrition. We strongly recommend that a member of the team review the resident's previous psychiatric records (especially regarding hospitalization, suicide attempts, a history of aggression and violence, and responses to previous treatment interventions). We also recommend periodic education of the family and staff regarding primary psychotic disorders. Doses of antipsychotic medications used to treat primary psychotic disorders may need to be higher than those used to treat secondary psychotic disorders (e.g., severe psychotic symptoms associated with dementia).

Affective Psychoses

People with affective psychoses typically experience psychotic symptoms along with significant mood symptoms (most commonly depression, but also mania). Psychotic symptoms do not occur in the absence of mood symptoms, and the family history of those with affective psychoses is often positive for mood disorders. There may be a past history of an affective episode (depression, mania) with or without psychotic symptoms. Catatonic symptoms may develop in residents with bipolar disorder or recurrent major depression. Depression with psychotic features is more common in people whose first major depressive episode occurs later in life than in those who had early episodes. The delusions accompanying depressive episodes may include a hopeless content, themes of persecution, guilt, and punishment, and somatic delusions. For example, an individual might believe that he or she has an incurable illness or deserves punishment for "unforgivable sins," or that impending catastrophes will affect loved ones. Delusions associated with affective disorders can be distinguished from those associated with dementia in that the latter are less systematized and less congruent with affective disturbance. People who are psychotically depressed often have more pronounced agitation or retardation. The presence of delusions appears to run true through repeated episodes.

Older individuals with mania are rarely euphoric and more commonly present with irritability, paranoia, or mild confusion. Similar to middle-aged and younger adults, LTC residents who develop mania may also have delusions of possessing great wealth, exceptional talents, and supernatural powers. Affective psychoses are often undertreated, resulting in significant morbidity and increased mortality. The clinician should consider ECT as one of the first-line treatment options for affective psychoses, especially when one does not have the luxury of time for medications to work (e.g., a patient who is suicidal or has stopped eating). The treatment of major depression with psychotic symptoms (a single episode or recurrent ones) is usually with a combination of antidepressants and atypical antipsychotics. The treatment of bipolar disorder (a depressed, manic, or mixed episode) with psychotic symptoms is best managed by atypical antipsychotics alone or in combination with mood stabilizers (e.g., valproate). The clinician may consider psychosocial interventions (e.g., psychotherapy, family education, social rhythm therapy) for cognitively intact residents with affective psychoses.

CLINICAL CASE Mr. T, a 78-year-old divorced male, had been reporting fears of being put in jail because he has been living "illegally" in the nursing home. He had also been having impaired sleep and a loss of appetite, the latter resulting in a 15-pound weight loss over the previous three months (from 189 to 174 pounds, height 5' 8"), and he had been refusing to shave, change clothes, or bathe for the previous three weeks. He was referred to the psychiatrist because in the last week he had been stating that he would be better off dead. The psychiatrist noted that Mr. T had a history of mini-strokes in the past. Six months previously, he developed severe abdominal pain, requiring gallbladder surgery, and was admitted to the nursing home for rehabilitation. After completing rehabilitation, he was transferred to the LTC wing for a continued stay, as there was no one to take care of him at home. He also had a history of recurrent falls, cognitive impairment, and noncompliance with medications, and he required close monitoring for his unstable diabetes. His family reported that Mr. T had been disappointed when he was told he could not return home and had since become withdrawn, stopped smiling, and even stopped watching sports on television (one of his favorite activities in the past).

During the interview, Mr. T reported feeling nervous and explained that his reason for not shaving or bathing was his fear that his skin would somehow "infect" his roommate. He felt that he could not ask for a room change because he was there "illegally." Mr. T further explained that he had no money to pay for the high cost of the nursing home. (He had apparently seen the monthly charge for his nursing home stay, which was approximately $6,000.) Mr. T had a history of severe depression 15 years previously, when he had retired, but his daughters did not know the details and Mr. T could not give provide any, except to confirm that he was put on some "nerve pills." There was no obvious history of a prior manic or hypomanic episode. Mr. T had a family history of depression (sister) and suicide (brother). A medication review did not identify any medications that could cause or exacerbate Mr. T's psychiatric symptoms, and laboratory tests (including thyroid tests and vitamin levels) were unremarkable. On a mental status examination, Mr. T exhibited a depressed mood and affect, delusions of persecution, and passive suicidal ideas (he felt life was not worth living), but he denied any specific suicidal intentions or plans. His recall was one out of three, his MMSE score was 16, and his GDS score was 20/30.

Mr. T was diagnosed with recurrent major depression with psychotic features and probable vascular dementia. The psychiatrist recommended hospitalization, but Mr. T declined. There were insufficient grounds for involuntary commitment, as he had agreed to treatment at the nursing home. The psychiatrist then offered Mr. T a choice, recommending hospitalization and ECT as a first option, hospitalization and medications as a second option, and treatment at the facility with psychotropic medications as the third option. Mr. T opted to try psychotropic medications. He started taking sertraline 25 mg daily, and the dose was gradually increased every four days by 25 mg, up to 100 mg daily. He started taking risperidone 0.25 mg at bedtime, and it was increased to 0.5 mg at bedtime after one week. After four weeks, the family and staff reported that his appetite and sleep had improved, but that he was still refusing to shave or to come out of his room.

During a subsequent interview, Mr. T continued to express delusional thinking and had a depressed affect. Risperidone was further increased to 0.25 mg daily in the morning and 0.5 mg at bedtime for seven days, and then to 0.5 mg daily in the morning and 0.5 mg daily at bedtime. After four more weeks, Mr. T reported that he was feeling better; he started showing an interest in watching sports on television again and allowed the staff to shave him and help him bathe. After four more weeks, he was shaving and bathing regularly and did not voice any of the fears he had before. Mr. T still expressed sadness at not being able to go home and hoped that the psychiatrist would help him return home. Mr. T's repeat GDS score was 8/30 and his repeat MMSE score was 21.

TEACHING POINTS During the management of any severe psychotic disorder, the first consideration is the safety of the patient and his or her need for hospitalization in an inpatient psychiatric unit. ECT is the first-line treatment for psychotic depression, although psychotic depression may respond to a combination of antidepressants and atypical antipsychotics. The full therapeutic effects of medications may take 12 or more weeks. Although risperidone has been associated with a slightly increased risk of strokes in people with dementia, the benefits of treating a potentially fatal illness, such as psychotic depression, usually outweigh this risk. The use of other SSRIs (such as citalopram or escitalopram) in place of sertraline, and other atypical antipsychotics (such as aripiprazole, quetiapine, or olanzapine in place of risperidone) may also have been appropriate.

Schizophrenia

Schizophrenia is a chronic psychotic disorder that usually starts in one's late teens or in young adulthood, although approximately 15 percent have an onset after age 40 (termed *late-onset schizophrenia* for an onset between 40 and 60 years old and *very late-onset schizophrenia* for an onset after age 60). The number of persons aged 55 or older who have a diagnosis of schizophrenia is projected to double (from 500,000 to 1 million) over the next 20 years (C. Cohen et al. 2008). Four subtypes have been described: paranoid, disorganized (also called *hebephrenic*), catatonic, and undifferentiated. There is remarkable heterogeneity among people with schizophrenia in their symptom presentations, everyday functioning, responses to treatment, and the course of the illness.

Delusions and hallucinations are the hallmarks of schizophrenia and occur in the absence of affective symptoms, although up to 40 percent of older adults with schizophrenia develop major depression. Depressive symptoms are associated with worse functioning in older people with schizophrenia. The presence of bizarre delusions (e.g., that a stranger has removed one's organs and replaced them with someone else's organs), persistent auditory hallucinations (e.g., hearing voices of people commenting on one's actions, or voices telling one what to do), an inappropriate affect, and negative symptoms (e.g., apathy, inattention) help differentiate schizophrenia from other psychotic disorders. Delusions are well systematized and complex in people with schizophrenia. People with late-onset schizophrenia have a higher prevalence of the paranoid subtype, have less severe negative symptoms, are more likely to be women (versus the greater number of men among those with earlier-onset schizophrenia), and require lower doses of antipsychotic medications than people with earlier-onset schizophrenia. Some residents with schizophrenia may have comorbid dementia. We recommend close monitoring for suicide risk. Aging is associated with a complete remission of social deficits in more than 25 percent of those with early-onset schizophrenia (onset before age 40), while another 40 percent show a marked improvement in their symptoms, especially positive symptoms. For some individuals with schizophrenia, negative symptoms may increase with age.

Approximately 13 percent of older persons with schizophrenia are in nursing homes (C. Cohen et al. 2008). Nursing home residents with a diagnosis of schizophrenia are more likely than other residents to be younger and nonwhite (especially African American) (Cano et al. 1997; McAlpine 2003). In addition, they have resided in nursing homes for longer periods (often more than five years and even up to 10 years for some). They report significantly lower levels of disability, as measured by problems in ADLs (McAlpine 2003). Most of the LTC residents with schizophrenia receive Medicaid and live in state-owned facilities, yet almost half of the nursing home residents with schizophrenia receive inadequate mental health services. As the population aged 65 or older increases in the coming decades, meeting the needs of persons with schizophrenia in LTC settings will be even more difficult.

The treatment of schizophrenia involves the use of atypical antipsychotic drugs and psychosocial interventions (e.g., supportive psychotherapy, education of family and staff). The clinician may consider prescribing the short-term use of benzodiazepines for residents with schizophrenia who are experiencing severe anxiety, agitation, insomnia, or catatonic symptoms. ECT is a reasonable choice for catatonic symptoms of schizophrenia and the severe depressive symptoms associated with suicidal behavior. Many residents with schizophrenia may have been taking high doses of conventional antipsychotic drugs for decades. These residents may benefit from a gradual reduction (over months) in their antipsychotic medication, with close monitoring for emergent tardive dyskinesia. If a resident with schizophrenia who has been taking conventional antipsychotics for most of his or her life is showing significant EPS (parkinsonism, drooling, recurrent falls due to hypokinesia), the clinician may consider switching medications. Some clinicians recommend that residents who are stable taking low doses of conventional antipsychotics and are tolerating the medication well should not be switched to atypical antipsychotics, but instead be closely monitored for tardive dyskinesia. Many residents with schizophrenia have mild to moderate tardive dyskinesia, so the clinician should cautiously consider reducing the dose of antipsychotics for these patients, due to the high risk of worsening their tardive dyskinesia, which in turn may adversely affect their quality of life. A small but significant group of people with schizophrenia show a reduction in or clearing of delusions and hallucinations in later life, and they may remain stable without antipsychotic medications.

Schizoaffective Disorder

With schizoaffective disorder, the criteria for a major depressive episode or a manic episode occur at the same time as symptoms that meet the diagnosis of an active phase of schizophrenia. The psychotic symptoms must be present for at least two weeks in the absence of prominent mood symptoms. We recommend close monitoring for suicide risk. The prognosis is intermediate between schizophrenia and bipolar disorder. The treatment of schizoaffective disorder involves pharmacological interventions (e.g., atypical antipsychotics, antidepressants, mood stabilizers [e.g., valproate, lamotrigine]) and psychosocial interventions (e.g., supportive psychotherapy, education of the family and staff). The clinician may consider prescribing the short-term use of benzodiazepines to treat severe anxiety symptoms, agitation, insomnia, or catatonic symptoms. We recommend ECT for the treatment of severe affective symptoms, especially if the resident poses an imminent danger to him- or herself or to others, or if the symptoms are refractory to medications.

> **CLINICAL CASE** Ms. S was a 69-year-old single woman living in a nursing home for the last two years due to sequelae of severe arthritis, obesity, congestive heart failure, chronic kidney disease, chronic pain, diabetes requiring insulin, poor mobility, and osteoporosis. She had a long history of schizoaffective disorder with multiple past hospitalizations for serious suicide attempts, had severe psychotic symptoms (paranoid delusions and auditory hallucinations), but was stable for the last seven years

on a medication regimen that included olanzapine 10 mg at bedtime, mirtazapine 30 mg at bedtime, and lorazepam 0.25 mg four times daily. A psychiatrist was consulted regarding management of her increased agitation (yelling instead of using the call light, calling her roommate "the devil"), paranoia (accusing staff of stealing her clothes), and insomnia. Ms. S was cognitively intact (MMSE 28) and was able to give a detailed history of her psychiatric illness. She reported that the current medication regimen had, for the first time, helped her tremendously compared with all other medications she had been taking since she was in her 20s, and she had avoided hospitalization for the last seven years. The psychiatrist also noted that Ms. S had a history of recurrent UTI and had started taking antibiotics two days previously for another UTI. On a mental status examination, Ms. S was found to be anxious and eager to please. She denied any suicidal or homicidal ideas and any current auditory or visual hallucinations. She acknowledged that she had called her roommate "the devil" but reported that she was angry with the roommate because the roommate would have her television on until late in the night and Ms. S liked to go to sleep by 8 p.m. The staff acknowledged to the psychiatrist that this was an ongoing conflict between Ms. S and her roommate. Ms. S denied feeling that the staff were taking her belongings, but she felt that certain staff members were "not nice" to her.

The psychiatrist made a provisional diagnosis of schizoaffective disorder but thought that Ms. S's psychotic symptoms were not severe and hence did not recommend any change in her antipsychotic dosage. The psychiatrist recommended that the nursing home's social worker address the conflicts between Ms. S and her roommate. The consulting psychiatrist also requested records from previous psychiatrists. He recommended adding lorazepam 0.25 mg twice a day as needed for anxiety and seeing if treatment of Ms. S's UTI would also improve her agitation and paranoia. The social worker, over the course of three meetings with Ms. S and her roommate, brokered an agreement that Ms. S's roommate could watch television until 9 p.m. and then could go to a family room that had a television if she wanted to continue.

After four weeks, the staff reported that Ms. S's agitation was much better. Ms. S also reported feeling less anxious and irritable. She was given as-needed lorazepam once almost daily in addition to her scheduled dose for the first week, but after that the staff were able to manage her anxiety without requiring any as-needed lorazepam. The psychiatrist considered switching olanzapine to another atypical antipsychotic with a lower risk of metabolic complications (e.g., weight gain, risk of hyperglycemia and hyperlipidemia), such as aripiprazole or ziprasidone, and discussed this with Ms. S. Previous psychiatric records indicated that Ms. S had tried risperidone, quetiapine, haloperidol, thiothixene, sertraline, fluoxetine, and venlafaxine without an adequate response. Previous records also confirmed that she had made several serious suicide attempts (primarily by overdose) in the past, requiring repeated hospitalizations, and had severe psychotic symptoms that had incapacitated her for several years. Ms. S was nervous about any change in her medications and expressed awareness of the metabolic risks with olanzapine and mirtazapine. The psychiatrist agreed that the risks of switching from olanzapine or mirtazapine (destabilizing the psychiatric illness, a relapse of severe depressive and psychotic symptoms, a need for hospitalization, and suicide) outweighed the benefits (lower risk of weight gain, better control of diabetes and hyperlipidemia, improved mobility).

TEACHING POINTS Residents with a severe persistent mental illness (e.g., schizoaffective disorder) are as likely to become agitated due to medical issues and/or environmental causes as residents who do not have such illnesses. The clinician should consider these factors before assuming that an exacerbation of the underlying psychiatric illness is the cause of increased psychiatric symptoms. If the resident has been stable on a psychiatric drug regimen, it would be advisable to avoid any major changes in this regimen, because obtaining a similar good therapeutic response from a different drug regimen is not predictable. The clinician should decide to switch antipsychotics or antidepressants only after thoroughly reviewing the patient's history and feelings (and those of his or her involved family) about the changes. Although drugs like olanzapine and mirtazapine carry substantial metabolic risks (especially for people who are obese), for some people (e.g., Ms. S), these risks may not outweigh the benefits of stabilization of a serious psychiatric illness.

Delusional Disorder

Delusional disorder is characterized by nonbizarre delusions involving situations that could occur in real life (e.g., being poisoned, infected, followed or loved at a distance, deceived by a spouse or lover, or having a disease). The delusions are usually not associated with prominent auditory or visual hallucinations. Residents with delusional disorder may become aggressive toward their supposed persecutors; some may lock themselves in their rooms and live a reclusive life. These delusions often have been present for many years or even decades. The clinician can consider prescribing antipsychotic medications and supportive psychotherapy for residents with this disorder who develop significant agitation due to their delusional thinking, although delusional disorder does not respond as well to antipsychotics as do many other psychotic disorders.

Brief Psychotic Disorder

Brief psychotic disorder is characterized by a sudden onset of delusions and/ or hallucinations that develop within one month of a major stressor (e.g., the sudden death of a loved one, an unexpected loss of money or health, a newly diagnosed terminal illness). The treatment of brief psychotic disorder may involve the short-term use of atypical antipsychotics, benzodiazepines for the management of severe anxiety and insomnia, and psychosocial interventions (e.g., supportive psychotherapy, family and staff education). An eventual full return to premorbid social and interpersonal level of functioning occurs when the stressors subside and the resident's coping skills are restored.

Hallucinations During Bereavement

Hallucinations may occur during bereavement in people with intact cognition, and they typically are visual in nature; however, both auditory and tactile hallucinations have been described in people who recently lost a spouse. The widow/widower reports seeing, speaking to, or even touching the deceased spouse. The majority of these experiences occur at night. The widow/widower acknowledges that the spouse looks different or "ghostlike"; additionally, she or he does not believe the deceased spouse is present. In most cases, the widow/widower describes the hallucinatory event as a positive experience. Treatment involves psychosocial interventions (e.g., emotional support, reassurance, and education of the family and staff).

Secondary Psychotic Disorders

Secondary psychotic disorders are characterized by the presence of psychotic symptoms due to a general medical or neurological condition or to medications. Most LTC residents with psychotic symptoms have secondary psychotic disorders. Visual hallucinations in the absence of auditory hallucinations are suggestive of secondary psychotic disorders rather than schizophrenia. Psychotic symptoms due to an acute general medical or neurological condition typically occur in the context of delirium, although sometimes psychotic symptoms may be the only manifestation of a general medical condition. Failure to identify secondary psychotic disorders may result in the inappropriate administration of antipsychotics, which may further obscure underlying medical conditions causing the psychotic symptoms. Secondary psychotic disorders may be part of the clinical manifestation of life-threatening medical conditions and thus, if not recognized and treated promptly, can be fatal.

Although the treatment of primary psychotic disorders usually requires atypical antipsychotics, the treatment of secondary psychotic disorders can often be managed with psychosocial interventions and either treatment of the underlying medical condition or removal of the offending medication. The use of atypical antipsychotics to manage psychotic symptoms due to secondary psychotic disorders is associated with a high risk of adverse effects, so the clinician should prescribe them cautiously, preferably with input from a geriatric psychiatrist. People with secondary psychotic disorders are at higher risk of serious adverse effects (e.g., EPS and tardive dyskinesia) from conventional antipsychotics than are those with primary psychotic disorders. Many secondary psychotic disorders are iatrogenic (e.g., caused by a failure to recognize the correct diagnosis or by the administration of inappropriate medications, such as anticholinergics), especially for people with dementia. Appropriate therapeutic choices may decrease the incidence of psychotic symptoms in LTC populations.

Dementia with Psychotic Symptoms

Psychotic symptoms are one of the most serious complications of dementia. The presence of visual hallucinations, more concrete or perseverative thought processes, a gradual cognitive impairment before the onset of the psychotic symptoms, and the absence of a long psychiatric history suggest psychotic disorder due to one of the dementias. Psychotic symptoms are common in people with Alzheimer disease, especially in its moderate and severe stages. More than 50 percent of the people with AD have some form of psychosis at some point during the course of the illness (Paulsen et al. 2000). Delusions are much more common (33% point prevalence) than hallucinations (7% point prevalence) (Chen et al. 1991; Deutsch et al. 1991; Mizrahi et al. 2006). Most residents who have hallucinations associated with AD also have delusions. Anosognosia (a lack of awareness of one's cognitive impairment) and depression often accompany delusions in AD (Mizrahi et al. 2006). An elevated mood often coexists with expansive delusions in AD. Aggression and agitation are the most common behavioral concomitants of psychosis in AD. Residents with AD and spontaneous EPS have twice the frequency of psychosis as residents with AD but no EPS. Residents with AD who have a sibling with AD and psychosis may be twice as likely to develop psychotic symptoms (Sweet et al. 2002).

Vascular dementia may be associated with paranoid psychotic features, with a prevalence ranging from 9 to 40 percent. Complex delusions are more likely in VaD than in AD. Vivid recurrent visual hallucinations are the characteristic features of dementia with Lewy bodies and are seen in up to 75 percent of the people with DLB. Visual hallucinations occur early in the course of DLB, whereas they typically occur in the moderate to severe stages of AD. Other types of hallucinations, as well as systematized delusions, are supportive features for a diagnosis of DLB (McKeith et al. 2005). More than 50 percent of the people with DLB have delusions. These delusions are of persecution and theft, television characters in the room, spousal infidelity, and delusional misidentification (i.e., Capgras syndrome). Psychotic symptoms are rare in frontotemporal dementia (Mendez et al. 2008). This may be due to a limited temporal-limbic involvement in this disorder. When psychotic symptoms are present in FTD, they usually take the form of delusions. Paranoid, bizarre, and grandiose delusions may be seen in people with FTD. Visual hallucinations in a person with dementia may be indicative of a co-occurring delirium. The psychotic symptoms associated with dementia wax and wane and are less persistent than those linked with schizophrenia. A significant number of residents with dementia develop transient psychotic symptoms that may remit spontaneously over time or with cholinesterase inhibitor therapy.

The most common delusions are of people stealing from, breaking into the room of, or having intentions to persecute the resident, or of the resident's food being poisoned. Often the delusional ideas in dementia have an ad hoc quality: a purse is misplaced, and the delusion arises that someone is stealing the resident's personal items. Delusions consisting largely of misconceptions or misidentifications are common. A mistaken suspicion of marital infidelity, the belief that other residents or caregivers are trying to hurt the resident, and the belief that characters on television are real are also common. Delusions of misidentification (Capgras syndrome) may be seen in people with dementia, especially DLB (Josephs 2007). This syndrome is characterized by the belief that other people, usually ones closely related to the resident, have been replaced by exact replicas or doubles who impersonate the original persons but are imposters (e.g., a wife would say, "He is not my husband, although he looks like my husband"). The presence of Capgras syndrome with visual hallucinations may indicate DLB rather than AD. As cognitive impairment increases, the complexity of the delusions is reduced. Many people with dementia experience visual agnosia, in which they do not recognize a person or believe that the person is someone else (e.g., a spouse is identified as a father, a daughter is identified as a sister).

Hallucinations are also found in residents with dementia. Visual hallucinations are the most common, followed by auditory hallucinations. Typical visual hallucinations include persons from the past (e.g., deceased parents), intruders, animals, complex scenes, or inanimate objects. Most of the auditory hallucinations seen in people with dementia tend to be simple (e.g., hearing dead spouses and other relatives) rather than persecutory ones, although the latter sometimes occur. A resident with advanced dementia may not be able to verbalize the hallucinations but may show hallucinatory behavior (e.g., reaching out to touch or grab imaginary people, objects, bugs). Agitation and aggression (verbal and physical) frequently co-occur with psychotic symptoms in residents with dementia. Psychosis is often a trigger for agitation and aggressivity, which may, in turn, be a response to frightening visual hallucinations. Depressive symptoms also frequently co-occur with delusions in residents with dementia.

The treatment of psychotic symptoms in residents with dementia includes a careful evaluation and treatment of their general medical condition (e.g., a UTI, an offending medication) and of environmental or psychosocial problems that may be precipitating or causing psychotic symptoms. Psychotic symptoms are often transient. If such symptoms persist, we recommend psychosocial-environmental interventions. If the resident is an imminent danger to him- or herself or to others, we recommend hospitalization in an acute inpatient psychiatric unit (preferably a geriatric psychiatry unit). Antidementia drugs (ChEIs) do not help acute psychotic symptoms, but the clinician may consider prescribing them to treat mild to moderate psychotic symptoms, particularly for residents with DLB but also for residents with AD or PDD. Antidepressants (e.g., citalopram) are also a good treatment option for the agitation and anxiety associated with psychotic symptoms in residents with AD, especially if depressive symptoms are also present.

For residents with dementia, the clinician may consider prescribing antipsychotics to treat the psychotic symptoms that cause severe emotional distress and are not responding to psychosocial-environmental interventions, or if the psychotic symptoms pose a high safety risk for the resident or others.

Deciding which antipsychotic to use is based on the relationship between the adverse effects profile of the various agents and the characteristics of the individual resident. While atypical antipsychotics carry a black box warning about a risk of death in elderly people with dementia, the typical or conventional antipsychotics carry an even higher risk of death and adverse effects (Broadway and Mintzer 2007). Hence we prefer atypical antipsychotics over conventional ones for residents with dementia. Besides a small increased risk of mortality, all antipsychotics carry a small increased risk of stroke. One of the suggestive features for a diagnosis of DLB is sensitivity to antipsychotic medication (both conventional and atypical agents). People with dementia (especially DLB and PDD, but also AD and FTD) may develop sedation, immobility, rigidity, postural instability, falls, and increased confusion, due to the antidopaminergic and anticholinergic properties of antipsychotics. If residents with any of the severe psychotic symptoms associated with DLB need antipsychotic medications, either aripiprazole or quetiapine is the drug of first choice. All antipsychotics should be started at low dosages, preferably given at night, and at the lowest possible effective doses. The goal is not to resolve psychotic symptoms, but to reduce the resident's distress and agitation and reduce behavior that is dangerous to the resident or to others (table 6.2). The clinician must weigh the potential benefits and risks of antipsychotics and discuss them with the resident and the family. Treatment-emergent sedation and constipation are associated with all antipsychotics. To minimize the risk of daytime sedation and falls, the clinician should discourage the concomitant use of benzodiazepines and antipsychotics or limit it to short periods with careful observation.

For a resident who has psychotic symptoms and dementia but is stable, it is prudent to attempt to taper off and then discontinue the antipsychotic after two to eight months. For residents who have problems with compliance or swallowing pills, the clinician may consider the use of liquid preparations (e.g., liquid risperidone) or orally dissolvable preparations of atypical antipsychotics (available for risperidone, olanzapine, and aripiprazole). Most atypical antipsychotics can be given as once-a-day dosing, but quetiapine has a short half-life and may need to be given twice or three times a day (unless one is using the newly available long-acting quetiapine formulation). The clinician may consider using behavioral observation scales, such as the CMAI or the NPI-NH, to monitor the resident's response to treatment (Cohen-Mansfield 1986). We recommend periodic monitoring (e.g., every three to six months)

TABLE 6.2
Potential benefits and risks in the use of antipsychotic medication to treat severe psychotic symptoms for residents with dementia

Potential benefits
Prevent serious injury to oneself (e.g., falls and hip fractures due to severe agitation)
Prevent serious injury to others (e.g., pushing another frail resident, with a subsequent fall and hip fracture or a head injury sustained by that resident)
Prevent hospitalization by reducing agitation and aggressive behavior
Prevent suicide or mortality due to other self-harmful behaviors (e.g., going out of the facility in cold weather in response to psychotic symptoms, refusing life-sustaining medications, refusing to eat)
Prevent fatal injury to others
Decrease emotional distress and thus improve the resident's quality of life
Allow staff to better meet the resident's basic needs (bathing, personal hygiene) after a reduction in the agitation and aggression caused by psychotic symptoms
Decrease the caregivers' (family and professional) stresses and burdens

Risks
Death due to heart-related events and infection, particularly pneumonia (2% increased risk on average)
Cerebrovascular adverse events (e.g., stroke) (2% increased risk on average)
Falls and serious injury (e.g., hip or vertebral fracture, skin tear, head injury)
Neuroleptic malignant syndrome (rare)
Tardive dyskinesia (especially with conventional antipsychotics)
Daytime sedation (and its attendant risks, such as aspiration pneumonia)
Accelerated cognitive and/or functional decline
Akathisia
Parkinsonian symptoms
Postural hypotension
Hospitalization due to falls and/or a decline in physical health

using the Abnormal Involuntary Movement Scale (AIMS) for the development of tardive dyskinesia due to the use of antipsychotics.

⁝ **CLINICAL CASE** Ms. L, an 84-year-old widow with dementia, was admitted to an assisted living facility because of increasing problems with agitation, incontinence, lack of self-care, and wandering out of her home. She had been in the facility for more than six months. Her family had noticed that even when Ms. L was living in her home, she talked about children coming into her house and bringing cats and dogs. Over the last four months, Ms. L was having periods of agitation and anxiety over "little children" going through her belongings and saying "yack, yack, yack." She also complained of being upset with the staff because they would allow cats and dogs to roam freely into her room. Ms. L was referred to the psychiatrist for management of hallucinations.

An evaluation revealed that Ms. L was not taking any medications that could have caused hallucinations (e.g., dopaminergic drugs or anticholinergic drugs), nor was she exhibiting any physical aggression or depressive symptoms. Ms. L was taking memantine 10 mg twice daily and donepezil 10 mg daily, in addition to medications for hypertension (hydrochlorothiazide and atenolol) and hyperlipidemia (simvastatin). She did not complain of any new physical health problems, and her family and the staff stated that the episodes of agitation and hallucinations occurred once or twice a week. The staff reported that Ms. L did participate in activities, slept well, and had a good appetite. When the psychiatrist inquired how the staff and family dealt with Ms. L's complains, they reported that they would try to convince Ms. L that she was imagining things and that no children or animals were coming to her room. The staff and family also said that often this would agitate Ms. L even more. The psychiatrist also inquired about Ms. L's personality before her dementia, and her family said that Ms. L had been an active person all her life, liked to be busy, and was always "on the go." During the interview, Ms. L denied having any problems, denied being in any physical pain, reported feeling "fine," said "yes" to becoming bored and lonely, but reported good sleep and appetite. Her mental status examination showed significant short-term memory loss (recall was 0/3), and her MMSE score was 12.

The psychiatrist explained to the family and staff that visual hallucinations were a symptom of dementia, and that currently Ms. L's symptoms were best managed with psychosocial-environmental interventions. The psychiatrist recommended that the family and staff not correct or argue with Ms. L, but try to reassure her and then try to distract her. The psychiatrist, together with the family and staff, devised a daily activity schedule that would involve more activities in which the staff and family could engage Ms. L (e.g., reminiscence with old photos, listening to music that she liked, reading the Bible to her) and a short nap in the afternoon. Ms. L continued to have transient visual hallucinations, but her agitation during those periods gradually decreased and the staff became more adept at distracting Ms. L after an initial reassurance that they would "take care of" the problem promptly.

TEACHING POINTS Many residents with dementia (due to AD or other causes) often develop visual hallucinations and agitation, but these can be safely and effectively managed by family and staff education and psychosocial-environmental interventions. Pharmacological interventions (e.g., antipsychotic drugs) are not necessary in such situations, because the severity of the psychotic symptoms is not high and physical aggression is absent.

CLINICAL CASE Mrs. S was a 78-year-old woman with dementia who lived in an assisted living facility. Over several months, she had been expressing concerns that men were in her "home" and were telling her to do inappropriate acts, such as taking down her pants. Mrs. S would start yelling from 3 p.m. onward, stating that she could see "the man" in the trees looking into her room. She was not sleeping well and she used foul language toward the staff during personal care. In the last four weeks, Mrs. S had become physically aggressive toward the staff (hitting, slapping, kicking, and biting). Psychosocial-environmental interventions had initially been successful, but in the last four weeks her behavior was not manageable. She was referred to the consulting psychiatrist.

On examination, the psychiatrist found that Mrs. S had mild muscle stiffness, an unsteady gait, a restricted affect, and persecutory delusions. A review of her medications did not identify any of them as having a potential etiology. She was taking rivastigmine 3 mg twice daily with meals. She had a history of not tolerating a higher dose of rivastigmine, and she could not tolerate memantine. Laboratory tests (electrolytes, renal function, TSH, vitamin B_{12} levels) were within normal limits and a urine analysis was negative for infection.

The staff and her family were counseled to use various psychosocial-environmental interventions to reduce Mrs. S's agitation. For example, the staff would engage Mrs. S from 2 p.m. onward and close her window curtains, so that when Mrs. S would go to her room she would not see the trees outside. Also, only female staff members were allowed to provide personal care. Mrs. S's family was informed about the risk of strokes and premature death associated with the use of atypical antipsychotic medications, as well as the risk of not giving her an antipsychotic (table 6.2). The family agreed to a trial of low-dose quetiapine.

Mrs. S started taking quetiapine 12.5 mg in the morning and at bedtime daily. She developed daytime sedation, so the quetiapine was shifted to 25 mg daily at bedtime. After one week her sleep had improved, but her agitation and aggression persisted; the quetiapine was increased to 37.5 mg daily at bedtime and, after four days, to 50 mg daily at bedtime. She had mild daytime sedation but it resolved after five days. Physical therapy was also initiated to improve her muscle strength and balance. Over the next two weeks her agitation and aggression improved significantly, she allowed most ADL care, and she felt that the men who had come into her room had left the place, so she was relieved. She still expressed periodic concern that the men were going through her belongings, but she could be reassured and distracted most of the time. After three months the quetiapine was tapered off, and then it was discontinued over a four-week period. Mrs. S did not show any worsening of her symptoms.

TEACHING POINTS For many residents who have dementia with severe psychotic symptoms associated with physical aggression and/or severe agitation, psychosocial-environmental interventions, when combined with trial of an atypical antipsychotic drug, may substantially improve their agitation and aggression. We recommend the lowest possible therapeutic dose. Close monitoring for adverse effects, such as daytime sedation and falls, is vital. The clinician should consider discontinuing the prescribed antipsychotic drug for residents whose symptoms are stable.

Psychosis Associated with Parkinson Disease

Parkinson disease is a common neurodegenerative disease affecting up to 1 percent of the elderly population (Weintraub and Hurtig 2007). Hallucinations are the most common form of psychotic symptoms (18%), followed by hallucinations with delusions (4%), and then by delusions only (2%). The presence of cognitive impairment (e.g., dementia, delirium) dramatically increases the prevalence of hallucinations in people with PD (up to 55%). The onset of psychotic symptoms in a resident with PD should prompt an evaluation for underlying dementia or delirium. Persistent psychotic symptoms in people with PD (PDPsy) are associated with an increased risk of admission to LTC, greater functional impairment, caregiver burden, and death (Ravina et al. 2007). PDPsy is associated with exposure to PD medications, the duration of PD, an increasing severity in executive function impairment, global cognitive impairment, poor visual acuity, depression, anxiety, Lewy body disease, older age, an imbalance of monoaminergic neurotransmitters, and deficits in visuospatial processing. NMDA antagonists (e.g., memantine, methadone, ketamine) may also precipitate psychosis in residents with PD (Chan, Cordato, and O'Rourke 2008). Psychotic symptoms can be more disabling than motor symptoms.

Visual hallucinations are mostly complex (vivid scenes involving people and animals); preserved or disturbed insight relative to the nature of hallucinations is a major prognostic factor, although eventually all hallucinations will present with reduced insight (Onofrj, Thomas, and Bonanni 2007). Initially, the hallucinations are usually friendly (i.e., benign hallucinosis). Residents often see vivid, colorful, and sometimes fragmented figures of beloved (deceased) persons and/or family pets. They talk to them and try to caress them or prepare food or drink for them, only later displaying insight into the unreality of these figures. Visual hallucinations are often preceded by sleep disturbances, mild changes in visual perceptions (e.g., the sensation of a presence or a sideways passage), or visual illusions. In due time, however, reality testing further decreases and the content of the hallucinations may change. Frightening insects, rats, and serpents may predominate, inducing anxiety. Delusions involving themes of persecution, spousal infidelity, or jealousy may also develop. More than 50 percent of the people with PDPsy have an additional psychiatric condition, such as depression. PDPsy may infrequently present as part of a manic episode. Psychotic symptoms are rare in people with PD when the disease is not treated. Psychotic symptoms occurring early in the course of PD suggest a diagnosis of DLB or a coexisting psychiatric illness that, before the onset of PD, was not recognized and has been unmasked by dopaminergic therapy (Poewe and Seppi 2001).

The treatment of PDPsy initially involves a thorough evaluation and treatment of various potential etiological factors, such as general medical conditions (e.g., dehydration, infection), environmental problems, and psychosocial problems. If the psychotic symptoms are mild and not bothersome to the resident, reassurance and education of the resident and the caregiver (family and professional) is sufficient for treatment. If psychotic symptoms are moderate to severe, the clinician should try reducing the anti-PD drugs. If the resident is taking multiple dopaminergic drugs, the drug with the greatest psychosis-inducing potential and the least antiparkinsonian activity should be discontinued first. The anti-PD drugs should be eliminated in the following order: (1) adjunctive drugs (anticholinergics, amantadine, selegiline), (2) dopamine agonists (pramipexole, ropinirole, rotigotine), and (3) levodopa/carbidopa. Anti-PD drugs should be reduced to a point at which psychotic symptoms are diminished without a drastic worsening of motor symptoms. A reduction or discontinuation of medication taken in the evening and at bedtime may alleviate agitation in the evening, nocturnal hallucinations, and insomnia.

If the psychotic symptoms do not improve with a reduction in anti-PD drugs or if the reduction significantly worsens the person's motor symptoms, the clinician should consider prescribing a trial of antipsychotic drugs with the least likelihood for parkinsonian adverse effects, such as aripiprazole, quetiapine, or clozapine (Weintraub and Hurtig 2007). Clozapine, aripiprazole, and quetiapine, at lower dosages, do not appear to worsen motor symptoms, although higher dosages may cause excessive sedation or confusion. The clinician may consider ziprasidone before clozapine to treat PDPsy in residents who cannot tolerate quetiapine or aripiprazole. We do not recommend conventional antipsychotic medications (e.g., haloperidol). Olanzapine and risperidone have not been found to be beneficial (Weintraub and Hurtig 2007). Although clozapine has the best evidence for treating psychotic symptoms in people with PD, it is not the drug of first choice. The weekly blood draw to monitor a person's white blood cell count (because of the risk of agranulocytosis) that is needed for clozapine use is a significant burden for the resident. In addition, the use of clozapine is associated with a risk of myocarditis, seizures, and orthostatic hypotension. We recommend clozapine primarily for the treatment of severe psychotic symptoms not responding to quetiapine, aripiprazole, or ziprasidone, or if the resident cannot tolerate these drugs. It is possible and reasonable to switch a psychiatrically stable resident with PDPsy from clozapine to quetiapine, provided a previous quetiapine treatment has not failed.

The clinician should cautiously consider attempting to wean stable residents off antipsychotics, due to a high risk of recurrence of the psychosis. Symptoms may be worse during recurrence than in the initial presentation (Fernandez, Trieschmann, and Okun 2004). If a resident with PDPsy also has dementia, cholinesterase inhibitors (especially rivastigmine, as it is the only ChEI approved by the FDA for the treatment of PDD) may help reduce the psychotic symptoms (especially hallucinations) or decrease the risk of worsening these symptoms (Emre et al. 2004). The clinician should consider prescribing ECT for the treatment of severe persistent psychotic symptoms not responding to psychosocial interventions and atypical antipsychotics. ECT should be considered the first-line treatment for people with PD and psychotic depression. ECT may also improve some of the motor symptoms of PD.

Delirium with Psychotic Symptoms

Psychotic symptoms are common in delirium, and they may be the predominant manifestation of delirium. Hallucinations are typically visual and accompanied by illusions (visual misinterpretation of things in the environment), and paranoid delusions may be present. Hallucinations are often vivid, elaborate, and frightening. Delusions are transient and poorly systematized. The treatment for this condition involves finding and treating the cause of the delirium. The clinician may consider antipsychotic drugs for a short-term treatment of severe agitation and aggression accompanying psychotic symptoms during delirium (Seitz, Gill, and van Zyl 2007).

Psychotic Symptoms Due to a General Medical Condition

On occasion, psychotic symptoms may be the only or the initial manifestation of underlying medical conditions (e.g., a UTI, thyroid dysfunction, electrolyte imbalance, epilepsy, dehydration, sleep apnea, a brain tumor), especially for people with preexisting dementia (Desai and Grossberg 2003a). Visual hallucinations among people with a retinal disease (e.g., macular degeneration) are common, underdiagnosed, and not associated with cognitive deficits, abnormal personality traits, or a family or personal history of psychiatric morbidity (Scott et al. 2001). Visual hallucinations and illusions may also accompany other ocular pathologies and decreases in visual acuity (e.g., cataracts, glaucoma). The hallucinations may be well formed and vivid, be miniaturized or distorted, and include perceptions of animals, people, or geometric shapes. The occurrence of such persistent, complex visual hallucinations with preserved insight in people with visual impairment and an absence of other etiologies (e.g., dementia) is known as the Charles Bonnet syndrome (Mahgoub and Serby 2007). Among people with relatively good vision, hallucinations are associated with increased emotional distress and a decreased quality of life. For all residents who have visual hallucinations, the clinician should consider the need for eyeglasses (or a change in glasses) or cataract surgery and suggest a referral to an ophthalmologist. We recommend close monitoring for cognitive decline, because the onset of complex visual hallucinations in elderly people with impaired vision may be an indication of early dementia (especially DLB).

Psychotic symptoms due to deep brain lesions (e.g., basal ganglia disease) resemble schizophrenia more closely than those seen with dementia (Desai and Grossberg 2003a). Vivid, elaborate, and well-formed visual hallucinations (called *peduncular hallucinosis*) may occur with disease (e.g., a stroke) in the upper brain stem. Psychosis can be a rare but devastating consequence of traumatic brain injury. In people with neurological deficits (e.g., due to a stroke or a tumor), delusional thinking may be associated with a denial of illness (anosognosia), a denial of blindness (Anton syndrome), or reduplicative paramnesia (in which a person claims to be present simultaneously in two locations). Aging people with AIDS may develop central nervous system manifestations that often result in psychosis.

A careful consideration of various etiologies is critical for an early and accurate diagnosis. The treatment of psychotic symptoms due to a general medical condition involves the identification and treatment of the underlying medical condition. When psychosis develops in the context of epilepsy, the clinician's first step is to maximize anticonvulsant therapy in an effort to reduce the possible contribution of electrophysiologic disturbances. The clinician may consider prescribing benzodiazepines for ictal and postictal psychotic symptoms and agitation. Antipsychotics can lower the seizure threshold, so the clinician should prescribe them cautiously to treat chronic psychotic symptoms in residents with epilepsy.

Medication-Induced Psychotic Symptoms

Drugs used to treat Parkinson disease, anticholinergic drugs, benzodiazepines, and steroids often cause psychotic symptoms. Withdrawal from anxiolytics and sedative-hypnotics may also be associated with psychotic symptoms (especially visual hallucinations along with illusions, but occasionally tactile hallucinations as well) (table 6.3). Compared with levodopa, dopamine agonists (e.g., ropinirole, pramipexole, rotigotine) have a much greater propensity to cause mental confusion, disorientation, and hallucinations, especially in people with dementia. So for residents with PD and cognitive impairment, we recommend avoiding the use of dopamine agonists as much as possible and using levodopa (with or without entacapone) and/or rasagiline to treat motor symptoms.

Psychotic Symptoms Associated with Alcoholism

Psychotic symptoms typically occur during alcohol intoxication and withdrawal. Psychotic symptoms can also occur as a separate syndrome of alcohol-induced psychotic disorder, with delusions (e.g., of infidelity) and/or hallucinations. A diagnosis of this condition requires that the clinician maintain a high index of suspicion, as many LTC residents consume alcohol. For residents who have dementia or are frail, even a small amount of alcohol may be sufficient to cause problems (intoxication or withdrawal). The treatment for alcohol withdrawal may require benzodiazepines, and, if there is risk of withdrawal seizures (e.g., a past history of withdrawal seizures) and/or delirium, the clinician should consider hospitalization. The treatment for benzodiaz-

TABLE 6.3
Medications commonly implicated in psychotic symptoms of long-term care residents

Anticholinergic drugs / drugs with high anticholinergic activity	
Diphenhydramine	Meclizine
Metoclopramide	Dimenhydrinate
Trihexyphenidyl	Atropine
Biperiden	Hyoscyamine
Benztropine	Cyproheptadine
Orphenadrine	Hydroxizine
Scopolamine	Meperidine
Anti-Parkinson disease drugs	
Ropinirole	Levodopa (L-dopa)
Pramipexole	Bromocriptine
Rotigotine	Amantadine
Cardiovascular drugs	
Digitalis	
Antiarrythmics (e.g., lidocaine, quinidine, procainamide)	
Steroids	
Corticosteroids (e.g., prednisone, dexamethasone)	
Gastrointestinal drugs	
Cimetidine	
Sedative-hypnotics (intoxication or withdrawal)	
Benzodiazepines (intoxication or withdrawal)	
Barbiturates	
Chloral hydrate	

epine intoxication involves a gradual tapering off and then discontinuation of benzodiazepines.

Psychotic Symptoms Associated with the Use of Street Drugs

Although it is rare, some LTC residents may be using cocaine, cannabis, or other street drugs. They usually have a past history of drug abuse. A high index of suspicion is crucial for an accurate diagnosis, and a urine drug screen usually confirms the diagnosis. The treatment may involve hospitalization (e.g., if delirium is present).

Mixed Psychotic Disorders

Many residents have two secondary psychotic disorders (e.g., dementia with psychotic symptoms and superimposed delirium with psychotic symptoms) or a primary psychotic disorder (e.g., schizophrenia) comorbid with a secondary psychotic disorder (e.g., psychotic symptoms due to dementia or delirium). Inadequate psychiatric care in an LTC facility may result in the development of dementia going unrecognized in residents with schizophrenia (Grossberg and Desai 2003a). A high index of suspicion and a comprehensive assessment are key to the accurate identification and appropriate treatment of mixed psychotic disorders.

Conclusion

Psychotic disorders are prevalent in long-term care populations, cause considerable suffering, and are associated with increased morbidity and mortality. Residents with psychotic symptoms may develop severe agitation and aggression and thus may pose a considerable danger to the staff and other residents. A thorough assessment (including for the risk of suicide) and treatment of the underlying reversible cause (if found) is the first step. Pharmacological and psychosocial-environmental interventions are usually effective in treating psychotic disorders in LTC populations and can greatly improve the quality of life for residents with psychotic disorders.

CHAPTER 7

Anxiety Disorders and Sleep Disorders

Anxiety and sleep disorders are common among residents in long-term care facilities, cause significant emotional distress to residents, increase family and caregiver stress, and may be associated with an increased risk of falls, injury, hospitalization, and excess disability.

Anxiety Disorders

Anxiety is defined as a vague, uneasy feeling, the source of which often is nonspecific or unknown to the individual who is experiencing it. Fear is anxiety related to a specific object, event, or situation. Anxiety disorders are less prevalent in elderly people than in young adults, but rates of subsyndromal anxiety disorders are nearly as high in elderly persons as in younger cohorts (Salzman 2004). The most common late-life anxiety disorders are mixed anxiety-depression and generalized anxiety disorder (GAD). In our experience, the majority of LTC residents experience anxiety symptoms during a depressive disorder, during bereavement, as adverse effects of medications, or due to dementia or delirium. The prevalence of anxiety is reported to be 15–69 percent in people with dementia (Jost and Grossberg 1996). Hence the clinician should include an assessment of anxiety in the routine evaluation of LTC residents. For residents with the ability to communicate, asking about their reactions to stress may help the clinician screen for anxiety symptoms. Pharmacological intervention for anxiety disorders may take at least four weeks to show noticeable benefits, and maximal benefits may take as long as one year. The clinician should keep the potential for drug-drug interactions in mind, as they may adversely affect the management of anxiety disorders.

The following are some examples of clinically relevant drug-drug interactions: (1) when a drug (e.g., clarithromycin) that inhibits the hepatic cytochrome P-450, 3A4 enzyme system is administered to a resident who is taking alprazolam (metabolized by 3A4 cytochrome P450 liver enzymes), the resident may experience increased sedation (due to the reduced metabolism of alprazolam); (2) when a resident with obsessive-compulsive disorder (OCD) who is stable taking fluvoxamine develops an exacerbation of his or her OCD after resuming cigarette smoking; (3) when the addition of fluoxetine for a resident who is taking digoxin causes anorexia, anxiety, and confusion due to digoxin toxicity. In example two, cigarette smoking causes the induction of 1A2 liver enzymes and thus lowers the level of fluvoxamine, which is metabolized by this enzyme. In example three, fluoxetine inhibits the P-glycoprotein transporter and thus increases the level of digoxin, which is a substrate of the P-glycoprotein transport protein. The addition of fluoxetine significantly impairs the ability of the P-glycoprotein transporter to extrude digoxin from enterocytes back into the gut lumen. Because more digoxin is retained in the enterocytes, there is greater bioavailability and absorption of digoxin from the gut, leading to an increase in the blood level of digoxin (Sandson 2007).

A variety of conditions can cause anxiety symptoms in LTC residents. Table 7.1 shows the differential diagnosis of symptoms of anxiety.

Primary Anxiety Disorders

Primary anxiety disorders are less prevalent in older adults than in younger adults (Dada, Sethi, and Grossberg 2001; Flint and Gagnon 2003; Flint 2005). Generalized anxiety disorder and phobias account for most cases of primary anxiety disorders in older adults (Flint 1998; Dada, Sethi, and Grossberg 2001; Lenze et al. 2005). Up to 48 percent of elderly persons with major depressive disorder also have a current, comorbid anxiety disorder (Beekman et al. 2000). Likewise, severe anxiety symptoms have been seen in as many as half of the people with late-life MDD. The combination of anxiety and depression in older adults is often more severe and resists treatment. Comorbid anxiety disorder and late-life depression may also predict future dementia. Anxious elderly people may experience anticipatory dread about the adverse effects of prescribed antianxiety medications, may be vigilant about potential adverse effects, and may have a tendency to catastrophize about these. Some family and professional caregivers may share these fears. Thus we recommend counseling residents, their families, and staff members in advance about the potential adverse effects of medications and reassuring them that

TABLE 7.1
Differential diagnosis of symptoms of anxiety

"Normal" anxiety

Anxiety during bereavement

Primary anxiety disorders: including generalized anxiety disorder, panic disorder, post-traumatic stress disorder, agoraphobia, social phobia, fear of falling, adjustment disorder with an anxious mood, and anxiety symptoms during a mood disorder

Secondary anxiety disorders: including anxiety disorders due to dementia, medications, medical conditions, substance abuse, and delirium

Mixed anxiety disorders: including a combination of one or more primary and one or more secondary anxiety disorders (e.g., generalized anxiety disorder with dementia and anxiety)

you will closely monitor the resident for adverse effects. The clinician may often need to minimize the dose of medications and make the upward titration even slower for residents with anxiety disorder than is recommended for residents with depression.

Generalized Anxiety Disorder

Generalized anxiety disorder is characterized by at least six months of excessive, uncontrollable worry accompanied by symptoms of motor tension and vigilance. With LTC residents, the disorder may manifest as excessive worries, agitation, pacing, restlessness, verbal and/or physical aggression, irritability, and insomnia. GAD has a high level of comorbidity with other psychiatric disorders (major depression being the most common), although pure GAD occurs in approximately 1 percent of community-dwelling elderly people (Flint 2005). Early-onset (before age 50) GAD constitutes a slightly higher proportion (57%) of GAD in late life than late-onset (after age 50) GAD (43%) (Le Roux, Gatz, and Wetherell 2005). Older adults with early-onset GAD have a higher rate of psychiatric comorbidity, a greater use of psychotropic medications, and severe worry. Older adults who have late-onset GAD have more functional limitations, due to physical problems. Elderly people who have GAD usually have chronic symptoms lasting for years to decades without interruption (Lenze et al. 2005).

The treatment of GAD involves psychosocial interventions, such as reassurance, a patient and gentle approach, and, in severe cases, the use of medications (e.g., SSRIs, venlafaxine, buspirone, or pregabalin) (Salzman 2004; Bandelow, Wedekind, and Leon 2007). If the clinician initiates medications, he or she should inform the resident, the family, and the staff that it may take several weeks to a few months after therapeutic dosages are reached for beneficial effects to occur. In severe cases, the clinician may consider prescribing low-dose benzodiazepines for the first few weeks. Many residents with GAD have been taking benzodiazepines for decades before their admission to the LTC facility. For these residents, the clinician should consider tapering off the benzodiazepines, due to the risk of cognitive impairment, falls, and fracture. If the clinician decides to do so, the taper should be extremely slow (over several months). A small group of LTC residents with severe GAD may need low-dose benzodiazepines for the rest of their lives. For these residents, the clinician should prescribe the lowest possible dose of benzodiazepine and monitor these individuals closely for adverse effects.

> **CLINICAL CASE** Mrs. U was a 96-year-old widow who was admitted to a nursing home several years previously because of frailty, blindness due to macular degeneration, and recurrent falls. She had a sister who was two years younger and in good health, a son, three grandchildren, eight great-grandchildren, and one great-great grandchild. For eight to nine months, she had been experiencing increased anxiety and nervousness, using her call light excessively, shouting "help, help" for long periods of time, and grabbing passersby and wanting them to help her. Mrs. U had always been somewhat anxious, but these symptoms were much more severe and apparently triggered by a UTI nine months previously. The staff was initially able to manage her anxiety with psychosocial interventions, such as taking her to church services twice a day (Mrs. U was a religious Methodist, but she also enjoyed attending church services of different denominations), hand massages, and soothing music. But for the last five months, the symptoms had become severe and difficult to manage. Mrs. U usually slept well and, although she was eating less in the last few weeks, had not lost weight. The family started decreasing their visits, because they felt Mrs. U would become more agitated when they would visit and ask her how she was feeling. The family would also grow distraught and feel helpless after each visit, particularly when they could not calm Mrs. U and the staff told the family that Mrs. U was having "another bad day." Mrs. U's primary care physician had prescribed citalopram and mirtazapine, but Mrs. U could not tolerate either of these. Hence the primary care provider referred Mrs. U to a psychiatrist.
>
> The psychiatrist found Mrs. U to be pleasant, talkative, and anxious about her "vision worsening in the last two weeks." She described herself as being a "worrier," and her son confirmed that she had always been nervous and impatient, would become "easily stressed," and thought and

feared the "worst outcome" in any situation. Mrs. U denied any depressive symptoms, and the son confirmed that Mrs. U had not had any significant depressive symptoms in the past. Mrs. U's primary care provider had evaluated her for a UTI, constipation, pain, electrolyte imbalance, thyroid dysfunction, and vitamin deficiency and did not find any problems. The pharmacist had reviewed Mrs. U's medications and had recommended discontinuing propoxyphene (which the primary care provider subsequently discontinued), but he did not find any other medications that could cause anxiety. Mrs. U's MMSE score was 24 (indicating fair cognitive functioning) and her GDS score was five (suggesting minimal depression).

The psychiatrist diagnosed Mrs. U as having GAD and a mild cognitive impairment, and ruled out early dementia. He prescribed buspirone 5 mg twice daily, which, after one week, was increased to 10 mg twice daily. After two weeks, the dose was further increased to 15 mg twice daily. The psychiatrist also recommended that the family visit as often as possible and have an active visit, rather than asking questions, and he counseled the family regarding some of the activities they could do with Mrs. U. The family would sit with Mrs. U and encourage her to tell stories about her younger days on the farm. The family would also take Mrs. U for a 10-minute walk each time they visited, listen to her favorite music and reminisce, or watch baseball games on television and keep Mrs. U informed about the game. The staff were encouraged not to tell the family that Mrs. U "was not doing well" but instead to reassure them that with time and treatment, Mrs. U should start feeling better. After four more weeks, the family and staff noticed that her anxiety decreased. Over the next three months, Mrs. U continued to show improvement, with only one to two episodes of anxiety and yelling per week.

TEACHING POINTS The clinician may need to prescribe multiple medication trials to identify a psychotropic drug that the patient tolerates and that is effective. Although antidepressants are the first-line agents for pharmacotherapy of GAD, the clinician should also consider prescribing buspirone. The full effect of medications for anxiety disorders may take a few months. Specific guidance and counseling for family and staff regarding individualized psychosocial interventions has a much higher success rate than nonspecific recommendations regarding psychosocial interventions.

Panic Disorder and Agoraphobia

Panic disorder involves recurrent panic attacks associated with a persistent concern about having more attacks and/or about the implication of the attack. A panic attack involves discrete periods of intense fear or discomfort that develop abruptly and reach a peak within 10–15 minutes. During these periods, the person may experience heart-pounding, sweating, trembling, chest pain or discomfort, nausea or abdominal distress, dizziness, unsteadiness, lightheadedness, faintness, fear of losing control or going crazy, fear of dying, numbness or tingling sensations, chills or hot flashes, and/or a feeling of choking. Panic disorder occurs less frequently in elderly people than in younger adults. Residents with panic disorder usually have a long-standing history of episodic anxiety attacks that have significantly impaired their daily functioning. The anxiety symptoms of residents with panic disorder usually have been treated with medications (antidepressants and/or benzodiazepines). Panic disorder may have an onset in late life, with the typical presentation being an older woman who has been recently widowed (in the last year) and experiences chest pain, although no evidence of coronary artery disease is found (Beitman, Kushner, and Grossberg 1991). Elderly people may have fewer and less severe symptoms and exhibit less avoidant behavior (Flint and Gagnon 2003).

Panic disorder in older adults may be accompanied by agoraphobia. Agoraphobia involves anxiety about being in places or situations from which escape might be difficult (or embarrassing) or in which help may not be available in the event of having an unexpected panic attack. Agoraphobia may also occur in the absence of panic disorder and it, too, may have its onset in later life. Most individuals with late-onset agoraphobia do not have a history of panic attacks, and the illness often starts after a traumatic event (Flint 1998).

Panic attacks occurring for the first time in elderly people are often due to conditions other than panic disorder. Bereavement, alcohol withdrawal, benzodiazepine withdrawal, caffeine withdrawal, cardiac arrhythmia, and pheochromocytoma are some of the conditions that may cause panic attacks for the first time in elderly people.

In most cases the management of panic disorder requires medication (SSRIs or venlafaxine and, occasionally, low doses of benzodiazepines). Residents with panic disorder should be started on a low dose of an antidepressant medication to avoid an initial exacerbation of their anxiety, but then the dosage should be gradually increased to the therapeutic range. Given the delayed onset of action for antidepressant medications (four to eight weeks), the short-term use of an adjunctive benzodiazepine (e.g., lorazepam) in the first few weeks of treatment may be helpful for selected residents. Residents with long-standing panic disorder who are stable taking antidepressants should continue at the same dose but periodically be evaluated to detect any adverse effects that may occur due to a change in the pharmacodynamic and pharmacokinetic physiologic processes related to aging, advancing dementia, and worsening medical comorbidity. Residents with panic disorder who have been taking benzodiazepines for decades and are stable may need to continue taking these drugs because of the high morbidity associated with poorly controlled panic disorder. We recommend close monitoring for any potential adverse effects of benzodiazepines (e.g., falls, sedation, cognitive impairment) and a gradual dose reduction as the resident ages or develops frailty or reduced clearance (due to progressive kidney and/or liver disease). The clinician should consider psychotherapy (e.g., cognitive behavior therapy, relaxation exercises) for residents who are relatively cognitively intact or have mild cognitive impairments.

CLINICAL CASE Ms. F was a 70-year-old resident who had a long history of severe panic disorder with agoraphobia. She had been stable for "decades" taking 5 mg of diazepam twice daily, along with 0.25 mg of alprazolam as needed once a day and imipramine 25 mg daily at bedtime. She was admitted to a nursing home for rehabilitation after receiving a second kidney transplant. The primary care provider who had prescribed her psychiatric medications had recently passed away and a young family practitioner took over. He felt that Ms. F was subject to a high risk of falls and confusion due to the diazepam, alprazolam, and imipramine. He also felt that Ms. F had become "addicted" to diazepam. He scheduled a withdrawal regimen. Within a few weeks, Ms. F was severely agitated and required hospitalization in a psychiatric unit. The psychiatrist discussed treatment options with Ms. F, including switching to an SSRI or mirtazapine or nortriptyline versus reinstating her original medications. Ms. F chose to restart her original medications, as they had helped her for years and she was willing to risk the potential adverse effects, including falls and cognitive impairment. The psychiatrist in the unit reinstated Ms. F's original medication regimen, and Ms. F was back to her baseline level of functioning within a few weeks. The psychiatrist also collaborated with the new primary care provider, explaining the severity of Ms. F's panic disorder and the plan for frequent outpatient follow-up visits to closely monitor the risk of falls and cognitive impairment.

TEACHING POINTS For a resident with a history of severe psychiatric disorder (e.g., severe panic disorder with agoraphobia), it may be prudent to continue the benzodiazepines and/or tricyclic antidepressants if the resident is tolerating them well and has been stable. Close monitoring and a thorough discussion of the risks and benefits of benzodiazepines and tricyclic antidepressants (including the risk of falls and fracture, delirium, cardiac toxicity, etc.) is necessary. The clinician should also discuss alternative treatment options, such as SSRIs, mirtazapine, and cognitive behavioral therapy.

Obsessive-Compulsive Disorder

Obsessions involve recurrent and persistent thoughts, impulses, or images that are intrusive and inappropriate and cause marked anxiety. Compulsions are repetitive behaviors (e.g., hand washing or checking objects) or mental acts (e.g., praying, counting, repeating words silently) that the person feels driven to perform in response to an obsession or according to rules that must be applied rigidly. People with obsessive-compulsive disorder have obsessions and/or compulsions lasting for at least six months that cause significant suffering and an impairment in daily functioning. OCD usually starts in young adulthood and persists into later life. Thus residents with OCD have a long-standing history of obsessions and compulsions that have significantly affected their daily life for decades before admission to the LTC facility. Up to 83 percent of the individuals with OCD improve after several decades, including a complete recovery in 20 percent and recovery with subclinical symptoms in 28 percent (Skoog and Skoog 1999). Elderly people with OCD have a later age at onset and have fewer concerns about symmetry, a need to know, and counting rituals than younger people with OCD (Kohn et al. 1997). Hand-washing and fear of having sinned may be more common in elderly people with OCD than in younger people with this condition. Symptoms of OCD appearing for the first time in someone who is elderly are rare, and they are often due to neurological disorders, such as a stroke in the basal ganglia.

The treatment of OCD is primarily with one of the SSRIs. Although clomipramine is often used as a first-line agent for treating young adults and middle-aged people with OCD, the clinician should avoid prescribing it for LTC residents, due to its high anticholinergic property, which puts residents at risk of additional cognitive impairment. Fluvoxamine, an SSRI, is also commonly used to treat OCD in younger adults, but the clinician should avoid prescribing it for older adults because of the high risk of a drug-drug interaction. The clinician should educate the staff about OCD and the need to accommodate the resident's compulsive behaviors.

Post-Traumatic Stress Disorder

An individual with post-traumatic stress disorder has a history of being exposed to a traumatic event or events that involved actual or threatened death or serious injury or a threat to the physical integrity of oneself or others. Examples of such traumatic events include being in a war (as a civilian [e.g., holocaust survivor] or as a soldier [in active combat and/or as a prisoner of war]), physical abuse, sexual abuse or rape or another violent crime, domestic violence, a terrorist attack, a mass shooting, a natural disaster, or a motor vehicle accident.

Symptoms of PTSD involve persistently re-experiencing the traumatic event—through recollections of images, thoughts, or perceptions, or through distressing dreams of the event—or acting as if the traumatic event were recurring (a sense of reliving the experience [e.g., a resident who is a war veteran acts as if bombs are falling and people are dying]); persistently avoiding stimuli associated with the trauma (e.g., avoiding conversations about the trauma, attempting to avoid places or people that arouse recollections of the trauma); and displaying symptoms of severe anxiety (irritability, outbursts of anger, sleep impairment). PTSD is a severely debilitating disorder. Events in later life may awaken long-suppressed memories and feelings in residents and yield emotional or behavioral problems that are evidence of an early traumatic experience. These residents may underreport their PTSD symptoms, or their symptoms may be masked by other diagnoses. PTSD is often associated with MDD, substance-related disorders, panic disorder, GAD, and social phobia.

World War II and Korean War veterans aged 65 or older now number approximately 1.2 million, and about 25 percent of these men served in combat. This means approximately 60,000 veterans are at risk of or are already diagnosed as having dementia. World War II veterans exposed to moderate or heavy combat were found to have a 13.3 times greater risk of having PTSD symptoms than noncombat veterans (Spiro, Schurr, and Aldwin 1994). Thus many World War II and Korean War veterans living in LTC are likely to have dormant or partially controlled PTSD. Alternatively, residents may have a history of PTSD that was under fairly good control until the onset of dementia, with the neurodegeneration of memory pathways possibly disinhibiting symptoms of PTSD. Acts of terrorism and war may be particularly disturbing for residents who survived traumatic events (e.g., World War II) in the past. Thus the clinician should screen all LTC residents who have a history of being in active combat for PTSD.

Dementia may present with PTSD symptoms in combat veterans (Johnston 2000), and residents who have more severe trauma (e.g., prisoners of war) are at high risk of developing paranoia. A violent outburst related to PTSD symptoms in residents with dementia may precipitate an emergency room visit or police involvement. Many residents who have recently been in intensive care units may have PTSD-like symptoms, especially if they had been in physical restraints without sedation, were in deep sedation, or could recall delusional memories (e.g., interpreting a simple injection as an attempted homicide) (Griffiths et al. 2007). Residents who had a past history of psychological problems may also be at increased risk of PTSD after a stay in intensive care. For a considerable number of elderly people, losing a spouse in late life appears to be a traumatic experience, so some of these bereaved elders may experience PTSD-like symptoms (Elklit and O'Connor 2005).

The treatment of PTSD involves a combination of antidepressants and psychosocial-environmental interventions. Benzodiazepines may be needed for a short-term treatment of severe anxiety, as well as antipsychotics if the resident develops severe psychotic symptoms with agitation. Residents with PTSD who are cognitively intact may benefit from psychotherapy. The clinician should consider recommending that residents with history of being in a war or of having witnessed terrorist attacks avoid news from television, radio, or newspapers. The clinician may also consider recommending group therapy if several cognitively intact residents with PTSD are living in one LTC facility (e.g., LTC facilities for veterans).

> **CLINICAL CASE** Mr. M was an 89-year-old man living in a nursing home.
> He had been experiencing nightmares, verbal and physical aggression,
> anxiety, and hypervigilance, as well as shouting "Bombs are falling. Run,
> run," thereby agitating other residents. He was also isolating himself.
> These symptoms began after Mr. M watched the terrorist attacks of September 11, 2001, on television. The staff at the nursing home felt that
> Mr. M should be hospitalized in a psychiatric unit, as he was "psychotic."

The consulting psychiatrist was asked to facilitate the hospitalization. The psychiatrist made an emergency psychiatric evaluation of Mr. M.

Mr. M's wife stated that her husband was an Army infantry man from 1940 to 1945 and had been in prolonged, intense combat in Sicily and Normandy. He had experienced mild PTSD symptoms and severe depression from 1946 to 1949. His symptoms gradually decreased after he started meeting regularly with a group of friends who were also in World War II.

Mr. M was married for 57 years and had four children and 11 grandchildren. His wife reported that Mr. M was an easygoing person who seemed to have enjoyed life until he was admitted to the nursing home in the year 2000, due to multiple medical problems. He had a successful career as a banker and he never abused drugs or alcohol. He developed severe peripheral vascular disease, resulting in bilateral above-knee amputation of his legs for the treatment of gangrene. He subsequently developed severe congestive heart failure and was admitted to a nursing home when his wife could no longer take care of his increasing physical needs at home.

After an evaluation, the psychiatrist counseled the family and staff that Mr. M's symptoms could be managed in the LTC facility if everyone collaborated in helping Mr. M; hospitalization carried its own risks of increased confusion and other iatrogenic problems. The psychiatrist prescribed sertraline 25 mg daily and increased it every seven days to a total of 100 mg daily. The psychiatrist also prescribed clonazepam 0.25 mg in the morning and at bedtime but, due to daytime sedation, later discontinued the morning dose. After two weeks, Mr. M was less agitated but continued to have nightmares, aggression, and nighttime agitation. The psychiatrist increased the dose of clonazepam to 0.5 mg at bedtime, but Mr. M had two falls, so the dose was decreased to 0.25 mg at bedtime. The psychiatrist added mirtazapine 7.5 mg at bedtime, and Mr. M began sleeping better over the next two weeks. The psychiatrist also recommended that the family and staff to avoid any discussion of the terrorist attacks with Mr. M and have him avoid watching the news on television. A list of topics for conversation that did not involve war, politics, religion, or terrorist attacks was devised, in consultation with the staff and family. Over the next three months, Mr. M gradually become significantly less anxious and started sleeping better regularly, and his verbal and physical aggression resolved.

TEACHING POINTS The treatment of PTSD may involve multiple medications. Aggressive psychosocial-environmental interventions, close monitoring of adverse effects, and prompt changes in medications that cause adverse effects often allows the PTSD to be managed safely in a LTC facility and avoids hospitalization.

Social Phobia or Social Anxiety Disorder

Social phobia is a prevalent disorder in later life, with lifetime and 12-month prevalence estimates of 4.94 percent and 1.32 percent, respectively (Cairney et al. 2007). Individuals with this disorder have a long history of a marked and persistent fear of one or more social or performance situations in which they are exposed to unfamiliar people or to possible scrutiny by others. The resident fears that he or she will act in a way (or show anxiety symptoms) that will be humiliating or embarrassing. A resident with social phobia may avoid participating in the group activities in the LTC facility. Residents with this disorder are best managed by having one or two staff members (e.g., a social worker) establish a trusting relationship with the resident, as well as through reassurance, graded and gradual exposure to other residents and to group activity, and, in severe cases, a trial of one of the SSRIs.

Specific Phobia or Simple Phobia

Individuals with a specific phobia or simple phobia have a long history of a marked and persistent fear that is excessive or unreasonable and cued by the presence or anticipation of a specific object or situation (e.g., flying, heights, storms, water, animals, receiving an injection, seeing blood). These individuals may refuse blood tests or injections, or become agitated and anxious during such tests. These phobias are best managed by psychosocial-environmental interventions, such as helping the resident avoid the object (e.g., removing blood) or situation (e.g., animals) when possible; preparing the resident emotionally for blood tests or injections and holding the resident's hand, using a soothing voice and a gentle approach; and constantly reassuring the resident during the test or injection.

Fear of Falling

The fear of falling has been recognized as an important consequence of having experienced a fall. Between 30 and 73 percent of elderly people who have fallen acknowledge a persistent fear of falling. Fear of falling is more common in new LTC residents than in community-dwelling elderly people or in residents who have been in LTC for some time. This fear frequently leads residents to voluntarily restrict their activities, limiting their independence and their ability to engage in routines and participate in activity programs. This fear is best managed with psychosocial interventions such as reassurance, a soothing voice and gentle approach, encouragement, and positive reinforcement of desired behaviors (e.g., efforts to walk despite fears). Working actively with a physical therapist may be useful.

Adjustment Disorder with Anxious Mood

Individuals who have adjustment disorder with anxious mood develop significant anxiety symptoms (worries, muscle tension, nervousness, agitation, jitteriness) in response to an identifiable stressor or stressors. Anxiety symptoms usually occur within three months of the onset of the stressor(s). For example, a resident who becomes extremely anxious and agitated after being told that his or her spouse has been hospitalized may develop an adjustment disorder with anxious mood. The treatment for this disorder is usually reassurance. In severe cases, low-dose benzodiazepines as needed may be warranted for a few days.

Secondary Anxiety Disorders

Dementia with Anxiety Disorders

Symptoms of anxiety (e.g., tension, restlessness, irritability, a fear of being left alone, an anxious or worried expression, fidgeting, pacing, anger, agitation, apprehension) are common in individuals with dementia. Symptoms of GAD have been reported in 5–6 percent of those with AD. Residents with mild to moderate dementia may experience a sense of fear about an upcoming event (Godot syndrome) and therefore may ask repeated questions about it; or they may experience an excessive fear of being left alone and, as a result, shadow the caregiver. Expecting too much of people who have dementia or changing their routines may lead to anxiety. Anxiety in people with dementia may be a reflection of the caregivers' stress, because such people tend to mirror the emotions of those around them. Anxiety symptoms correlate with the severity of the cognitive impairment. Anxiety symptoms in residents with dementia are often comorbid with depression, hallucinations, delusions, aggressiveness, angry outbursts, and activity disturbances, such as wandering (Ferretti et al. 2001). Some individual symptoms of anxiety disorder can be easily confused with dementia. These symptoms include memory impairment and impairment in attention and concentration. Many residents with dementia may have undiagnosed premorbid anxiety disorders that may worsen after the resident develops AD. PTSD-like symptoms can develop for the first time after the onset of dementia if the resident was exposed to a traumatic event.

The treatment of dementia with anxiety disorders is primarily psychosocial (e.g., hand massage, soothing music, aromatherapy). As a result of short-term memory loss, every day is a new and potentially stressful experience for a person with dementia. However, procedural memory is retained longer than the ability to form new memories. Therefore rituals, consistency in routine, and consistency in caregivers help to prevent anxiety. We recommend that caregivers take a calm and patient approach, offer frequent reassurance, and avoid arguments. Reducing stress by modifying the environment (e.g., reducing the noise level by removing an anxious resident from an activity program with lots of sounds [singing and playing live music] to an activity that is relatively quiet [painting with water colors]) and reducing unrealistic demands on a resident with dementia (expecting the person not to become agitated in response to another resident's yelling or expecting a resident with receptive aphasia to understand simple spoken language) can also reduce anxiety. Bathing can be anxiety provoking for residents with dementia and can be better managed with towel baths by two staff members (one gently cleaning and the other soothing and distracting the resident), rather than a shower assisted by just one staff member.

Residents with severe anxiety, comorbid depression, or a past history of an anxiety disorder may benefit from a trial of antidepressants or buspirone (for GAD). For residents with dementia and severe anxiety symptoms, the clinician may prescribe low doses of benzodiazepine (short-acting ones such as lorazepam or oxazepam) during an acute anxiety attack or for short-term use, in order to give antidepressants or buspirone time to start helping. Catastrophic reactions, such as extreme anxiety before a visit to a dental clinic, can be aborted with a one-time use of low-dose benzodiazepine (e.g., 0.5 mg of lorazepam one hour before the visit).

> **CLINICAL CASE** Mrs. B was a 91-year-old woman admitted to an assisted living facility six months previously because of her increasing agitation and anxiety at home. Mr. B, who was 93 years old, could no longer take care of her. Mrs. B had been diagnosed as having dementia three years prior to her admission, could not tolerate cholinesterase inhibitors (ChEIs) due to nausea and diarrhea, and was taking memantine 10 mg twice daily

for the last two years. Over the past year, she would become increasingly anxious and agitated and start yelling for her husband if she was left alone even for a few minutes. Mrs. B would worry that something terrible might have happened to Mr. B. She did not want her husband to go anywhere, even if her three daughters agreed to stay with her. Mrs. B would try to leave the house to look for Mr. B and would become aggressive if someone tried to stop her. She showed the same behavior in the assisted living facility, and although lorazepam 0.5 mg three times a day started by her primary care provider had helped, she became more anxious when taking 50 mg sertraline also started by the primary care provider. The family was becoming increasingly frustrated because they would spend several hours with Mrs. B without any success in calming her. Her husband would grow irate at Mrs. B, and her daughters could not understand why Mrs. B was "so stubborn." A psychiatrist was consulted at this point.

The psychiatrist discovered from Mrs. B's sister that Mrs. B had lost her younger brother through accidental drowning when she was 10 years old. Mrs. B was the oldest of six children and did not have any part in the drowning. Mrs. B's mother was overwhelmed with working on the farm and raising six children and had put a lot of responsibility onto Mrs. B regarding housework and looking after her younger siblings. Mrs. B had expressed guilt off and on to her sister for several years and had always been an anxious and shy person who liked to be in her home and take care of her husband and three daughters. There was no history of her anxiety and shyness having caused a significant impairment in functioning. Mrs. B was otherwise in good health.

Mrs. B denied any depressive symptoms during the interview. She stated that she had a difficult life, said her worries about her husband were "normal," and denied her husband's report that she would become "belligerent." Mrs. B could not give a detailed history because of her dementia; her MMSE was 16 and her GDS-30-item was seven. The psychiatrist diagnosed Mrs. B as having severe anxiety disorder with dementia (with separation anxiety disorder–like symptoms) and prescribed 12.5 mg of sertraline, increasing it every two weeks to a total of 50 mg.

The psychiatrist informed the staff at the assisted living facility about Mrs. B's childhood trauma. The staff and family were also counseled that Mrs. B's dementia made her more susceptible to emotional disorders caused by her past trauma. The staff became more sympathetic, allowed the sertraline more time to work, and tried harder to distract Mrs. B. The family and staff were informed that SSRIs such as sertraline may cause an initial increase in anxiety, especially for someone who is already anxious, before reducing that anxiety. After eight weeks, the staff and family reported mild a improvement in Mrs. B's agitation and anxiety, especially the yelling episodes. The psychiatrist further increased the sertraline to 62.5 mg daily for two weeks and then to 75 mg daily. After eight more weeks, Mrs. B's anxiety and agitation were substantially less and her yelling episodes were occasional and easily managed. The lorazepam was gradually decreased and changed to an as-needed dosage. Mrs. B used it once or twice a week on average.

TEACHING POINTS The starting dose of antidepressants (especially SSRIs, venlafaxine, duloxetine) for people with severe anxiety needs to be much lower and increased more slowly than for people with depression, and the response time may be much longer than with depression. Explaining the possible impact of an earlier trauma on the resident's current problems to the staff and family may help them view the resident with more empathy and patience.

Medication-Induced Anxiety Disorder

Many commonly prescribed and over-the-counter medications (including herbs and supplements) can cause anxiety symptoms and mimic an anxiety disorder (table 7.2). The treatment for this condition involves discontinuing the offending drug or lowering its dose. If this cannot be done, treating the anxiety symptoms with psychosocial-environmental interventions and, in severe cases, with medications (benzodiazepines, antidepressants) may be necessary.

Medical Conditions Causing Symptoms of Anxiety

Medical conditions causing anxiety disorders or anxiety symptoms include but are not limited to pain, hypoglycemia, hyperthyroidism, pheochromocytoma, hyperadrenalism (Cushing disease), cardiac arrhythmia, COPD, strokes, PD, and brain tumors. Residents with anxiety symptoms or an anxiety disorder due to medical conditions typically have other signs of these medical conditions and do not have a long-standing history of anxiety disorder. A thorough history and a physical exam, laboratory tests, and/or neuroimaging usually pinpoint these medical conditions. Anxiety disorders are seen in up to 40 percent of people who have PD (Richard 2005). The most common anxiety disorders in people with PD are panic disorder, GAD, social

TABLE 7.2
Medications that may cause symptoms of anxiety and/or sleep disturbances

Sympathetomimetics (anxiety and/or insomnia)
    Phenylephrine
    Phenylpropanolamine
    Pseudoephedrine

Medications for chronic obstructive pulmonary disease (anxiety and/or insomnia)
    Theophylline
    Beta-adrenergic inhalers

Thyroid supplements (anxiety and/or insomnia)
    Levothyroxine (T4)
    Tri-iodothyronine (T3)

Anti-Parkinsonian medications (anxiety and/or insomnia and/or excessive daytime sleepiness)

Medications used for Attention Deficit Hyperactivity Disorder (anxiety and/or insomnia)
    Nonstimulants (atomoxetine)
    Stimulants (methylphenidate, dextroamphetamine)

Antidepressants
    Selective serotonin reuptake inhibitors (anxiety and/or insomnia)
    Bupropion (anxiety and/or insomnia)
    Venlafaxine (anxiety and/or insomnia)
    Duloxetine (anxiety and/or insomnia)
    Mirtazapine (excessive daytime sleepiness)
    Nefazodone (excessive daytime sleepiness)
    Trazodone (excessive daytime sleepiness)
    Tricyclic antidepressants (excessive daytime sleepiness)

Antipsychotics
    Aripiprazole (anxiety and/or insomnia)
    Ziprasidone (anxiety and/or insomnia)
    Quetiapine (excessive daytime sleepiness)
    Olanzapine (excessive daytime sleepiness)
    Clozapine (excessive daytime sleepiness)
    Risperidone (excessive daytime sleepiness)
    All conventional/typical antipsychotics (such as haloperidol, fluphenazine) (excessive daytime sleepiness)

Antidementia medications
    Cholinesterase inhibitors (insomnia)
    Memantine (excessive daytime sleepiness)

Withdrawal of sedative hypnotic medications (anxiety and/or insomnia)
    Benzodiazepines
    Zolpidem
    Barbiturates

Sedative hypnotic medications (excessive daytime sleepiness)
    Benzodiazepines (short-acting [lorazepam, oxazepam, alprazolam] and long-acting [flurazepam, diazepam, clonazepam, chlordiazepoxide])
    Barbiturates
    Chloral hydrate

Analgesics
    Withdrawal of opiates (insomnia)
    Opiates and tramadol (excessive daytime sleepiness)

Other medications
    Corticosteroids (anxiety and/or insomnia)
    Antiepileptic drugs (such as topiramate) (anxiety and/or insomnia)
    Modafinil (anxiety and/or insomnia)
    Nicotine (anxiety and/or insomnia)
    Caffeine (anxiety and/or insomnia)

continued

TABLE 7.2 *continued*

Diuretics (may cause insomnia by causing nocturia or electrolyte imbalance)
Anticholinergic medications (such as diphenhydramine, hydroxyzine) (excessive daytime sleepiness)
Antiepileptic drugs (such as pregabalin, gabapentin, carbamazepine, phenytoin, oxcarbazepine, leviracetam) (excessive daytime sleepiness)
Antihypertensives (such as clonidine) (excessive daytime sleepiness)

phobia, and anxiety coexisting with depression. Assessing the timing of anxiety symptoms for people with PD is important. If anxiety symptoms occur during the on-off period of motor fluctuations, adjustment of their antiparkinsonian medications may reduce or resolve the symptoms.

An acute episode of anxiety attack for the first time in residents who have no prior history of anxiety disorder should prompt a thorough investigation to evaluate for medical causes if a review of their medications does not find any obvious etiology. This investigation can start with measuring their vital signs, oxygen saturation, and blood glucose levels. If necessary, the clinician may consider additional blood tests and other tests. The treatment for anxiety symptoms or anxiety disorder caused by medical conditions involves a treatment of the cause. For example, an acute attack of anxiety may be secondary to hypoglycemia due to antidiabetic agents or to an asthma attack. For some residents with severe anxiety symptoms due to medical conditions (e.g., hyperthyroidism), treating these symptoms with psychiatric drugs such as benzodiazepines (at the lowest possible dose, over the shortest possible time to treat acute severe anxiety symptoms) and/or antidepressants (especially for chronic anxiety symptoms) may be warranted.

Symptoms of Anxiety Due to Caffeine, Alcohol, or Street Drugs

Excessive caffeine intake, alcohol withdrawal, opiate withdrawal, the use of a stimulant (cocaine, amphetamine), and the use of cannabis can trigger anxiety or panic symptoms and mimic any of the anxiety disorders mentioned above. Management of these conditions involves having a high index of suspicion and administering benzodiazepines for a short period of time, with a gradual tapering off.

Symptoms of Anxiety Associated with Delirium

Symptoms of anxiety are common in people with delirium. Such symptoms usually occur along with illusions, visual or other hallucinations, and paranoia, but they can occur in the absence of all of these accompanying problems. A dramatic fluctuation in sensorium and an acute onset often help differentiate this condition from other anxiety disorders. The clinician should avoid prescribing benzodiazepines to treat anxiety and agitation associated with delirium, because of the high risk of exacerbating cognitive impairment in residents with delirium. Benzodiazepines may be prescribed in the last hours or days of their lives for anxious and agitated residents with delirium. Benzodiazepines are also the drugs of choice to treat delirium associated with alcohol and sedative-hypnotic withdrawal.

Sleep Disorders

Sleep disorders include disorders that cause insomnia and/or excessive daytime sleepiness, neither of which are a normal part of aging nor an accepted consequence of living in an LTC facility. Nonetheless, insomnia and excessive daytime sleepiness are prevalent in LTC residents (Martin and Ancoli-Israel 2008). The frequency of insomnia and daytime sleepiness in residents with dementia in assisted living facilities is similar to that found in those in nursing homes (Rao et al. 2008). Among LTC residents, self-reported difficulties with sleep are even more common and more severe than among older adults living in the community. The sleep of LTC residents is distributed across a 24-hour day rather than consolidated in the nighttime hours, as they are commonly asleep intermittently at all hours of the day, even during mealtime periods. LTC residents are rarely asleep or awake for a continuous one-hour period during the day or night.

Major causes of sleep disturbances in this population include physiological changes associated with aging (fragmented nocturnal sleep, increased daytime napping, and decreased slow-wave sleep), a pathological involvement of the suprachiasmatic nucleus (due to dementia, a stroke, etc.), the effects of co-occurring medical conditions (e.g., untreated pain, sleep apnea, RLS), psychiatric disorders (e.g., MDD, GAD), medications (e.g., diphenhydramine, ChEIs), and a variety of environmental factors. Environmental factors are probably the most important of these (table 7.3). Residents are usually exposed to less bright light and sunlight than younger community-dwelling adults and require more light to maintain a normal circadian rhythm (Martin et al. 2007).

Sleep disorders are associated with negative health outcomes (e.g., an increased risk of cardiovascular and cerebrovascular disease) and an increased risk of mortality among LTC residents (Martin and Ancoli-Israel 2008). Other consequences of persistently poor sleep include irritability, poor con-

TABLE 7.3
Factors affecting sleep

Medical illness (e.g., pain, sleep disorders [sleep-disordered breathing, also called obstructive sleep apnea, restless leg syndrome, REM sleep behavior disorder], infection, heart failure, chronic obstructive pulmonary disease)

Medications (see table 7.2)

Psychiatric illness (e.g., delirium, mood disorders, anxiety disorder, psychotic disorder)

Disruption in the circadian rhythm due to dementia or a lifetime of working evenings or nights

Environmental factors (e.g., inadequate exposure to light in the daytime [low daytime indoor illumination, little time spent outdoors], excessive exposure to light at night, excessive noise at night, uncomfortable bed, bedroom is too hot or too cold or there is problem with humidity), sleep interrupted by the staff or by another resident

Poor sleep hygiene or lifestyle factors (e.g., daytime napping, spending too much time in bed, keeping an irregular sleep-wake schedule, lying down in bed for activities other than sleep and sex [watching television, eating, worrying, reading], being inactive [inadequate social, intellectual, and physical stimulation], routinely using products that interfere with sleep [caffeine, nicotine, alcohol])

Change in one's living situation (a newly admitted resident, moving to a different long-term care facility, a change in room, a change in roommate)

Multifactorial

centration and memory, a slower reaction time, decreased ability to perform ADLs, fatigue, agitation, falls, accelerated cognitive decline, exacerbation of preexisting pain, and depressed mood (St. George et al. 2008). The effect on family caregivers, who are roused by an affected loved one with nighttime awakening and behavioral disturbances, often leads to admitting the person with dementia to LTC. Insomnia often plays a role in both the etiology and the presentation of delirium in some residents with dementia. The insomnia and resultant pharmacological treatment attempts are equally implicated in the potential sequelae, ranging from excessive daytime somnolence to falls, accidents, and injuries (e.g., hip fractures, subdural hematomas). Sleep disorders, in particular nighttime behavioral disturbances, can also have a negative impact on the quality of life for other residents (especially roommates) and increase the strain on LTC staff. Hence recognition and treatment of sleep disorders is important in improving the quality of life for LTC residents.

Simple or Primary Insomnia

A resident with simple insomnia cannot fall asleep or else wakes up early and is unable to go back to sleep, and typically has a long history of insomnia. He or she may also have a history of taking sedative-hypnotics for long periods of time. Even for residents with long-standing insomnia, we recommend evaluating them for secondary causes of insomnia. The main treatment for primary insomnia involves psychosocial-environmental interventions (e.g., sleep hygiene). The clinician may consider prescribing a short-acting seda-tive-hypnotic (e.g., zolpidem, zaleplon, or eszopiclone) at bedtime or when the resident wakens in the night. The clinician may also consider prescribing ramelteon to treat primary insomnia. We do not recommend prescribing an-tihistamines, because of the high risk of adverse effects.

REM Sleep Behavior Disorder (RBD)

REM sleep behavior disorder is a condition in which the central nervous sys-tem mechanisms that cause muscle paralysis during REM sleep cease to func-tion properly, and the sleeper acts out dreams. RBD precedes or accompanies many neurodegenerative disorders, especially synucleinopathies (e.g., DLB, PD, multisystem atrophy) and, less frequently, tauopathies (e.g., AD, cortico-basal degeneration, progressive supranuclear palsy, Pick disease) (A. Thomas, Bonanni, and Onofrj 2007). RBD also occurs in amyotrophic lateral sclerosis, limbic encephalitis, epilepsy, and PTSD. RBD is confirmed with a sleep study in which the individual has dream-enactment behavior associated with a loss of muscle tone (atonia) on polysomnographic electromyogram recordings. The main concern associated with RBD is safety. Residents can fall out of bed or engage in dangerous behavior during the night as a result of acting out dream-related behaviors while asleep. The treatment involves securing the sleep environment to ensure the resident's safety. The clinician may also con-sider prescribing a small dose of clonazepam (0.25-0.5 mg at night).

Restless Leg Syndrome (RLS)

Restless leg syndrome (also called Ekbom syndrome) is common in elderly peo-ple, with an estimated prevalence of 10 to 15 percent in individuals over 65 years old (Milligan and Chesson 2002). RLS is defined as an irresistible desire to move one's limbs, and it is usually associated with paresthesia and motor restlessness. The symptoms start or worsen when a person is at rest and im-prove with activity. Additionally, the symptoms worsen in the evening and/or night, which often results in sleep disturbances and daytime tiredness. Other symptoms and signs of RLS include pacing/walking excessively, a complaint of leg discomfort, flexing or stretching the legs, crossing the legs repeatedly, rubbing the legs, and general restlessness. RLS is confirmed by a finding of periodic limb movement in a polysomnographic sleep study. The pathophysi-ology of primary RLS is associated with a deficiency in dopaminergic neu-rotransmission. Secondary RLS occurs in association with iron-deficiency anemia, uremia, and polyneuropathies. Primary RLS is twice as prevalent in women and onset may occur before the age of 20 in up to 45 percent of all individuals. Those with primary RLS often have a family history of RLS. The syndrome is associated with iron deficiency. RLS is typically diagnosed by an interview, but residents with significant cognitive impairments may not be able to describe their symptoms of RLS reliably.

Individuals with poorly controlled RLS may develop depression. RLS may be responsible for some of the wandering, pacing, restlessness, agitation, and sleeplessness that occur in residents with dementia. The clinician should screen those residents whose insomnia and agitation improves with ambulation for RLS. A persistent sleep impairment can cause cognitive impairments and worsen a preexisting cognitive impairment. Treating RLS may improve cognition by improving sleep.

For residents with intermittent RLS, we recommend psychosocial-environmental interventions (e.g., scheduled walking, sleep hygiene), avoiding drugs that may worsen RLS (e.g., SSRIs), and avoiding factors that provoke symptoms (e.g., a sedentary lifestyle) (Hening 2007). Residents with daily RLS symptoms may need pharmacologic interventions. The pharmacologic treatment is iron supplementation if an iron deficiency is present and/or a small dose of a dopamine agonist (e.g., pramipexole, ropinirole). We do not recommend the use of levodopa to treat RLS, due to the risk of augmentation, in which the RLS symptoms begin appearing earlier during the day and involve new parts of the body with increasing severity. For severe or refractory cases of RLS, the clinician may consider prescribing gabapentin, carbamazepine, opiates, and clonazepam. For secondary RLS, the clinician should first treat the underlying illness, although dopamine agonists may also be useful. The prevalence of dental disease may be considerable in residents with RLS, because of a diminished salivary flow resulting from the medications used to treat RLS (Friedlander, Mahler, and Yagiela 2006). In this instance, educating the resident and the caregivers (family and professional) and using saliva substitutes and anticaries agents may be indicated.

Obstructive Sleep Apnea

Obstructive sleep apnea is a condition in which airflow during respiration is interrupted. This can occur because the airway collapses during sleep or because one's central nervous system signaling is impaired. These respiratory events can involve a complete cessation of airflow (apnea) or a partial reduction in airflow (hypopnea). Events are considered clinically significant when they last at least 10 seconds and occur 15 or more times per hour of sleep. This can lead to decreased oxygen saturation and an interruption of nighttime sleep. OSA is common and is an underrecognized cause of insomnia, daytime sleepiness, and cognitive impairment in LTC residents (Martin, Mory, and Alessi 2005). The clinician should suspect OSA in any overweight resident who has a history of snoring and/or daytime sleepiness. OSA can be screened by simple overnight oximetry. After a sleep study confirms the diagnosis, treatment with continuous positive airway pressure (CPAP) to deliver nasal oxygen at night may lessen cognitive impairments as well as improve sleep and reduce daytime sleepiness. The clinician may consider prescribing modafinil to treat excessive daytime sleepiness due to OSA.

Sleep Disorders in Individuals with Dementia

Nighttime behavioral abnormalities and sleep disturbances affect up to half of all individuals with dementia (Paniagua and Paniagua 2008). The severity of the disordered sleep pattern and the daytime napping tend to parallel that of the dementia as it progresses (Vitiello and Borson 2001; Boeve, Silber, and Ferman 2002). Sleep changes seen in dementia (especially AD) appear to be an exacerbation of normal age-related changes (e.g., an increased number of nighttime awakenings [sleep fragmentation], lowered sleep efficiency, increased daytime napping, difficulty initiating and maintaining sleep, a decrease in both slow-wave sleep and REM sleep, and a decrease in total sleep), which increase in magnitude with the progression and severity of the disease. Nighttime awakenings are usually more disturbing to the caregivers than daytime napping and early-morning awakening. Some residents with dementia may sleep up to 16 hours a day; others may sleep only two to four hours a night. The cycle of sleep and wakefulness may be reversed. Disruptive nighttime behaviors often develop in residents with moderate to severe dementia, including nocturnal wandering, agitation, and even combativeness. High rates of OSA may also contribute to daytime sleepiness and agitation in people with dementia (Ancoli-Israel et al. 1991; Gehrman et al. 2003). Other sleep disorders, such as periodic limb movement disorder and RLS, commonly occur in residents with dementia. REM sleep behavior disorder is not typically seen in AD, but it is characteristic of DLB, and its development may precede the onset of symptoms of dementia (Boeve, Silber, and Ferman 1998).

Sundowner syndrome refers to increased confusion after the sun goes down, often accompanied by agitation, in residents with dementia. It occurs mostly in the afternoon and evening. Sundowning is associated with a disruption of the circadian rhythm. In contrast with general agitation during other times of the day or night, sundowning correlates highly with rates of cognitive decline in affected patients. Depression may also manifest as sundowner syndrome, but other clinical signs of depression are usually present.

The treatment of sleep disturbances in residents with dementia follows the principles and recommendations described in a later section on the treatment of sleep disorders. Sundowner syndrome is managed primarily by using psychosocial-environmental interventions (e.g., providing short afternoon naps after lunch and calming activities in the late afternoon, controlling noise and traffic flow in the evening, frequently reassuring the resident, adjusting lighting in the environment to prevent the room from becoming dark in the evening). ChEIs can improve daytime alertness for residents with AD, DLB, or PDD, but it may contribute to insomnia.

Medication-Induced Sleep Disorder

All the medications listed in table 7.1 have the potential to cause insomnia. In addition, drugs used to treat dementia, such as ChEIs (donepezil, rivastigmine, galantamine), may cause insomnia. Some specific medications (e.g., sympathecomimetics, bronchodilators) can be particularly problematic when taken near bedtime. Also, the use of sedating medications during the daytime (e.g., benzodiazepines, certain antipsychotics [quetiapine, olanzapine], opiates, trazodone, certain antidepressants [mirtazapine, tricyclic antidepressants], mood stabilizers [valproate], anticonvulsants [gabapentin, pregabalin]) can contribute to a disrupted sleep/wake cycle by causing daytime drowsiness leading to daytime sleeping. Some medications used in the treatment of depression (e.g., SSRIs, venlafaxine, bupropion), Parkinson disease (e.g., levodopa, dopamine agonists [ropinirole, pramipexole, rotigotine]) can impair sleep and cause vivid dreams and nightmares. Sleep attacks (a sudden, irresistible onset of sleep without any awareness of falling asleep) have been described in individuals who are taking dopaminergic medication.

Medical Conditions Causing Sleep Problems

Pain (e.g., from arthritis), paresthesias, a nighttime cough, dyspnea, and gastroesophageal reflux are common causes of insomnia in LTC residents. Treating the underlying medical condition usually improves sleep. The clinician may consider prescribing the short-term use of sedative hypnotics (e.g., zolpidem) for insomnia due to certain medical conditions (e.g., UTI) until the medical condition is fully treated. Nocturia and urinary incontinence are common causes of insomnia and fragmented nighttime sleep. Nocturia is

typically seen in males with a prostate problem and in people who are taking diuretics (especially near bedtime), but it can be seen in any resident. The
treatment of nocturia involves a prompt voiding protocol in the daytime,
avoiding caffeine intake, and adjusting diuretics. Sleep disorders such as
insomnia (69%), OSA (23%), RLS (18%), and excessive daytime sleepiness
(12%) are highly prevalent in people with end-stage renal disease who are
undergoing dialysis therapy (Merlino et al. 2006). We recommend screening all LTC residents who are on dialysis for sleep disorders and instituting
the appropriate treatment. Due to a decrease in slow-wave deep sleep with
aging, even low-intensity pain or discomfort caused by the symptoms of a
medical condition, as well as other stimuli (e.g., a full bladder), may result in
disturbed sleep. Nightmares and excessive daytime sleepiness are seen in up
to 32 percent of the individuals with PD (Kumar, Bhatia, and Behari 2002).

Psychiatric Disorders Associated with Sleep Disturbance

Acute delirium of any etiology can have insomnia or excessive daytime sleepiness as a feature of its initial presentation. Nighttime agitation or insomnia
can also be a hallmark of untreated or undertreated (partially improved) depression. Nightmares are one of the key symptoms of PTSD, and RBD may
occasionally be seen in individuals with a history of PTSD. The treatment
of an underlying psychiatric disorder often improves sleep disorders, but the
short-term use of sedative hypnotics (e.g., zolpidem) to treat insomnia may
be necessary for residents with depressive or anxiety disorders.

Treatment of Sleep Disorders

Sleep problems in LTC residents require a broad approach, looking into
unique etiologies and consequences. A diagnosis of the underlying cause of
insomnia or daytime sleepiness is a necessary first step. This is done through
a comprehensive evaluation that includes complete medical, psychiatric, and
sleep assessments, in addition to a review of current medications (those given
by the LTC facility as well as medications [over-the-counter medications,
herbal remedies and supplements] taken by the resident [or given by a family
caregiver] without the knowledge of or documentation by LTC staff) and of
the timing of the doses. The clinician should also inquire about the resident's
daily use of caffeine, alcohol, or tobacco. Resident or caregiver reports or a
sleep diary for the preceding one to two weeks that includes the onset, duration, frequency, and severity of sleep disturbances, plus the total sleep time,
can be useful in determining a pattern of sleep disruption. For a resident who

had insomnia before admission to LTC or who is experiencing the onset of dementia, the clinician may also need to evaluate that person's lifestyle in relation to his or her sleeping habits (e.g., diet, the times for meals and snacks, the regularity of sleep and awakening times, the use of one's bed for activities other than sleep or sex [e.g., watching television, eating, reading], exercise late in the evenings).

The treatment of sleep disorders is a treatment of the cause (e.g., OSA or RLS). For residents with dementia who are suspected of having one of these disorders, the clinician may consider referral to a sleep disorders specialist (e.g., pulmonologist, neurologist) for an evaluation of OSA, RLS, or RBD through polysomnography, although this may not be practical for residents with severe dementia. For these residents, a tentative diagnosis after observation of their behavior at night and a trial of an appropriate treatment (e.g., CPAP for OSA, pramipexole or ropinirole for RLS, clonazepam for RBD) may be suitable. The clinician should consider prescribing modafinil to treat excessive daytime sleepiness in residents with dementia and OSA or narcolepsy.

Because sleep problems are the result of many underlying disturbances, any intervention needs to be multifaceted. Many researchers are investigating some basic questions: What is normal sleep in an LTC resident? What are the consequences of sleep disorders in this population? How do we evaluate sleep, and when and how do we intervene? Until further research clarifies the answers, we recommend the following approach. The first step is to review the resident's medications and discontinue any offending medication(s), or to reduce the dose (e.g., lowering the dose of memantine from 10 mg twice daily to once daily at bedtime [especially for residents with moderate to severe kidney insufficiency] may improve excessive daytime sleepiness) or replace it with a better alternative agent (e.g., replacing amitriptyline, which has high anticholinergic activity, with nortriptyline, which has much lower anticholinergic activity, may improve excessive daytime sleepiness). Changing the timing for administering some medications (e.g., changing the administration of donepezil from bedtime to the morning for residents who are experiencing insomnia and/or vivid dreams/nightmares) may improve sleep problems. However, in most situations more needs to be done, especially if the insomnia is chronic.

The next step is a multicomponent psychosocial-environmental intervention that includes daily exposure to at least 30 minutes of outdoor sunlight when feasible, daily exposure to at least 30 minutes of bright indoor light (using a bright light box if necessary) if outdoor sunlight exposure is not feasible (e.g., due to the weather), a standardized program to increase physical activity, the institution of a regular bedtime routine, and efforts to reduce nighttime noise and light in residents' rooms (Alessi et al. 2005; Martin, Mory, and Alessi 2007). Although this initially seems daunting for an already overburdened staff, conducting a mini-education session with the staff, enlisting the resident's family or volunteers when possible, and praising the staff for making an effort may provide successful outcomes. The clinician should also consider other psychosocial interventions for the treatment of insomnia (table 7.4). Some residents who experience sundowning may benefit from a short afternoon nap in addition to some of the psychosocial interventions mentioned above. If the resident is not disruptive at night and adequate supervision can be provided, the clinician should consider allowing the resident to sleep in the daytime and be awake at night.

The clinician may consider pharmacological interventions if psychosocial-environmental interventions fail and the potential benefits of the former outweigh the risk of their adverse effects. The use of sedative hypnotics and other pharmacological interventions (see table 7.4) has not been rigorously studied in LTC populations. The clinician may consider prescribing the short-term use of sedatives/hypnotics (e.g., zolpidem, zaleplon, or eszopiclone) for acute-onset insomnia related to a specific stressor (e.g., the death of a loved one) or while waiting for antidepressants to improve depressive or anxiety symptoms. The use of sedatives/hypnotics, especially for ambulatory residents, frail residents, and residents with severe cognitive impairment, should be minimized because of the risk of falls and cognitive impairment. Sedatives/hypnotics should be used for the shortest possible duration and follow the OBRA guidelines.

The clinician may consider prescribing ramelteon to treat insomnia. The clinician may also consider prescribing sedating antidepressants (e.g., low-dose mirtazapine or trazodone) to treat chronic insomnia in some residents (e.g., residents with low-grade depression or anxiety). The treatment of psychiatric disorders (e.g., antidepressants for a depressive disorder) may lessen a resident's insomnia without any need for sedatives/hypnotics. The clinician may consider prescribing the long-term use of sedatives/hypnotics for an occasional resident with chronic primary insomnia that is resistant to psychosocial-environmental interventions and sedating antidepressants. A combination of melatonin given at night and bright light treatment in the daytime may also help manage a disturbance in circadian rhythms for resi-

TABLE 7.4
Interventions for the treatment of insomnia in long-term care residents

---

Dietary

Restrict the intake of caffeine and chocolate, particularly in the evening.

Avoid a heavy meal late at night

Recommend a light snack (e.g., a glass of milk, crackers) if nighttime awakenings are caused by hunger

Avoid fluid intake in the evening by residents with nocturia and encourage maximum bladder emptying before retiring

Environmental

Increase exposure to natural light in the daytime

Increase exposure to indoor light in the daytime on cloudy, rainy, and snowy days

Recommend bright-light therapy

Ensure optimal room temperature and humidity

Reduce nighttime noise and nighttime exposure to bright light (using low-intensity nightlights for residents who have nightmares and/or other fears may promote sleep and increase safety during nighttime awakenings for toileting, etc.)

Change the room if conflict with a roommate or the location of the room is an issue

Activity-oriented

Limit daytime napping to a short period in the morning or early afternoon

Limit the time spent in bed in the daytime

Increase physical activity in the daytime (e.g., a regular exercise program)

Increase meaningful activity and socialization in the daytime

Employ a warm bath in the evening

Avoid excessive stimulation and exercise after dinnertime

Sleep hygiene

Recommend regular sleeping and waking times and a structured bedtime routine

Recommend calming bedtime rituals (e.g., soothing music, reading or listening to audio recordings of nonfiction books [such as spiritual and religious books])

Use one's bed for sleep and sexual activity (rather than watching television, eating, or reading)

Staff-oriented

Educate and train staff regarding the evaluation and treatment of insomnia and other sleep disorders

Have staff mediate differences between roommates (e.g., one resident wanting to watch television late at night, disturbing the roommate who wants to go to sleep early) or find a better pairing for residents living in one room

Minimize staff interruptions of a resident's sleep

Use massage therapy (e.g., back rubs and hand massages)

Use aromatherapy

Specific interventions for residents who are cognitively intact

Relaxation training

Cognitive behavior therapy

Stimulus control therapy

Sleep restriction therapy

Pharmacological

If a medication is suspected of causing or contributing to insomnia, discontinue the offending agent, reduce the dose, change the timing, or replace the medication with a better alternative

Restrict the use of alcohol and tobacco, particularly in the evening

Prescribe sedative hypnotics (e.g., zolpidem, zaleplon, eszopiclone)

Prescribe antidepressants with sedating properties (e.g., trazodone, mirtazapine) to treat insomnia in residents with depression

Prescribe atypical antipsychotics with sedating properties (e.g., quetiapine) to treat insomnia in residents with severe psychotic symptoms

continued

TABLE 7.4 *continued*

Prescribe a pharmacological treatment for underlying medical conditions (e.g., analgesics for the treatment of pain, continuous positive airway pressure for obstructive sleep apnea, dopamine agonists for restless leg syndrome, clonazepam for REM sleep behavior disorder, antibiotics for infection)

Prescribe other medications (e.g., ramelteon, melatonin, chamomile tea, valerian herbal remedies)

dents with dementia (Dowling et al. 2007). We do not recommend tricyclic antidepressants, antihistaminic agents (e.g., diphenhydramine), certain sedative hypnotics (e.g., triazolam, barbiturates, chloral hydrate), and antipsychotic medications for treating LTC residents with insomnia, due to the high risk of adverse effects, such as falls, daytime sedation, and a decline in cognition and functioning. The clinician may also consider prescribing modafinil or methylphenidate for some residents with dementia and excessive daytime sleepiness, especially if they also have OSA (Boeve, Silber, and Ferman 2002). OSA is a relative contraindication to the use of benzodiazepines and other agents that suppress respiratory drive.

Conclusion

Anxiety disorders and sleep disorders are prevalent in long-term care populations and are associated with significant morbidity and increased mortality. We recommend a thorough evaluation of all residents with significant anxiety and/or sleep disorders to identify one or more etiological factors. A variety of psychosocial and pharmacological interventions are available to treat anxiety and sleep disorders and thereby improve the resident's (and the caregiver's) quality of life.

CHAPTER 8

Personality Disorders, Somatoform Disorders, Substance Use Disorders, and Other Psychiatric Disorders

In the differential diagnosis of behavioral and psychological symptoms in long-term care populations (including comorbidity with more prevalent psychiatric disorders [e.g., dementia, depression, and anxiety disorders]), psychiatric disorders that clinicians need to consider include personality disorders, somatoform disorders, substance use disorders, impulse control disorders, and dissociative disorders.

Personality Disorders

Personality disorders are deeply ingrained, maladaptive patterns of behavior. A person is diagnosed with a personality disorder if he or she has shown an enduring pattern of inner experience and behavior involving cognition (i.e., ways of perceiving and interpreting oneself, other people, and events), affectivity (i.e., emotional responses), interpersonal functioning, and impulse control that is maladaptive, inflexible, and pervasive across a broad range of personal and social situations. The initial signs of personality disorders can be recognized in adolescence or earlier, and symptoms usually persist into late life. If personality is defined by an individual's adaptive style, then over time one's personality changes profoundly (Vaillant 2002). The prevalence of personality disorders in elderly people is essentially equivalent to that of younger groups, and approximates 10 percent (Agronin and Maletta 2000). Some 10 to 20 percent of older adults with MDD also have a personality disorder. An even larger percentage of older adults with chronic depression also have a personality disorder (Morse and Lynch 2000). Obsessive-compulsive personality disorders, dependent personality disorders, and mixed personality disorders (personality disorders with more than one type of personality trait) are the most frequently diagnosed personality disorders in older adults who are receiving treatment at mental health clinics (Abrams and Sadavoy 2004). Antisocial and borderline personality disorders may become less of a problem in late life, as symptoms such as impulsivity and sociopathic behaviors decrease with age (Black, Baumgard, and Bell 1995; Seidlitz 2001). A clue to the existence of a personality disorder in an LTC environment is when a resident is on his or her fifth roommate (i.e., cannot get along with anyone).

Preexisting personality disorders need to be differentiated from personality changes due to dementia or a general medical condition (e.g., a stroke, a brain tumor), where a persistent personality disturbance means a change from the individual's previous characteristic personality. Damage to the frontal lobes is the most common cause of such a change. Changes in personality due to dementia and a general medical condition include irritability, anger, aggression, and impulse control problems, as well as becoming apathetic, listless, mean or cruel, unreasonable, emotionally cold (lack of empathy, insensitive), averse to company, overly cautious, childish, and emotionally labile. Dementia may exacerbate a preexisting personality disorder, resulting in severe behavioral disturbances. Frontotemporal dementias may present with personality changes (especially social disinhibition) years before any cognitive impairment is evident. Apathy and passivity are common personality problems that develop in people with PDD or DLB.

Personality disorders may predispose an individual to anxiety and/or mood disorders and may complicate the course and treatment of the latter. Personality disorders in older adults are associated with a poor or partial response to antidepressants, refusal of or noncompliance with medical care, increased disability, disruption of interpersonal relationships, and suicidal behavior (especially with a narcissistic personality). Despite challenges, personality disorders are treatable psychiatric conditions, and treatment may improve the resident's quality of life and reduce the family's and professional caregiver's stress. Table 8.1 lists some strategies to help residents with personality problems. The treatment of personality disorders involves educating the staff and family regarding the diagnosis (so that their expectation that the resident will change is lowered), treating the symptoms (e.g., depression, anxiety, hostility) that are part of personality disorders, and treating any superimposed comorbidity (e.g., mood disorder, anxiety disorder, alcohol or drug use disorder). Residents with personality disorders may generate strong negative emotions in the staff and may cause the staff to split (some staff taking the side of the resident and others strongly opposing the resident). Despite such challenges, treatment should be respectful and relevant to the resident in order to produce relief of the person's symptoms, allow interdependence, accommodate change, and support healthy narcissism. Residents with personality disorders often have a history of a traumatic and difficult childhood, and awareness of such a history may enable the staff to have compassion for the resident despite his or her hostile behavior.

CLINICAL CASE Ms. L was a 64-year-old woman admitted to a nursing home for rehabilitation after a prolonged (three-month) hospital stay for nephrectomy and postnephrectomy complications (infection, bleeding, and delirium with agitation). Ms. L was taking sertraline 100 mg daily for depression. A psychiatrist was consulted to help manage Ms. L's "hostile and aggressive" behavior toward the staff. The staff expressed anger and resentment at having to provide personal care for Ms. L because of her persistent name-calling, as well as her yelling at the staff and demeaning them. Some staff members had started to call in sick if they found out that they had to care for Ms. L, and some flatly refused to care for her.

The psychiatrist found Ms. L to be an intelligent and cognitively intact person who was quick to take offense but also willing to accept help from "competent" professionals. Ms. L repeatedly expressed a wish to "get out of this miserable place." The psychiatrist then met with the staff to explain that Ms. L had been experiencing severe depression with an underlying long-standing personality disorder. Ms. L had confided to the psychiatrist that she had been severely physically and emotionally abused as a child and had had three "horrible" marriages. Ms. L had told the psychiatrist that "I hate everyone" and that she liked animals more than people; she had a number of pets that she took care of herself, and she also helped the humane society care for sick pets.

The psychiatrist increased the dose of sertraline from 100 to 150 mg. He also encouraged the staff to set firm limits but to express to Ms. L that her behavior prevented the staff from wanting to care for her. The psychiatrist gently helped Ms. L understand that her hostile behavior put her at risk of a prolonged stay in the nursing home, because the staff would be less likely to meet her needs. Ms. L agreed to be taken to an outpatient clinic for once-a-week counseling with a social worker. Over the next few

TABLE 8.1
Strategies to help residents with personality problems

General

Form a therapeutic alliance (a trusting, nonjudgmental, and supportive relationship)

Seek to understand the resident and not manipulate or control him or her

Develop a regard for the entire personality that we are trying to heal

Enhance the resident's social support (through family meetings, the help of volunteers and chaplains, etc.)

Psychological strategies for cognitively intact residents

A resident who is bitter (overcritical, blaming others, and harsh) may be helped by efforts to show that no one is trying to take advantage of him or her and that being overcritical may push the staff away

A resident who is acquiescent (blaming self, not assertive, overly trusting) may be helped to slowly become assertive (by practicing with the staff, a counselor, the psychiatrist) and needs to be reassured that one can be assertive without being harsh

A resident who is overanxious (brooding, pessimistic) may be helped by mind-body interventions (relaxation, breathing, and mindfulness exercises) and needs to be reassured that worrying less does not mean being careless

A resident who is hedonistic (careless, chaotic, never plans) may be helped to realize the potential benefits of thinking about a problem and solving it, as well as the costs of solving any difficulty by seeking pleasure (risk of injury, poorer health)

A resident who is fiercely independent (avoiding intimacy, avoiding help from family and friends) may be helped with a reassurance that one can be close to others without being engulfed or controlled

A resident who is overly dependent (always seeking nurturance from others) may be helped by addressing his or her fears of abandonment

An empathic manner can enhance the resident's capacity for balanced reflection about his or her own behaviors and the potential consequences of them

Pharmacological strategies

Antidepressants for depressive symptoms and anxiety symptoms

Mood stabilizers for symptoms of severe impulse dyscontrol

Low-dose atypical antipsychotics for transient but disabling psychotic symptoms

Staff education regarding relevant issues

Origin(s) of the personality disorder (e.g., traumatic childhood, neurological insult)

Ways to manage strong negative emotions and the splitting (i.e., taking sides for or against the resident) involved in caring for some residents with personality disorders, and to realize the potential for abuse (typically through neglect) if negative emotions are not recognized and managed

Importance of identifying the emotional strengths and resilience that all residents have, but which are not being recognized and can be tapped into, to improve the residents' psychosocial well-being

Importance of compassion and limit-setting in caring for all residents, especially for residents with personality disorders

Importance of staff rotation to avoid staff burnout in caring for residents with personality disorders, because caring for these residents can be emotionally draining

Vigilance for the pitfall of making some residents with personality disorders overly dependent or reliant on or emotionally close to the staff, as this may meet the emotional needs of the staff but may harm the resident in the long run weeks, the frequency and intensity of Ms. L's hostile comments decreased, the staff were able to meet more of her needs, and she made significant progress in physical therapy.

TEACHING POINTS Depressive disorders are common in people with a personality disorder (especially if the individual has relatively intact cognition) and are often undertreated. Also, a resident with a personality disorder generates strong negative feelings in others that may cause the staff to be less likely to meet the resident's needs. Interventions (e.g., antidepressants, staff education, counseling for the patient) should be designed to make at least a modest change in behavior possible (e.g., reduced namecalling by the resident toward the staff) to achieve the desired result (e.g., increased likelihood that the staff will be able to meet the resident's needs). Psychotherapy is useful in the management of cognitively intact residents with personality disorders.

Somatoform Disorders

Somatoform disorders are the repeated presentation of physical symptoms with persistent requests for medical investigations, in spite of negative findings and reassurances by health care providers that the symptoms have no physical basis. If any physical disorders are present, they are insufficient to explain the severity of the person's symptoms or distress. Somatization is not a normal part of aging. The trait of neuroticism, defined in part as the tendency to experience negative emotions, is a better predictor of somatic complaints than age. The majority of residents who have multiple physical complaints without an identifiable cause have depression and/or anxiety disorders. Comorbid somatization and depression are highly associated with suicide (Agronin 2004). A learned role of often complaining of sickness in childhood may predispose an individual to somatoform disorders later in life. Gender, education, ethnicity, and social class also influence somatoform disorders. In some residents, somatoform disorders may reflect aging-associated conflicts, such as fears of irrelevance and abandonment, sexual decline, and a repressed expression of helplessness and anger. Individuals with somatoform disorders may not express anger easily. Personality characteristics, such as alexithymia (the impaired ability to describe emotions), are also frequently seen with somatoform disorders. Hypochondriasis is characterized by a preoccupation with the belief that one has a serious illness, and it is frequently comorbid in older adults with severe depression (Rabinowitz, Hirdes, and Desjardins 2006). Residents with somatoform disorders (e.g., hypochondriasis) typically have a long-standing history of these disorders. The clinician should consider chronic pain in elderly people to be a sign of depression until proven otherwise.

The most important consideration in the treatment of any resident suspected of having somatoform disorders is to aggressively treat that person's comorbid anxiety and depression. Once a diagnosis of somatoform disorder is made (after a comprehensive psychiatric evaluation and the necessary medical testing), the clinician should forge a strong therapeutic alliance with the resident and avoid unnecessary or excessive testing to clarify the etiology of multiple somatic complaints. It is equally important to avoid excessive medical and surgical procedures to treat somatic symptoms in residents with somatoform disorders.

Substance Use Disorders

Clinical syndromes can occur as a result of using substances that act on the central nervous system (e.g., alcohol, cocaine, amphetamines, opiates, cannabis, caffeine). Substance use disorders (substance abuse and substance dependence) are diagnosed when an individual has a history of using the substance in excessive amounts, difficulty cutting back, and an impairment in his or her interpersonal and occupational functioning due to substance use. Men are at greater risk of substance use disorders than women. Substance use and abuse in later life is a growing public health issue. The prevalence rates of alcohol and substance abuse are lower in older adults than in younger adults. However, the prevalence of substance use disorders may be underestimated because of the limited applicability of DSM-IV-TR criteria for the geriatric population (Jeste et al. 1999). Currently, the prevalence of alcohol and illicit drug use disorders in LTC populations is low (Llorente, Oslin, and Malphurs 2006), but significantly higher rates of illicit drug and alcohol use and related mental illness are expected in future LTC residents because of the higher prevalence of these disorders in the baby boom generation. Substance use and abuse in LTC populations can result in accelerated cognitive and functional declines, falls and injuries, a lack of response to treatments for depression, sleep and anxiety disorders, harmful drug interactions, liver disease, cardiovascular disease, and increased mortality. Thus treatment of substance use and abuse is important to improve the psychosocial well-being of LTC residents.

Problems related to alcohol use are by far the largest class of substance use and abuse problems seen in older adults today. The one-year prevalence rate for alcohol abuse and dependence is 2.75 percent for elderly men and 0.51 percent for elderly women; prevalence rates are higher, however, in primary care settings, where at-risk drinking has been estimated to be 5 to 15 percent (Oslin 2005). The prevalence of a lifetime history of alcohol abuse or dependence is 1.5 times greater among older adults with dementia than among those with no cognitive impairment (George 1991). Alcohol problems are underrecognized in older men and women. Also, the prevalence of alcohol problems in older women may be increasing (Atkinson 2004). Residents with a past history of alcohol abuse or dependence have a high comorbidity of sleep disorders, depression, and anxiety disorders. A diagnosis of substance use disorders is best made through the use of interviews with the patient, the family, and caregivers. The geriatric version of the Michigan Alcoholism Screening Test, a physical examination, and laboratory tests may also be helpful in clarifying the diagnosis. Residents with a current or past history of alcohol use disorder have a high prevalence of comorbid tobacco use, nicotine dependence, and affective disorders. The clinician should routinely inquire about these comorbidities during the assessment and then treat them if present. Evening or nightly cocktail hours at LTC facilities (a recent trend) need to be supervised, and some residents should be limited to nonalcoholic drinks.

Many alcohol drinkers maintain steady consumption levels into later life. At-risk drinking may go unrecognized, because health care providers may not realize that the allowable intake for an elderly adult is different from that for a middle-aged adult. Older adults, especially those with cognitive impairments, have an increased sensitivity to alcohol. The National Institute on Alcohol Abuse and Alcoholism and the Center for Substance Abuse Treatment recommend that individuals aged 65 or older consume no more than one standard drink (one unit of alcohol or 8 grams of ethanol) per day or seven standard drinks per week; no more than two standard drinks on any drinking day; and less than one standard drink per day for women (National Institute on Alcohol Abuse and Alcoholism 1995; Oslin 2005). The standard definition of a unit of alcohol is one that contains 8 grams of ethanol or 10 ml by volume. One unit is contained in a 12-ounce bottle of beer, one 4-ounce glass of wine, 4 ounces of liqueur, or 1.5 ounces (a shot) of liquor (e.g., whiskey, vodka, rum, gin).

The consumption of one to two standard alcoholic drinks per day may be prevalent in LTC populations, and its negative health consequences are underrecognized. Therefore, the clinician should screen all residents for alcohol consumption and related problems. Although such consumption does not constitute abuse or dependence, the clinician should discourage it in residents with cognitive impairment and those with behavioral and psychological symptoms. Residents and their families should be educated regarding sensible drinking guidelines and what comprises a unit of alcohol. Each visit to a resident who consumes alcohol regularly can be an opportunity for providing such education. Polypharmacy is highly prevalent among LTC populations, and alcohol reacts negatively with more than 100 prescription and over-the-counter medications, as well as with many herbals and supplements. Therefore, interactions between alcohol and medications are possible among LTC residents who drink even one or two drinks regularly.

It is important to acknowledge issues of stigma and ambivalence, as well as cultural issues that may affect the resident's feelings about drinking behaviors and treatment. It is equally important to address negative health consequences in a consistent but nonjudgmental manner. The treatment of problems caused by alcohol use is usually psychosocial (e.g., educating the resident and family; replacing alcoholic drinks with nonalcoholic drinks that are similar in taste). Drugs approved for the treatment of alcohol dependence include disulfiram, naltrexone, and acamprosate. These drugs have not been well studied in LTC populations, so the clinician should prescribe them cautiously for this cohort, because of a significant risk of adverse effects due to high medical comorbidity. Acamprosate is excreted unchanged by the kidneys, and significant reductions in the dosage are required for residents with chronic renal insufficiency and alcohol dependence.

Many residents have chronically used benzodiazepines (daily use for more than a year, typically for several years or even decades). More than 10 percent of the older adults living in the community take benzodiazepines on a regular basis (Oslin 2005). They usually do not have a history of taking more than the prescribed doses or of using other substances (e.g., alcohol or street drugs), and they have a history of regularly seeing a physician (Llorente, Oslin, and Malphurs 2006). Older adults who chronically use benzodiazepines have a high prevalence of comorbid anxiety disorders (e.g., generalized anxiety disorder and/or panic disorder) and sleep disorders (chronic insomnia). Elderly people who are benzodiazepine-dependent often develop withdrawal symptoms, anxiety, sleeplessness, and agitation, conditions that are frequently overlooked or attributed to other medical illnesses. The continued use of benzodiazepines in an LTC setting may pose a high risk of falls and injuries (e.g., a hip fracture), cognitive impairments, and functional declines.

Most residents tolerate a dose reduction without any worsening of their anxiety symptoms or sleep impairments, and they may even show cognitive and functional improvements. Some residents may be able to be weaned off benzodiazepines completely by a slow tapering off over weeks to months.

The use and abuse of nicotine (typically cigarette smoking, but also chewable tobacco and snuff), like alcohol use, is underrecognized and undertreated in LTC populations. Smoking by older adults is associated with many deleterious health outcomes (e.g., chronic obstructive pulmonary disease, cardiovascular disease, a variety of cancers, an abdominal aortic aneurysm, peripheral arterial disease, nicotine-drug interactions, and accelerated cognitive and functional decline). Chronic smoking is associated with the induction of cytochrome P450 1A2 liver enzymes, which in turn can lower the levels of drugs metabolized by this enzyme system (e.g., clozapine, olanzapine, fluvoxamine). Like hospitals, almost all LTC facilities do not allow smoking in the facility, although some have arrangements for smoking outdoors. Psychosocial-environmental treatment strategies for nicotine use and abuse are similar to those for alcohol use and abuse. Pharmacological treatment strategies, such as nicotine patches, varenicline, nicotine gum, and inhalers, have not been well studied in LTC populations, so the clinician should prescribe them judiciously. The use of varenicline is associated with a small increased risk of suicidality; therefore the clinician should avoid prescribing it for residents who are at risk of suicide.

Some residents may be allowed the continued use of small amounts of alcohol and/or nicotine for daily consumption if, after a comprehensive assessment, the use of these substances is deemed critical for the resident's quality of life and the resident and family have been educated about the potential risks of a continued use of these substances.

Impulse-Control Disorders

This group of disorders is characterized by the failure to resist an impulse, a drive, or a temptation to perform some act that is harmful to oneself or to another. Impulse-control disorders—such as kleptomania (the inability to resist impulses to steal objects that are not needed for personal use or for their monetary value), pathological gambling (the inability to resist gambling or placing a bet), trichotillomania (an irresistible urge to pull one's own hair), intermittent explosive disorder (irresistible aggressive impulses), pyromania (deliberately setting fires), and compulsive buying (an irresistible urge to spend money on unnecessary items)—are uncommon in LTC residents.

Residents with these impulse-control disorders usually have a history of such behaviors for decades before their admission to an LTC facility. Most recently emergent impulse-control disorders in residents are secondary to dementing illnesses (e.g., frontotemporal dementia) and other causes of frontal lobe damage (e.g., a stroke, a head injury), and they manifest as impulsive verbal or physical aggression or impulsive sexually inappropriate behavior. Sexual impulse-control disorders are prevalent in LTC populations (see chapter 3). The treatment of impulse-control disorders involves psychosocial-environmental interventions (educating the staff about a lack of impulse control in residents with frontal lobe damage) and, in persistent and severe cases, pharmacological intervention (e.g., a trial of SSRIs, valproate).

Dissociative Disorders

Individuals with a dissociative disorder present with episodes during which they are unable to recall important personal information. These episodes of forgetfulness are too extensive to be explained by ordinary forgetfulness and can be easily differentiated from late-life cognitive disorders (e.g., dementia), as in the latter the forgetfulness is pervasive, persistent, and, in the majority of cases, irreversible. Residents with a dissociative disorder have a past history of such episodes, dating back for decades before admission to LTC, and they often have a history of childhood abuse. Dissociative disorders are rare in LTC populations, and in most situations an episode of amnesia regarding important personal information is due to an identifiable physical (e.g., hypoglycemia) or neurological condition (e.g., seizure).

Conclusion

Although dementia, mood and psychotic disorders, anxiety disorders, and sleep disorders are the most prevalent psychiatric disorders in long-term care populations, they are often comorbid with a variety of conditions, such as personality disorders, somatoform disorders, substance use disorders, and, to a smaller extent, impulse-control disorders and dissociative disorders. The early detection and treatment of these comorbid conditions is crucial to successful outcomes in the treatment of dementia, depression, anxiety, psychosis, and sleep disorders.

CHAPTER 9

Psychiatric Aspects of Nutritional Disorders, Frailty, and Failure to Thrive

Nutritional disorders, frailty, and failure to thrive are highly prevalent medical conditions in long-term care populations, and their prevalence is even higher in LTC populations with psychiatric disorders (e.g., dementia, depression, or delirium) (Robertson and Montagnini 2004; P. Thomas et al. 2004; Morley et al. 2006). Fortunately, these disorders are eminently treatable.

Psychiatric Aspects of Nutritional Disorders

In an elderly population, healthy dietary patterns are related to decreased total mortality and lower disease-specific mortality. While poor nutrition is not a natural concomitant of aging, older adults who experience several concurrent diseases are at higher risk of undernutrition or malnutrition. Within the overall older cohort, LTC populations are more likely to consume an unbalanced diet (P. Thomas et al. 2004). Under- or malnutrition can be defined as any insufficient dietary intake of essential nutrients (macronutrients [carbohydrates, fat, protein], micronutrients [vitamins, minerals], and fluid), and it is typically multifactorial in its etiology (Morley 2001; Amella 2004). Under- or malnutrition is a common, multidimensional, frequently undetected problem for approximately two out of every five nursing home residents, negatively influencing their health and quality of life (Kayser-Jones 2000). Obesity is the result of a form of malnutrition, with a caloric intake that exceeds energy expenditures. The consequences of malnutrition can be devastating and fatal (table 9.1).

Unintentional Weight Loss

Unintentional weight loss is prevalent in LTC populations. A low energy intake goes together with an insufficient supply of micronutrients. Elderly people in LTC tend to have both a lower energy intake—mainly due to a lower intake of fat—and a lower protein intake. In older adults, nearly all of their higher mortality risk is due to weight loss, independent of a person's initial body weight. Although depression is the most common cause of unintentional weight loss in LTC residents, the clinician should thoroughly evaluate residents with this problem to identify other causes (table 9.2).

Weight loss may be due to dehydration. Rapid and acute weight loss in excess of 3 percent of one's baseline body weight is most likely due to reduced total body water from dehydration. Residents with certain medical conditions (e.g., severe COPD, congestive heart failure) may be unable to consume a large meal at one sitting and may do better with multiple small meals. The clinician should use the Mini Nutritional Assessment, or MNA (www.mna-elderly.com), to assess both residents who are at risk of weight loss (have a poor appetite, feel full after eating only a small amount, report that the food tastes bad, eat one or less than one meal a day) and residents who already have weight loss, as well as to treat any reversible causes of weight loss (Vellas et al. 2006). Sarcopenia (excessive age-related muscle loss), a common cause

TABLE 9.1
Potential complications and consequences of malnutrition

Delirium (due to hypoglycemia, dehydration, electrolyte imbalance, drug toxicity from a reduction in serum protein binding, etc.)

Cognitive impairments

Functional impairments

Frailty

Failure to thrive

Acute renal failure

Falls and injuries (e.g., a hip fracture, a subdural hematoma)

Pressure ulcers, or *decubitii*

A compromised immune system leading to recurrent infections (e.g., urinary tract infections, pneumonia) and poor wound healing

Vitamin deficiency and its complications (e.g., dementia, peripheral neuropathy, depression)

Anemia

Electrolyte imbalance and its complications (e.g., seizure)

Oral ulcers

Sarcopenia (severe loss of muscle mass)

Exacerbation of chronic medical illnesses (e.g., diabetes, chronic kidney disease, osteoporosis)

Death

TABLE 9.2
Common causes of anorexia and weight loss in long-term care residents

Age-related changes in taste, smell, thirst recognition, and satiation

Environmental causes
Inadequate assistance with feeding; poor mealtime environment
Lack of opportunities for the resident to express satisfaction or dissatisfaction with the quality of the food or with the quality of care and the environment surrounding mealtimes
Trouble getting the meals ready on time
Interpersonal aspects of food service and the meal environment (e.g., being returned to one's room immediately after a meal; a lack of prompt help for toileting issues during meals, which may reduce the resident's willingness to consume adequate amounts of food and fluid)
Financial constraints of the long-term care facility

Quality of food issues
Therapeutic diets (e.g., low salt, low cholesterol, diabetic diet)
Poor-quality food (e.g., is too mushy, lacks variety, everything is cooked the same way, lacks flavor)
Food not in keeping with the resident's personal, cultural, or religious background

Psychiatric disorders
Alzheimer disease and other dementias
Dementia-related behaviors (e.g., apathy, wandering, pacing)
Depression
Psychotic disorders
Anxiety disorders

Dehydration

Medications: digitalis, amiodarone, cholinesterase inhibitors, stimulants, topiramate, selective serotonin reuptake inhibitors, venlafaxine, duloxetine, bupropion, theophylline, cimetidine, calcium, digoxin, polypharmacy, bad taste of medications (e.g., residents who take medications crushed)

Oral problems: ill-fitting dentures, loss of teeth, lesions in the mouth, gingival or periodontal disease

Gastrointestinal problems: swallowing problems (dysphagia), gallbladder problems (such as gallstones, cholecystitis), protein-wasting enteropathy and malabsorption syndromes

Sarcopenia (severe loss of muscle mass)

Cancer

Endocrine disorders: hypothyroidism, hyperthyroidism, hypercalcemia, hypoadrenalism

Chronic infections: tuberculosis, AIDS

End-organ failure: heart failure (cardiac cachexia), kidney failure, severe chronic obstructive pulmonary disease

Immobility

Tremors, especially affecting the dominant hand

Rheumatoid arthritis

Recent hospitalization or multiple hospitalizations in the recent past

Iatrogenic (prescription medications)

of weight loss in LTC populations, may be due to testosterone deficiency, peripheral vascular disease, inadequate protein intake, and a lack of physical activity. The clinician should address a loss of appetite, poor positioning while eating, and oral status concerns. Table 9.3 lists various tests and measurements we recommend for screening and assessing nutritional disorders and monitoring the response to treatment. We recommend a routine screening of all residents for nutritional disorders at the time of admission and then periodically (quarterly if possible) thereafter.

TABLE 9.3
Tests and measurements to assess various nutritional disorders

Test/Measurement	Reason
Body weight (measured frequently)	Monitor weight loss or gain
Body mass index	Diagnose obesity
Serum total protein, prealbumin, albumin	Low levels suggest undernutrition
Serum B_{12} and folate levels	Assess B_{12} and folate deficiencies
Serum calcium and vitamin D levels	Assess calcium and vitamin D deficiencies
Serum cholesterol level	Low levels suggest undernutrition
Serum blood urea nitrogen and creatinine	Assess for dehydration
Serum sodium and potassium	Assess for electrolyte imbalance
FoodEx-LTC questionnaire	Assess resident's satisfaction with meals
Mini Nutritional Assessment	Identify reversible causes of weight loss

The clinician should be aware that medical record documentation over-estimates the quality of care, assistance with feeding, supplements offered, and oral intake of meals. Thus it is important to train staff to provide better assistance with feeding, make keener observations, and have better documentation of food and fluid intake. Some of the key areas for nutritional assessment include, but are not limited to, an assessment of alertness; cognitive and functional impairments; the condition of the teeth and oral health; the ability to see, hear, and follow instructions; the ability to speak clearly; the presence or absence of saliva in the mouth; the ability to seal one's lips and move one's tongue in a coordinated way; and the ability to cough.

The treatment of unintentional weight loss is a treatment of all possible treatable causes, identified with the help of an interdisciplinary team (table 9.4). An interdisciplinary team ideally involves the resident, the family, the physician, physician extenders, nurses and nurses aides, registered dieticians, pharmacists (to review medications causing nutritional disorders), the housekeeping staff (to encourage food and fluid intake between meals), and social workers (to address psychosocial issues). Best practice requires an individualized care plan with the dual objectives of providing adequate food and fluid intake and maintaining the resident's self-feeding abilities to the extent possible (Amella 2004). A resident's eating and feeding behaviors may change during an acute illness or with the progression of dementia or other disease(s), requiring the staff to assess the plan regularly and adjust it as needed.

The amount and quality of feeding assistance provided to residents is one of the most powerful determinants of daily food and fluid intake. Instituting a staff training program on feeding skills increases the eating time for residents with dementia. The clinician should note the staffing levels during feeding

TABLE 9.4
Strategies to increase nutrient intake

Assess nutritional status using an interdisciplinary approach

Discontinue medications that may cause anorexia and/or unintentional weight loss

Institute person-centered care practices, such as
  Provide individualized schedules
  Provide preferred food and fluids
  Provide meals at preferred times
  Provide food in the preferred amount
  Provide meals in the preferred place
  Provide meals at the preferred frequency
  Provide ethnic food options

Increase daily physical activity

Provide hand feeding when necessary

Increase feeding assistance time (with the help of feeding assistants, family, and/or volunteers)

Enhance the flavor of foods

Liberalize a diet prescription

Improve meal ambience

Provide verbal cuing (e.g., "pick up your spoon," "take a bite," "chew," "swallow"), simulate eating
  motions so that the resident can imitate them, and provide frequent verbal encouragement

Provide a hand-over-hand technique as appropriate to initiate and guide self-feeding

Encourage social interactions during meals

Provide soothing music during mealtimes

Increase lighting at the meal location

Help the resident sit in a comfortable chair (not a wheelchair) with good posture, and have the staff
  member sit at the resident's eye level to provide assistance as necessary

Use bright and contrasting colors for tableware and placemats

Reduce distractions (turn off the television; avoid interruptions and people entering the dining room)

Ensure that the resident has dentures and/or eyeglasses as needed and can see and reach the food
  plate or tray

Simplify the meal presentation; serve one food item at a time if necessary; remove unnecessary
  utensils as appropriate

Provide finger foods if the resident experiences difficulty managing eating utensils

Remove items that should not be eaten and hot items that may be spilled

Assess and manage medical and psychiatric conditions that may cause anorexia and/or unintentional
  weight loss (e.g., depression, pain)

Provide nutritional supplements between meals

Prescribe vitamin and mineral supplements (e.g., vitamin B_{12}, folate, thiamine, vitamin D, calcium)

Use specialized utensils (weighted spoon, rocker-bottom knife, side-cutter fork) and other assistive
  devices as recommended by an occupational therapy evaluation

Obtain the routine input of registered dieticians for residents with nutritional problems as well as for
  facility-wide directives to improve the nutritional status of all residents

Refer the resident to a speech therapist for suspected dysphagia

Provide a separate feeding area for disruptive residents

Provide smaller, more frequent meals for certain residents (e.g., residents with a lifetime history of
  multiple small meals, residents with severe chronic obstructive pulmonary disease)

Consider prescribing appetite stimulants as appropriate (e.g., cannabinoids [dronabinol, marinol,
  nabilone], megestrol)

continued

TABLE 9.4 *continued*

Consider prescribing anabolic steroids as appropriate (e.g., nandrolone [for cachectic residents with AIDS], oxandrolone [for weight loss in residents with an HIV infection, cachectic residents with chronic obstructive pulmonary disease, and residents with cancer and weight loss or delayed wound healing)

Consider prescribing testosterone as appropriate (for male residents with a testosterone deficiency and malnourishment)

Consider prescribing a growth hormone as appropriate

Consider prescribing antidepressants (especially mirtazapine) for residents with depression and anorexia and/or unintentional weight loss

Institute appropriate palliative care and provide referral to a hospice for residents who are in the terminal stages of dementia or another progressive disease

---

time. Expert panels recommend a ratio of five residents to one nurse aide during mealtimes (Rahman and Simmons 2005). Staffing below a 5–7:1 level (one staff member for five to seven residents) may require targeting residents who are most in need or assigning nonnursing staff for some daily mealtime tasks. Along with adequate staffing, an increase in the feeding assistance time (from 10 minutes to 30 minutes), verbal cuing, and social interaction can dramatically improve the residents' oral intake of food and fluids. Staff or volunteers should offer feeding assistance to groups of three to four residents three times per day between meals (10 a.m., 2 p.m., 7 p.m.) for about 15–20 minutes per snack period.

Verbally prompting residents to drink on four to eight occasions between meals, offering residents their beverages of choice, offering an enhanced between-meal snack program with appropriate feeding assistance, and actively encouraging residents to eat and drink several times a day are some of the interventions we recommend to prevent and treat dehydration and weight loss. The staff should consider family-style meals, especially for residents who do not have dementia. Encouraging residents to take extra food at mealtimes (with verbal prompts, physical assistance) over a period of time, rather then allowing them to eat at their own volition, can promote weight gain (Yeh, Lovitt, and Shuster 2007). Having a social happy hour with snacks and beverages being offered helps improve food and fluid intake for some residents, and it may add an element of fun to their lives. Although offering food and fluids is time consuming and requires special knowledge of physiological changes and empathy for persons whose behavior might be objectionable at times, it may be one of the few times during the day when an individual with dementia receives normalized social interaction.

The staff should offer a variety of snack foods during each snack period. Morning and afternoon snack periods are more successful than evening snack periods, and snack periods that are offered three times a day are more successful than those offered twice a day. The staff should present snacks on a moveable, attractive cart so that the residents can see them. Juices, yogurt, ice cream, fresh fruit, pudding, cookies, pastries, and cheese or peanut butter and crackers are good snack choices for most residents. Snacks should also be available for diabetic residents and others who have special diets. We recommend that the staff and the family casually converse or otherwise socially interact with a resident throughout the snack period. The clinician should consider liberalizing the diet of all residents with anorexia, poor oral intake, and unintentional weight loss. According to the American Diabetes Association (2002), the imposition of dietary restrictions on elderly LTC residents with diabetes is not warranted. Specialized diets do not appear to be superior to standard (regular) diets in LTC settings. Therefore, we recommend that LTC residents with diabetes be served the facility's regular (unrestricted) menu, with consistency in the amount and timing of carbohydrates. There is no evidence to support diets such as "no concentrated sweets" or "no sugar added," which are often served to elderly people in LTC. It may often be preferable to change medications to control blood glucose rather than to implement food restrictions for residents with diabetes.

Nutritional supplements not only may promote gain weight, but they may also improve immune functioning and have other clinical benefits (e.g., less fever, fewer prescribed antibiotics, cognitive improvements) (Langkamp-Henken et al. 2006). Nutritional supplements are most effective when given between meals (more than 60 minutes before the next meal), not with them. When given with meals, supplements may have a suppressant effect on the appetite. Providing nutritional supplements with a wide variety of sweets and carbohydrates may be helpful as the second step in the treatment of weight loss. Residents who are less cognitively and physically impaired respond better to between-meal snack programs, and more cognitively and physically impaired residents respond better to improved mealtime assistance with feeding.

Inadequate food intake in LTC populations may be due to the type of food served. More than 50 percent of LTC residents are regularly served food they dislike and that lacks variety (B. Evans and Crogan 2005). Most residents do not complain because of cognitive impairments, feared retribution from the staff, or a perception that complaining in public is socially inappropriate.

Some of these barriers can be overcome by the use of questionnaires (such as FoodEX-LTC) administered privately, away from the dining room and the food service staff (B. Evans and Crogan 2005). Financial constraints may prevent a resident from living in an optimal LTC facility in terms of staff who are trained and available for feeding assistance. Financial constraints of the LTC facility may limit the purchase of fresh fruits and vegetables, and the facility may use outdated preparations and food-storage techniques (resulting in folate undernutrition). Some LTC facilities may have a registered dietician present in the facility only for as long as it is mandated by law.

The treatment of choice for sarcopenia is resistance exercise and increased protein intake. We recommend a trial of testosterone replacement for male residents with a testosterone deficiency. Feeding alone has little effect on the outcome of cachexia. After ruling out other treatable causes, the clinician may consider prescribing an appetite stimulant (e.g., megestrol, mirtazapine) for some residents with weight loss due to cachexia. A combination of testosterone and megestrol may be particularly useful for malnourished male residents with anorexia, unintentional weight loss, and sarcopenia. Dysphagia may be due to medications such as antipsychotics, as well as neurological conditions such as cerebrovascular disease. Metoclopramide is often used for gastroparesis and regurgitation or vomiting, but its use is associated with drug-induced parkinsonism (which may cause dysphagia), apathy, depression, confusion, and daytime sedation. For residents with anorexia and unintentional weight loss, a trial of discontinuing their medications (e.g., metoclopramide, antipsychotics) may be necessary to clarify if these medications provide any therapeutic benefit. Parenteral nutrition and tube feeding should be restricted to residents who are not in the terminal stage of dementia or another medical condition, such as a resident who had a recent stroke and swallowing difficulties but seems to be otherwise healthy and is benefiting from rehabilitative interventions. For residents with unintentional weight loss who are in the terminal stage of dementia or another progressive disease, the clinician should provide appropriate palliative care and referral to a hospice.

Cachexia

Cachexia is a complex metabolic syndrome associated with an underlying illness and characterized by a loss of muscle with or without a loss of fat mass. The prominent clinical feature of cachexia in LTC residents is recent weight loss. Cachexia is also called *wasting disease*, and it is associated with anorexia, inflammation, insulin resistance, increased mortality, deterioration in ADLs, and an increased breakdown of muscle protein (W. Evans et al. 2008). Common causes of cachexia are cancer, chronic infections, heart failure, kidney failure, and COPD. Approximately half of the residents admitted from a hospital to a skilled nursing facility have cachexia (D. Thomas et al. 2002).

The cornerstone of managing cachexia is a comprehensive nutritional approach. The initial approach to treatment involves caloric nutritional supplements rich in amino acids and creatine given twice a day between meals, along with multivitamins, omega-3 fatty acids, and probiotics. We recommend vitamin D replacement therapy if vitamin D levels are below 30 ng/dl (Morley and Thomas 2008). The clinician may consider prescribing the short-term use of megestrol (preferably the nanocrystal form) for residents with loss of appetite. The clinician should avoid prescribing megestrol for completely immobile residents, as it may increase the risk of deep vein thrombosis. Megestrol is poorly absorbed when not taken with food. Comorbid depression is common in residents with cachexia and may be treated with mirtazapine. The clinician should consider recommending ECT if the resident has cachexia and severe depression, as it can be life saving. Short-term peripheral parenteral nutrition may be needed for residents who are not eating or are eating less than 25 percent of their necessary daily caloric intake. Severe muscle loss (sarcopenia) may be treated with testosterone enanthate or nandrolone (Morley and Thomas 2008). Cachexia during end-of-life care may be treated with dronabinol.

Loss of Appetite / Anorexia

Appetite is crucial to maintaining nutrition. On average, food intake is about 30 percent lower in elderly people than in young adults, secondary to a physiological decrease in appetite. This is called the *anorexia of aging* and may predispose individuals to undernutrition. Anorexia is a common problem among LTC residents, and it is one of the most common reasons for a psychiatric consultation. It should be differentiated from a reduced oral intake of food and fluids due to factors other than anorexia (e.g., swallowing problems, dental problems). The assessment of anorexia needs to address not only depression (the most common reversible cause of anorexia in LTC populations), but also a host of other causes (see table 9.2). Anorexia is of particular concern in residents with diabetes (especially brittle diabetes), because of the high risk of potentially serious and even fatal hypoglycemia.

The treatment of anorexia is a treatment of its cause(s). Good nutritional practices (described in the section on unintentional weight loss) may enhance a person's response to the treatment of anorexia. Because losses of taste and smell are common in elderly people, the use of flavor-enhanced food may improve their appetites. The clinician should consider discontinuing medications that suppress the appetite and address residents' complaints regarding meal service and meal quality. Liberalization of one's diet and less-rigid mealtimes may also improve a person's appetite. Other appetite-improving strategies include allowing families to bring the residents fast foods or their favorite meals or snacks, and allowing residents to eat when they want to eat. The potential negative impact of a diet high in saturated fats on cholesterol levels is not usually an issue for the majority of LTC residents.

Dehydration and Electrolyte Imbalance

Adequate nutritional care includes monitoring for sufficient fluid intake. Dehydration refers to the loss of body water, with or without salt, at a rate greater than the body's replacement of it. There are two types of dehydration: water-loss dehydration (hyperosmolar, due to increased sodium or glucose), and salt-and-water-loss dehydration (hyponatremia). Although dehydration is a sentinel event thought to reflect poor care, it is rarely due to neglect from formal or informal caregivers, but rather results from a combination of physiological and disease processes (D. Thomas et al. 2008). Older adults are at risk of dehydration because of both reduced fluid intake and increased fluid loss. As a rule, fluid intake among LTC residents is well below the recommended daily requirement of 1,500–2,500 ml/day (D. Thomas et al. 2000; Feinsod et al. 2004).

Body weight and body water decrease with age, which, together with the well-known deterioration of thirst perception in old age, may give rise to dehydration and its potentially lethal complications (circulatory collapse, acute renal failure). In addition, there is a decline in the glomerular filtration rate with increasing age, which may contribute to an impaired ability to conserve water. Reduced skin integrity due to subcutaneous dehydration may result in xerosis, pruritus, recurrent skin infections, and pressure ulcers in an immobile resident. A urinary tract infection may result from the irritant effect of highly concentrated urine on the vesical mucosa. Thickened oral and gastrointestinal secretions can lead to constipation, impaction, xerostomia, periodontal disease, and mouth ulcers. Neurological dysfunction in dehydrated residents may present as delirium, dizziness, recurrent falls, and subsequent complications (e.g., hip fractures, a traumatic brain injury).

Dehydration is present in up to one-quarter of older people, and individuals with dementia are likely to have an even higher risk (Archibald 2006). Other common causes of dehydration include infection, delirium, and the use of diuretics. During the warmer months and in warm climates, increased ambient temperatures should prompt careful attention to fluid intake. In addition, residents with fevers, burns, vomiting, diarrhea, or draining fistulas may need additional fluid. Residents with chronic lung disease, decubitus ulcers, excessive tremors, or movement disorders are likely to have increased amounts of insensible fluid loss and thus may need more than the usual daily fluid intake. Increased fluid intake may also be necessary for residents with poorly controlled diabetes mellitus or who are taking laxative therapy. Dehydration is a common problem in LTC populations, often due to a failure to detect and appropriately manage it.

The detection of dehydration depends largely on a high threshold of suspicion. A clinical diagnosis of dehydration in LTC populations is unreliable. Serum osmolality greater than 300, blood urea nitrogen greater than 20, and a BUN:creatinine ratio greater than 20 are useful indices to detect dehydration. Dehydration can be accompanied by hypernatremia (typically due to restricted water intake) or hyponatremia (typically due to the use of diuretics). Excessive fluid loss due to diabetes insipidus (due to a stroke, neurosurgery, etc.) may cause hypernatremia. Hypernatremia in elderly people carries a poor prognosis, with mortality in excess of 40 percent when plasma sodium exceeds 150 nmol/l.

The treatment of dehydration is a treatment of its cause. Common causes of dehydration in LTC populations are preventable and easily treatable. However, an early diagnosis and intervention are key. We recommend encouraging oral ingestion of at least 1.5 liters of fluid daily if the resident's cardiac and renal status allow it. Yet an aggressive and rapid replacement of fluid and electrolytes may lead to fluid overload and neurological complications. The availability of water fountains, circulating water or juice carts, the encouragement of fluid intake at medication rounds, and frequent drinking prompts or assistance are simple strategies to reduce the prevalence of dehydration in LTC populations. With the availability of recombinant hyaluronidase, a subcutaneous infusion of fluids (hypodermoclysis) provides a better opportunity to treat mild to moderate dehydration in LTC populations (D. Thomas et al. 2008).

Micronutrient Deficiency

Many residents have a micronutrient deficiency with or without a macronutrient deficiency (D. Thomas 2004). Table 9.5 lists risk factors for micronutrient deficiencies. Elderly people have higher requirements for vitamins D, B_6, and B_{12} than do younger people. Vitamin B_{12}, folate, and vitamin B_6 are needed for homocysteine metabolism, and deficiencies result in elevated levels of homocysteine, which has been associated with cognitive decline and osteoporotic fractures. Vitamin B_{12} deficiency is highly prevalent (25%–35%) in LTC populations. Atrophic gastritis (prevalent in elderly people) reduces the absorption of several nutrients, which, especially for vitamin B_{12}, leads to a deficiency state. B_{12} levels decline during prolonged use of a proton pump inhibitor in older adults (Dharmarajan et al. 2008). Pernicious anemia is a rare but serious disorder associated with vitamin B_{12} deficiency. Vitamin B_{12} deficiency may also result in a cognitive decline, depression, and, in severe cases, peripheral neuropathy, dementia, and subacute combined degeneration of the spinal cord. These neuropsychiatric complications due to vitamin B_{12} deficiency can be seen in the absence of anemia or of an elevated mean cell volume.

Folate deficiency is much less prevalent than vitamin B_{12} deficiency in elderly people, although up to 95 percent of the foliate in foods is destroyed by excessive cooking. Folate deficiency is associated with anemia, fatigue, glossitis, and cognitive impairment. Folate supplementation in the presence of a vitamin B_{12} deficiency may cause cognitive decline; folate supplementation in the presence of adequate levels of B_{12} may improve cognition. Vitamin B_2

TABLE 9.5
Common risk factors for micronutrient deficiencies in the long-term care population

Increased requirements in elderly people compared with younger people
Part of general malnutrition (along with anorexia, weight loss, and/or obesity)
Diabetes mellitus
Alcohol abuse
Smoking
Liver disease
Chronic diarrhea
Chronic total parenteral nutrition
Inflammatory diseases of the gastrointestinal tract
Certain medications (e.g., methotrexate, triamterene, phenobarbital, phenytoin, theophylline)
Certain diets (e.g., vegan, vegetarian)

(riboflavin) deficiency is seen in conjunction with other vitamin B deficiencies. Vitamin B_2 deficiency may manifest as cheilosis, glossitis, and anemia. Residents with a low fruit and vegetable intake and those who smoke (and are not taking vitamin C supplements) may have low vitamin C serum levels. Vitamin C deficiency may result in excessive bleeding from minor cuts, bleeding gums, poor wound healing, poor bone health, and, in severe cases, bleeding disorders.

Approximately one-third of one's vitamin D requirements can be obtained from one's diet; the rest is synthesized in the skin under the influence of sunlight. Vitamin D deficiency is highly prevalent (30%–40%) in LTC populations, because of the residents' limited exposure to the sun and a fourfold reduction in the skin's capacity to produce vitamin D due to aging-related changes in the skin. Calcium deficiency may develop in residents who have few or no dairy products in their diet. Vitamin D deficiency and calcium deficiency may result in osteomalacia, fractures, neuromuscular irritability, musculoskeletal pain, neuropathy, cognitive impairments, depression, and hyperesthesia. The daily intake of vitamin D in older adults should be at least 800 IU, with at least 1,200 mg of elemental calcium in the diet or as a supplement, with the goal of a serum vitamin D level of 30–50 ng/dl.

Other populations at risk of micronutrient deficiencies include residents with a partial gastrectomy (vitamin B_{12} deficiency), bacterial overgrowth (vitamin B_{12} and folate deficiencies), celiac disease (folate deficiency, vitamin A or D deficiency), pancreatic insufficiency (vitamin A, D, E, and calcium deficiencies), terminal ileum diseases (vitamin A, D, E, B_{12}, and calcium deficiencies), alcoholism (folate deficiency, thiamine deficiency), and chronic liver and gallbladder diseases (vitamin A, D, E, K deficiencies).

Medications are an important cause of micronutrient malabsorption (e.g., antacids and H2 blockers may decrease vitamin B_{12}; diuretics can cause electrolyte imbalance [hypo- or hyperkalemia, hypo- or hypernatremia]; calcium and iron absorption from the stomach and the use of broad-spectrum antibiotics [e.g., neomycin] are associated with decreased absorption of vitamin K and folate, due to changes in one's intestinal bacterial flora; high doses of aluminum or magnesium hydroxide antacids may deplete phosphate and potassium stores). Folate deficiency may worsen depression and decrease cognition. Other micronutrients that may have psychiatric significance (e.g., an increased risk of cognitive impairments and/or depression) include copper, selenium (especially in residents with diabetes mellitus or chronic total parenteral nutrition), zinc, vitamin B_1 (especially in residents with diabetes mellitus or a past or current history of alcohol abuse), B_5, B_6, and B_7. Maintaining normal zinc levels may be an important factor in reducing the risk of pneumonia in LTC populations, as well as reducing the risk of vision loss in elderly people who are at high risk of macular degeneration.

Micronutrient deficiencies may present atypically or they may be masked by coexisting diseases or a general failure to thrive. Thus the clinician should maintain a high index of suspicion for these deficiencies, leading to an early diagnosis and treatment. Older adults are often subject to syndromes that present with early manifestations in the oral cavity (e.g., tongue changes due to nutritional anemias, reactions to medications [such as dry mouth], and deficiency diseases such as scurvy [a vitamin C deficiency causing excessive bleeding from the gums]). Low fiber intake may worsen certain gastrointestinal conditions, such as chronic constipation, diverticulosis, gallbladder disease, and celiac sprue (Baker 2007).

We recommend that the clinician test all residents (unless a resident is in a hospice) for serum vitamin B_{12}, folate, calcium, and 25(OH)D3 levels, ideally at the time of admission (if these levels had not been tested recently). Some elderly people may have cellular B_{12} deficiency, but their B_{12} levels may still be in the normal range (usually at the lower end of the range). If the clinician suspects B_{12} deficiency, he or she may consider measuring serum methylmalonic acid and homocysteine levels for a resident with a vitamin B_{12} level in the lower range of normal. Residents at high risk of one micronutrient deficiency may need additional tests to detect other micronutrient deficiencies. Even if a resident's folate levels were within normal limits in the past, recently developed malnutrition should prompt the clinician to recheck folate levels, as folate levels drop quickly once a person's dietary intake is decreased. This is in contrast with vitamin B_{12} deficiency, which takes months to years to develop because vitamin B_{12} is stored in the liver.

Although food remains the best vehicle for nutrient consumption, many LTC residents may need vitamin and/or mineral supplements. We recommend vitamin B_{12} supplements (500–1,000 mcg/day) for residents with vitamin B_{12} deficiency and for those with depression and vitamin B_{12} levels at the lower end of the normal range. Residents with vitamin B_{12} deficiency due to pernicious anemia may need vitamin B_{12} injections (1,000 mcg subcutaneously once a month). Besides vitamin D supplementation, we recommend increased exposure to the sun and/or the use of sunlamps for residents with vitamin D levels below 30 ng/ml. Vitamin D also has the beneficial effect of reducing the risk of falling, which is explained by its improvement of muscle function. We recommend vitamin C supplementation for residents at risk of vitamin C deficiency. Malnourished residents usually need a host of vitamin and mineral supplements in addition to an increased intake of nutritious food and fluids. A subgroup of LTC residents who do not have dementia may also benefit from multivitamin and mineral supplementation (Liu et al. 2007). For instance, residents with depression and low serum selenium levels may show an improvement in mood after taking selenium supplementation (Gosney et al. 2008). We recommend involving a registered dietician for all residents at risk of or suspected to have micronutrient deficiencies.

We do not recommend vitamin E supplements for LTC populations, because of inconclusive data regarding the benefits of these supplements and their potential risks (e.g., increased all-cause mortality, increased risk of bleeding [especially with the concomitant use of blood thinners such as warfarin]) with a high-dose (more than 400 IU/day) vitamin E intake. Vitamin A deficiency is rare in the United States and other industrialized countries (although common in poorly developed countries). We discourage vitamin A and beta-carotene supplementation for all elderly people, due to a lack of data examining their clinical benefits and possible adverse effects (e.g., osteopenia, fractures). The clinician should evaluate all residents who are taking vitamin and mineral supplements to see if these supplements are necessary, both because many residents may not need some or all the supplements they are consuming and because of the risk of adverse vitamins/minerals-drug interactions. Also, some residents may be consuming potentially toxic amounts of vitamins and minerals by supplementation.

Obesity

Obesity is defined as a body mass index of 30 or greater (the normal range is between 19 and 25; an overweight person has a BMI between 25 and 29.9). Central obesity means having a large waist circumference. Obesity is a common problem in elderly people, although its prevalence decreases in extreme old age (Kennedy, Chokkalingham, and Srinivasan 2004). Some 25 percent of adults older than 50 are obese. Today's obese elderly experience more impairment in their functional abilities related to movement and to ADLs than those from previous generations. Weight gain among community-dwelling elderly people is primarily caused by a decline in physical activity rather than by eating more or consuming energy-dense food. The prevalence of obesity in LTC is also increasing: 25 percent of newly admitted residents in U.S. nursing homes were obese in 2002, compared with 15 percent in 1992 (Lapane and Resnik 2005). Nearly 30 percent of residents who have a BMI of 35 or greater are younger than 65, and a much higher percentage of obese residents are African Americans.

In LTC populations, excessive food consumption and a sedentary lifestyle also contribute to increasing rates of obesity. Residents identified as obese have a higher likelihood of comorbid conditions (e.g., diabetes mellitus, arthritis, hypertension, depression, chronic pain, allergies) (Lapane and Resnik 2005). Obesity can occur either along with protein malnutrition, sarcopenia, and micronutrient deficiency or in their absence. Because elderly people (especially those with frontal lobe impairments [e.g., individuals with FTD]) are not able to adjust their food intake after a period of overfeeding; they will continue exceeding their eating needs and thus gain weight.

Obesity in the elderly is associated with a poor perception of one's health, poor physical functioning, and poor social functioning. Elderly people who are obese are more likely to become disabled and thus be admitted to a nursing home. Obesity in the elderly is a major predictor of a loss of independence, and it exacerbates an age-related decline in physical functioning. Residents who are obese may reduce or stop their ambulating (due to pain or the need for greater physical effort), and they may have chronic pain due to osteoarthritis. Slight excess weight may be helpful when a resident is ill and in a catabolic state, as the immune system faces increased wear and tear then. Excess weight stresses the skeleton and thus reduces the loss of bone mass, so overweight elderly people are less likely to have hip fractures. However, the health risks of excess weight and obesity in elderly people are greater than any advantages (Villareal et al. 2005). Obese residents may increase the risk of workplace injuries among LTC staff, who already face high workplace injury rates. Special equipment (e.g., chair lifts) may be needed to safely transfer a resident who is obese (especially one who is morbidly obese [BMI greater than 40]), and for ambulation, bathing, and physical therapy. LTC facilities may not have the specialized supplies (e.g., blood pressure cuffs to accommodate larger arms) and equipment (e.g., beds and wheelchairs to accommodate persons weighing more than 300 pounds) or adequate space (e.g., larger rooms with wider doorways to accommodate larger equipment and wider wheelchairs) to provide care for residents who are obese (Felix 2008).

The primary purpose of the treatment of obesity in elderly people is to increase their physical functioning and quality of life, not to prevent disease. The focus of treatment should be on reducing weight and preserving muscle mass and strength without contributing to frailty. This is achieved through increased physical activity (exercise and increased leisure activity) and judicious nutritional strategies. We recommend progressive resistance training (which helps conserve lean body mass, strengthens bone, and increases energy expenditure) and low-intensity physical activity (e.g., walking) to treat obesity in residents who do not have medical contraindications to exercise (Kennedy, Chokkalingham, and Srinivasan 2004). The clinician should remind residents and their families that most popular diets are nutritionally unacceptable (Baker 2007). The goal is to reduce caloric intake, not nutrients. A decrease of 500 calories daily will result in the loss of one pound of body weight weekly, but a daily intake of less than 800 calories should not be prescribed. Simple dietary modifications include decreasing the person's saturated fat intake, using lean cuts of meat and lowfat or skim milk, and limiting (as much as possible) or avoiding candy, ice cream, pastries, pies, and cakes. We recommend fruit for dessert. Broiling and baking food, instead of frying, is also helpful. The staff should encourage residents to increase the proportion of fruits and vegetables in their diets, especially dark green leafy vegetables. Portion size should be controlled, and residents should feel under no obligation to clean their plates. Their intake of beverages with a high caloric and sugar content (sodas, alcoholic beverages) should be limited as much as possible. Nonetheless, all of these changes need to be individualized and implemented at a level that does not significantly compromise the person's existing quality of life.

Elderly people who are obese and intentionally lose weight may not have the risks of weight loss (e.g., increased morbidity and mortality) seen in elderly people with unintentional weight loss. We do not recommend using medications such as phentermine, orlistat, and sibutramine to treat obesity because of the high risk of adverse effects (e.g., insomnia and agitation). For many obese residents, their long-term quality of life is expected to improve with weight reduction, due to improved physical and cognitive functions, a decrease in musculoskeletal pain, and other potential benefits. The clinician should carefully consider decisions about whether or not to institute a weight-loss intervention for obese residents and then make choices on an individualized basis, with special attention to each resident's life expectancy, weight history, and medical condition (Bales and Buhr 2008). Residents who are obese and in the terminal stage of dementia (or in other disease states) need appropriate palliative care and referral to a hospice rather than weight-reduction strategies.

CLINICAL CASE Mr. W was an 81-year-old resident of an assisted living facility. He was doing well taking 40 mg daily citalopram for the treatment of his depressive and anxiety symptoms due to dementia. Over the last two years he had gained 50 pounds, and in the last three months he added another 14 pounds (for a final BMI of 42), primarily due to a sedentary lifestyle and excessive eating during and between meals. Mr. W had struggled with obesity for most of his life and intermittently went to Weight Watchers to reduce his weight and eat healthier. Due to dementia, he had stopped going to Weight Watchers for the last five years. Mr. W's health care provider ordered a program of exercise (five minutes of strength training and 15 minutes of assisted ambulation daily) and nutritional strategies. The nutritional strategies involved a portion-controlled diet (smaller portions given during the three daily meals), replacing Mr. W's consumption of unhealthy snacks (crackers, candies, ice cream) with fruits and vegetables (carrots, celery with a vegetable dip), and replacing his intake of cola and coffee with diet cola and water. Mr. W initially resisted this change in his diet, but with staff support and positive reinforcement, he acquiesced. Over the next eight weeks, not only did Mr. W lose seven pounds, but he appeared to have more energy, began getting out of chairs on his own (previously he needed assistance to do this), and began walking around the facility. The staff also noticed that Mr. W seemed to carry on a longer conversation and showed less agitation.

TEACHING POINTS For some individuals who are obese, simple nutritional changes can lead not only to a modest but significant weight loss, but also to functional and cognitive improvements.

Nutritional Disorders Associated with Dementia

Nutritional disorders (anorexia, unintentional weight loss, abnormal eating or appetite behaviors, obesity) are common in residents with dementia, because cognitive impairment and behavioral disturbances can prevent residents from meeting their nutritional needs or from being able to express them to the staff. In fact, an inability to maintain adequate nutritional status may be one of the reasons for admission to LTC. Neurotransmitter abnormalities may also play a role, in that levels of neuropeptide Y and norepinephrine (potent stimulators of food intake) have been found to be reduced in various brain regions of people with AD (Morley, Flood, and Silver 1992). Weight loss in late life is associated with dementia, and those categorized as underweight are also at a greater risk of dementia (Whitmer 2007). Individuals with advanced cognitive impairments may also be at risk of dehydration, due to a loss of protective thirst responses (Albert et al. 1994). Thus it may be harder to recognize dehydration in residents with dementia.

Approximately 90 percent of all persons with AD lose weight. In the early stage of dementia, the person may forget to eat, and his or her appetite may also diminish as a result of depression. Affected persons may become distracted and leave the table without eating. In the middle stages of dementia, individuals may have difficulty initiating the eating process or they may start eating, become distracted, and fail to finish. They may not be able to sit long enough to finish a meal or they may forget that they have just eaten. At this stage, additional calories may be required for residents with dementia who develop symptoms of wandering, pacing, or motor restlessness. In the severe and terminal stages of AD, the resident may fail to recognize food, eat things that are not food, no longer have the oral-motor skills for chewing and swallowing, or not be able to coordinate activities to self-feed. Thus a resident in the moderate to severe stages of dementia needs to be given adequate assistance during feeding and a sufficient increase in caloric intake, especially if he or she has increased motor activity. Residents who have had a stroke or have Parkinson disease or dementia with Lewy bodies often develop a slowing of their motor functions (bradykinesia) and a slowing in their thinking (bradyphrenia), and hence may require assistance with feeding for a much longer time period (30–60 minutes) to achieve an adequate intake of nutrition (calories and nutrients).

In the severe and terminal stages of dementia, advanced neurodegeneration may severely impair the resident's ability to maintain an adequate food and fluid intake to sustain life, despite adequate feeding assistance, the administration of nutritional supplements, and the treatment of other factors contributing to weight loss. These residents are essentially in the process of dying. Tube feeding does not improve the quality or quantity of life for them, and it may even worsen their quality of life, due to associated complications (e.g., pain, discomfort, aspiration). We recommend hand feeding to address anorexia and weight loss in the severe to terminal stages of dementia. Cachexia and dehydration are common causes of death among residents with terminal-stage dementia. We recommend that the clinician use the Edinburgh Feeding Evaluation in Dementia Questionnaire, or EdFED-Q (http://consultgerirn.org/uploads/File/trythis/issue11_1.pdf), an observational instrument, to identify eating and feeding difficulties and determine the level of assistance needed (R. Watson and Dreary 1997). Residents with dementia who have eating difficulties may have swallowing disorders that are often unrecognized. These residents are sometimes labeled as combative, uncooperative, and difficult to feed when they try to refuse food they cannot swallow. If an assessment suggests an undiagnosed swallowing disorder, the clinician should refer the resident to a speech pathologist for further evaluation.

Obesity, central obesity, and excess weight in middle age are associated with an increased risk of AD and VaD, independent of diabetes and cardiovascular-related morbidities (Whitmer 2007; Whitmer et al. 2008). Many residents with dementia develop abnormal eating or appetite behaviors. These are seen more often with FTD, but they can also be seen with AD. These behaviors include odd eating habits, a tendency to place nonfood objects in the mouth, an increase in appetite (hyperphagia), overeating, eating between meals, a preference for sweets and soft drinks, a desire to eat at the same time every day, and a decline in table manners. The presence of irritability, agitation, and disinhibition may result in shifts in eating patterns toward carbohydrates and away from protein, placing these residents at increased risk of protein malnutrition (Greenwood et al. 2005). Research has shown shifts in the circadian patterns of intake in LTC residents with dementia, with a lower food intake consistently observed at lunch and dinner, but not breakfast, in individuals with higher levels of functional disability. These behavioral problems are best managed with psychosocial-environmental interventions, such as redirecting them, replacing high-calorie food items (e.g., desserts) with low-calorie food items (e.g., fruits and vegetables) to prevent obesity due to hyperphagia, and allowing residents to eat in smaller groups with greater monitoring.

Depression and Malnutrition

Weight loss is more prevalent in older people with depression than younger ones. A loss of appetite is one of the most common symptoms of depression in LTC residents. Death by starvation can be a method by which a depressed resident may attempt suicide. Most antidepressants (except mirtazapine, which is associated with an increased appetite and weight gain) have the potential to cause anorexia and even weight loss, although more often antidepressants improve appetite and weight by alleviating depression. Possible causes of high mortality in residents with severe depression and severe malnutrition include their protein needs not being met at a time of increased nitrogen turnover (stress) and/or an increased release of tumor necrosis factor (cachectin) with an increase in lipoprotein lipase and a subsequent weight loss. The convergence of depression and malnutrition is a psychiatric or medical emergency, because these patients are also immune-compromised and susceptible to potentially life-threatening infections. Treating undernutrition and depression aggressively (with antidepressants and/or ECT) may be life saving. Depression often leads to poor fluid intake, resulting in dehydration. If the resident is also taking diuretics, dehydration can quickly become severe and potentially fatal. In such a situation, eliminating drugs that may cause or exacerbate dehydration and anorexia (e.g., diuretics, calcium [it may cause constipation and nausea]) and treating the depression, as well as improving the oral intake of fluids with psychosocial interventions, are necessary for a successful outcome.

Healthy Nutrition

We recommend that cognitively intact residents who are interested in eating a healthy diet and residents with moderate dementia for whom family members would like healthy nutritional strategies (as compared with a diet with no restrictions) pursue a modified food guide pyramid for people over 70 years old (Russell, Rasmussen, and Lichtenstein 1999). This includes consuming at least four glasses of water; six servings of bread, fortified cereal, rice, or pasta; two servings of fruit; three servings of vegetables; two servings of meat, poultry, fish, dried beans, eggs, or nuts; and three servings of milk, cheese, or yogurt daily. In addition, we recommend calcium and vitamins D and B_{12} supplements. Saturated fats and sweets are to be consumed sparingly. We recommend that residents pursuing a diet that may promote cognitive well-being and slow cognitive decline increase their consumption of fruits, vegetables, food rich in omega-3 (oily fish [e.g., salmon, sardines, herring, black cod], walnuts, flaxseed, canola oil, omega-3 enriched eggs or cereals), food rich in monounsaturated fatty acids (e.g., avocados, olive oil), whole grains, and spices (e.g., turmeric). The clinician should adjust these recommendations for the individual's medical conditions and personal preferences.

Frailty

Frailty is a syndrome of decreased reserve and resistance to stressors, resulting from cumulative declines across multiple systems and causing vulnerability to adverse outcomes. Frailty status is based on the presence of three or more of the following: unintentional weight loss, muscle weakness (as shown by weak grip strength), exhaustion, slow walking speed, and low physical activity levels (Espinoza and Fried 2007). Frailty is a form of predis-ability. Frail residents are at increased risk of becoming disabled and are more likely to fall, to be hospitalized, and to die within several years. Frailty is a common condition in older people (Morley et al. 2006). About 7 percent of the population older than 65 and 20 percent of the population older than 80 are frail. Frailty among older persons is a dynamic process, characterized by a frequent transition between frailty states over time. Thus there may be an opportunity for the prevention and remediation of frailty (T. Gill et al. 2006). The presence of only one of the five criteria denotes prefrailty, which often leads to frailty. A cognitively capable resident who displays only one criterion for frailty may be a target for intervention.

An assessment and treatment of frailty is best done by an interdisciplinary team, because of the complexity of the person's coexisting social, spiritual, psychological, and medical needs. Ongoing dialogue with the resident and the family is critical to deciding what level of testing and treatment to implement in keeping with the resident's wishes. The clinician should screen all frail residents for pain, depression, nutritional deficiencies (e.g., serum albumin, prealbumin, vitamin D and B_{12} levels), medication issues (adverse drug reactions, inappropriate or unnecessary medication prescriptions), and anemia. Frail residents with comorbid behavioral and psychological symptoms are at higher risk of adverse effects from all medications, including psychotropic medications, than nonfrail residents. Thus the doses of psychotropic drugs that are used for frail residents may need to be even lower than those for the elderly population as a whole, and the dose increase even slower. When in doubt about whether a medication may be causing behavioral and psychological symptoms or physical symptoms (tiredness, anorexia), the clinician should err on the side of reducing or discontinuing the suspected offending drug.

In treating frailty, we recommend initiating regular physical exercise (especially muscle-strengthening exercise and balance exercises [tai chi], but also endurance exercises), improving nutritional status (with a combination of macronutrients and micronutrients [enriched or fortified foods] at recommended daily doses), reducing pain, and discontinuing unnecessary medications (Best-Martini and Botenhagen-DiGenova 2003). The clinician should consider prescribing vitamin and mineral supplements (e.g., vitamin D and/ or B_{12}) for all frail residents. The clinician may also consider referring such individuals for physical therapy. Testosterone replacement therapy for hypogonadal males (free testosterone levels below the normal range) who are frail and/or have sarcopenia may improve their muscle strength and lead to functional improvements. The appropriate management of underlying diseases (e.g., anemia, diabetes mellitus, congestive heart failure, hypothyroidism) is important in the management of frailty. Such comprehensive treatment strategies may lead to constraining the downward spiral of disability in frail residents and improving their quality of life. The quality of the time spent with family may also improve with a reduction in frailty. Comprehensive treatment strategies for residents exhibiting prefrailty may even prevent the development of frailty in some cases. Even small improvements in their frailty may result in improved mobility and reduced disability in ADLs. Frail elderly people often show improvements in cognition, the ability to perform ADLs, the ability to participate in leisure activities, strength, stamina, flexibility, and balance after participating in multimodal interventions that address frailty.

Many frail residents in LTC populations may be in the terminal stage of dementia or another chronic disease. For these residents, we recommend appropriate palliative care and referral to a hospice, in contrast with a comprehensive assessment and treatment of all factors contributing to their frailty.

Failure to Thrive

In older adults, a failure to thrive involves an insidious yet significant decline in their physical, emotional, and functional status (Robertson and Montagnini 2004). Key features of the failure-to-thrive syndrome include progressive functional decline, social withdrawal, depression, cognitive impairment, weight loss, and nutritional deficiencies. Failure to thrive typically follows a bout of acute illness, such as pneumonia or a hip fracture. The treatment for failure to thrive involves a thorough evaluation to identify and treat overlooked acute (e.g., UTI) or chronic conditions (e.g., congestive heart failure, hypothyroidism). We also recommend correcting nutritional deficiencies (e.g., a vitamin B_{12} deficiency), treating depression and pain, encouraging exercise, discontinuing unnecessary medications, and addressing social isolation. The treatment of failure to thrive for residents in the terminal stage of dementia or another medical condition involves appropriate palliative care and referral to a hospice.

Conclusion

Psychiatric disorders such as dementia, depression, and delirium predispose residents to nutritional disorders, frailty, and failure to thrive, which, in turn, predispose them to psychiatric disorders. Besides improving their quality of life, the early identification and treatment of nutritional disorders, frailty, and failure to thrive in all residents may prevent many psychiatric disorders and accelerate the improvement of psychiatric disorders that are being treated concomitantly.

CHAPTER 10

Abuse and Neglect, Ethical Dilemmas, and Medicolegal Issues

Old age is an authentic period of life, and integrating the unity of one's life is one of the tasks of old age. The majority of the residents in long-term care facilities are weak and diminished due to multiple medical and psychiatric disorders and thus need help to achieve this integrating task. All health care providers should strive to keep our elderly people in caring LTC facilities. Ageism should not be a factor in allocating resources, and when attempting to evaluate the quality of life of an older individual, one must be aware of the limitations of a purely professional assessment.

Abuse and neglect are prevalent in LTC populations and may cause serious setbacks to residents' efforts to live with dignity. Ethical and medicolegal issues may also pose barriers to the residents' ability to live their last years meaningfully. Efforts to prevent abuse, neglect, and unethical professional conduct are necessary, but far from sufficient, for residents to work toward integrating and unifying the elements in their lives. Every LTC facility needs to focus on ways to promote the need for all residents to reach their spiritual and psychological goals.

Abuse and Neglect

Because of their significant dependence on others for their care, LTC residents are vulnerable to abuse and/or neglect (Lindbloom et al. 2007). Elder abuse is a common problem with serious consequences for the health and well-being of older people (Lachs and Pillemer 2004), and it is even more common among older people at the end of their lives (Jayawardena and Liao 2006). Elder abuse and neglect also occur frequently among people referred to geriatric psychiatry services (Vida, Monks, and Rosiers 2002). Elder mistreatment is a significant problem in LTC facilities. More than 30 percent of the nursing homes in the United States were cited for abuse violations that had the potential for significant harm to residents (House Committee on Government Reform 2001). Some of the key reasons elderly people are fearful of residing in LTC facilities are concerns involving mistreatment (Gibbs and Young 2007). Elderly men and women of all socioeconomic and ethnic backgrounds are vulnerable to abuse and neglect, and most often it goes undetected.

Elder abuse or mistreatment means an intentional act of commission or omission that results in harm or threatened harm to the health or welfare of an elderly person. Table 10.1 defines abuse in LTC facilities. Abuse and neglect include the intentional infliction of physical or mental injury; sexual or financial abuse; or the withholding of necessary food, clothing, monetary resources, and medical care to treat the physical and mental health needs of an older person by another person having responsibility for that older adult. Undue influence that harms the older adult should also be considered a form of abuse. Physical abuse is most recognizable, yet neglect is most common.

TABLE 10.1
Definitions of abuse in long-term care facilities

Abuse	The willful infliction of injury, unreasonable confinement, intimidation, or punishment with resulting physical harm, pain, or mental anguish. This also includes deprivation by an individual, including a caretaker, of goods or services that are necessary to attain or maintain physical, mental, and psychosocial well-being. This presumes that instances of abuse of any resident, even one in a coma, cause physical harm or pain or mental anguish.
Verbal abuse	The use of oral, written, or gestured language that willfully includes disparaging or derogatory terms directed toward residents or their families, or within their hearing, regardless of their age, ability to comprehend, or disability. Examples of verbal abuse include, but are not limited to, threats of harm or saying things to frighten a resident, such as telling a resident that he or she will never be able to see his or her family again.
Sexual abuse	This includes, but is not limited to, sexual harassment, sexual coercion, and sexual assault.
Physical abuse	This includes hitting, slapping, pinching, pushing, and kicking. It also includes controlling the resident's behavior through corporal punishment.
Mental abuse	This includes, but is not limited to, humiliation, harassment, threats of punishment, or deprivation.
Involuntary seclusion	The separation of a resident from other residents or from his or her room, or confinement to his or her room (with or without roommates), against the resident's will or the will of the resident's legal representative.

Source: Data from American Health Care Association 2001.

TABLE 10.2
*Some key questions useful in screening for and eliciting
information on elder abuse*

Has anyone at the [name of the long-term care facility] ever hurt you?

Have you ever been struck, slapped, or kicked?

Has anyone ever touched you without your consent?

Has anyone ever made you do anything you didn't want to do?

Has anyone ever taken anything that was yours without asking?

Has money or have your belongings ever been stolen from you?

Has anyone ever scolded or threatened you?

Have you ever signed any document that you didn't understand?

Are you afraid of anyone at [name of the long-term care facility]?

Are you alone a lot?

Has anyone ever failed to help you take care of yourself when you
needed help?

Do you lack aids such as eyeglasses, hearing aids, or dentures?

Are your needs being neglected?

Source: Data from Aravanis and American Medical Association 1994; Carney,
Kahan, and Paris 2003.

Psychological and financial abuse may be more easily missed. An awareness of risk factors (cognitive impairments, depression, frailty, caregiver stress, admission to LTC, aggressive residents) and clinical manifestations (e.g., bruises, fractures, malnutrition) allow health care personnel to provide early detection of and intervention for elderly abuse and neglect (Levine 2003). Interdisciplinary collaboration among physicians, social workers, and mental health professionals is crucial.

Health care providers should have a high index of suspicion regarding abuse and neglect in residents at risk. We recommend that the clinician routinely ask a few screening questions during each assessment (e.g., Are you being treated well? Is anyone trying to hurt you? Do you feel safe?) for the early detection of abuse and neglect (table 10.2).

Nursing assistants report low confidence in their ability to prevent agitation or aggression in LTC residents, and they report even lower confidence in their ability to decrease residents' agitation and aggression once they become agitated or aggressive (Gates et al. 2004). This issue may be one of the key reasons that predisposes residents who express their needs through aggressive behavior to be victims of abuse and neglect. Staff members may respond to a resident's anger, verbal abuse, or physical aggression with anger, disrespect, hostile distancing, and passive-aggressive behavior (not responding to the resident's yelling or calling).

Neglect of a resident typically involves the failure to provide life essentials, such as food, water, medication, comfort, safety, personal hygiene, clothing, and other necessities as required by the individual's physical condition. Other allegations include improper handling, delayed assistance, lack of care planning, contractures, pressure sores, and unattended symptoms. Incidents of neglect are underreported, due to the difficulties inherent in defining and recognizing this type of treatment. LTC staff members commonly hide drugs in food and beverages without the resident's knowledge or consent. Drugs are concealed more frequently for residents with severe cognitive impairments, reduced function in ADLs, and aggressive behavior. This practice should be discouraged, because it encourages both secrecy and poor documentation.

Dementia and Elder Abuse

Because of the impairments consequent to dementia, residents with dementia may be particularly at risk of elder abuse. Often heath care providers are not aware of the special vulnerabilities of a resident with dementia and fail to recognize elder abuse (Hansberry, Chen, and Gorbien 2005). Residents with advanced dementia may not be able to report abuse and may express distress caused by abuse in the form of agitation, aggression, or depression. Thus the clinician should maintain a high index of suspicion regarding the abuse of residents with dementia.

Differential Diagnosis of Neglect

Self-neglect in residents is different from neglect related to abuse or mistreatment. Neglect is caused by others, but self-neglect is self-imposed, and in some cases a particular lifestyle is involved (Reyes-Ortiz 2001). Other terms for self-neglect in elderly people are *Diogenes syndrome* and *squalor syndrome*. Primary Diogenes syndrome involves premorbid personality traits and precipitant factors, rather than a mental disorder; secondary Diogenes syndrome may be due to dementia, depression, or schizophrenia. Bruises due to falls may be mistaken for physical abuse, and vice versa. Health care providers should have a high index of suspicion regarding the coexistence of abuse and neglect with accidental falls and injuries, self-neglect, and other conditions that may mimic abuse.

Preventing Elder Abuse in Long-Term Care Populations

One important strategy to prevent the mistreatment of elders is to increase the bridging-and-bonding social capital available to professional and family caregivers (Donohue, Dibble, and Schiamberg 2008). The facility's leadership team should consider consulting an elder-law attorney, geriatrician, and/or geriatric psychiatrist to help develop rigorous, high-quality practices for hiring staff, high-quality staff training programs, and risk-management procedures for the prevention and prompt treatment of elder abuse. Key strategies to prevent elder abuse in LTC facilities includes screening all employees (e.g., criminal background checks), verifying credentials, and conducting ongoing staff training in areas such as language, communication, and sensitivity. The staff should be encouraged to be vigilant about problems in the facility and to report problems. Communication among the staff, residents, and family members is important. Everyone needs to know how to initiate a complaint. Residents and their families should have a way to lodge complaints with multiple levels of staff, and not just with the direct care providers. We strongly recommend educating caregivers regarding the clinical manifestations of dementia, implementing psychosocial-environmental interventions to manage agitation, and improving support for professional and family caregivers to reduce the abuse of residents with dementia.

Long-Term Care Ombudsman Program

The Long-Term Care Ombudsman Program resolves the problems of individual residents; assists resident councils, family councils, and citizen organizations; and represents residents' needs and interests to public officials. The Administration on Aging of the U.S. Department of Health and Human Services is responsible for the national program. Each state has a Long-Term Care Ombudsman Program operated through, or by, that state's Area Agency on Aging. Each state program is headed by a state LTC ombudsperson. Throughout the state, paid staff and volunteer ombudspeople serve residents. Thus an LTC ombudsperson is an advocate for the residents of nursing homes, board-and-care homes, and assisted living facilities. The ombudsperson plays an important role in educating consumers and LTC providers about residents' rights and good care practices. The ombudsperson addresses many concerns related to the violation of residents' rights or dignity, such as physical, verbal, or mental abuse, poor quality of care, and inappropriate use of chemical or physical restraints.

Treatment of Elder Abuse

Health care providers have an ethical and legal responsibility both to report and to work to prevent suspected abuse in all elderly people. Physicians are in an ideal position to recognize, manage, and prevent elder abuse. Elder abuse is multifactorial and needs individual medical, psychiatric, and social intervention strategies, preferably in the context of a multidisciplinary team (Lachs and Pillemer 2004). Health care providers must be visible and available to residents, their families, and staff members to answer questions related to resident care. Although there are multiple gray areas in suspected abuse cases, much of the obvious abuse is being missed. If any health care provider suspects elder abuse, neglect, or exploitation, he or she needs to call the national Eldercare Locator, a public service of the U.S. Administration on Aging (800-677-1116). In case of emergency, health care providers should call the local police station or dial 911. All potential modifiable factors that predispose the resident to abuse (e.g., cognitive impairments, depression, hearing and/or vision deficits, a lack of family to act as advocates) and to the emotional (e.g., verbal and/or physical aggression, agitation) and physical complications of abuse (e.g., depression, pressure ulcers) should be identified and aggressively treated.

Ethical Dilemmas

Clinical medical ethics attempts to address the identification, analysis, and resolution of moral problems that arise in the care of a particular patient (Hayley et al. 1996). Autonomy, beneficence, nonmaleficence, and distributive justice are four core principles of clinical medical ethics in LTC settings. Autonomy, or self-determination, is fundamental in the daily lives of most Americans. Privacy and the confidentiality of personal information are closely related to autonomy, and health care providers need to vigorously protect them. Attention to small details may make a big difference in the residents' sense of autonomy. For example, a resident's life-long habit (and joy) of reading the morning newspaper with a cup of coffee may not fit with a regimented schedule, but this habit could be relatively easy to accommodate. The principle of beneficence involves the intention and acts to do good, and the principle of nonmaleficence entails the intention and acts to do no harm. Distributive justice consists of the equitable treatment in the distribution of resources.

Ethical dilemmas are encountered frequently in LTC facilities, encompassing a myriad of concerns related to end-of-life care, hospitalization, artificial hydration and nutrition, one's capacity for decision making, the use of sedation, and how to handle conflicts that may arise among those caring for and about the resident (Fleming 2007). The majority of these dilemmas are linked to the high prevalence of dementia and other disorders that affect a person's decision-making capacity. Health care providers have an ethical responsibility to defend the best interests of the resident at all times and to act as his or her advocate when required. For instance, this may mean resisting pressure to provide futile treatment that is not in keeping with the resident's wishes (expressed in a living will) because the family is not ready to "let go." Beneficence (i.e., doing good for the resident) and nonmaleficence (i.e., doing no harm to the resident) must be balanced against autonomy (i.e., the resident's right to take risks). The dignity of the resident is upheld through informed consent and opportunities for choice and risk taking. The clinician should keep in mind that the presence of a Do Not Resuscitate order may affect his or her willingness to order a variety of treatments not related to CPR. Thus the clinician should elicit additional information about the resident's treatment goals to inform these decisions (Zweig, Kruse, and Binder 2004).

People have unconditional worth and dignity, which supports a strong argument for the maintenance of autonomy (e.g., by not restraining them in order to prevent falls), even in the event of possible harm from an injury (e.g., fracture). The widely divergent cross-cultural differences and varying religious views in a pluralistic democratic society require that all professional staff (including physicians) approach treatment decisions with openness and sensitivity. In encounters with the resident, the physician should listen to, adapt, and, if possible, adopt the resident's perspective. Such an approach may help resolve many ethical dilemmas that are commonly encountered in caring for frail LTC populations. Every LTC facility is a community, albeit an artificial one, in which strangers come and live together. Ethicists are now giving thought to the nature of such communities and the obligations of people within it to each other. Often a formalized means of sorting through difficult cases is not readily available in LTC facilities that have limited staffing and lack access to physicians with expertise in geriatrics (especially geriatricians and geriatric psychiatrists) and ethicists from tertiary care centers. Some centers (e.g., the Center for Health Ethics, University of Missouri–Columbia) provide innovative statewide consultation services on request through video conferencing (tele-ethics), telephone conferencing, and e-mail.

We recommend that in an LTC facility, a mechanism should be made available on site to effectively address complex ethical issues in a timely fashion. This process can be instrumental in sustaining the dignity of the resident and maintaining the quality and safety of resident care. Such a mechanism has been proposed, involving five steps (Fleming 2007). The first step is to clarify the facts that relate to the organizational, medical, and social circumstances of the case. This also includes obtaining as much information as is feasible regarding the resident's personal values and beliefs, his or her degree of suffering, and the spiritual and psychological goals that are important to the resident. The second step is to clearly identify ethical concerns and differentiate them from legal concerns and issues related to miscommunication. The third step is to frame the issue in ethical terms, so that it can be critically discussed. The fourth step is to identify and resolve the conflict. The fifth and final step is to make a decision regarding the issue that raised the ethical conflict.

LTC facilities should be seen as communities promoting caring and interdependence. The goal should not simply be to eliminate or minimize dependence whenever possible, but to make creative and nurturing use of the dependence that is an inevitable reality for most LTC residents (Collopy, Boyle, and Jennings 1991). LTC facilities may be places for rehabilitation and recovery for some, but for most they need to be places of healing—of making whole—where frail and disabled elderly persons with a terminal illness are able to use their dependence to grow as human beings.

Research Ethics

The position statement of the Alzheimer's Association regarding ethical issues in research on individuals with dementia (www.alz.org) provides reasonable but not excessive protection for the people who participate in this research. The threat that medical, psychiatric, and environmental conditions pose on the well-being of the large (and growing) LTC population requires that research efforts not be hampered by excessive restrictions. We recommend adopting the following key features of the Alzheimer's Association position statement on this issue, with minor modifications.

For minimal-risk research, all residents (with their consent) should be allowed to enroll in a research project, even if there is no potential benefit to the individual. In the absence of an advance research directive, proxy consent is acceptable for residents who do not have the capacity to consent to research.

For greater-than-minimal-risk research where there is a reasonable potential benefit to the individual, all residents should be allowed to enroll based on the consent of the resident or the proxy. The proxy's consent can be based on either a research-specific advance directive or the proxy's judgment regarding the individual's best interests.

For greater-than-minimal-risk research where there is no reasonable potential benefit to the individual, only those individuals who (1) are capable of giving informed consent or (2) have executed a research-specific advance directive should be allowed to participate. In the latter case, and for residents who have dementia but retain the capacity to give consent, a proxy must be available to help monitor the resident's involvement throughout the duration of the research.

Truth Telling

Truthfulness is the foundation of all relationships. Without honesty and truthfulness, trust cannot be established and established trust can quickly erode. Without trust, family and professional caregivers may not be able to meet the emotional and physical needs of the residents and may even cause emotional harm. Most residents do not have the ability or the resources to find a different environment in which caregivers are honest and truthful. Yet truth telling, especially to residents with moderate to severe dementia, causes ethical dilemmas for many caregivers (family as well as professional).

All methods of discourse with residents should be truthful, with rare exceptions. Residents (whether they have dementia or not) are resilient, and even cognitively impaired residents can quickly detect a lie (e.g., caregivers telling a resident who wants to go home that he or she is at the facility "for only a few days" and soon will be able to go home). Benevolent deception should be an exception, rather than the rule, in caring for vulnerable LTC populations.

Truth telling is not synonymous with being bluntly honest. Blunt honesty in some situations may be harmful to the resident. Strict adherence to the virtues of truthfulness and candor in some situations (e.g., giving a diagnosis of a terminal illness [e.g., metastatic cancer] to a resident who made a recent serious suicide attempt) risks violating the core ethical principles of beneficence and nonmaleficence. In daily practice such situations are rare, but the frequency of lying and dishonesty in dealing with LTC populations (especially for those with dementia) is far from rare. This culture of dishonesty is fueled by the irrational fears of the caregivers (professional and family) and by their discomfort in addressing a resident's grief and loss.

Truth telling needs to be done with utmost sensitivity to the resident's emotional state and to the individual circumstances, and efforts should be made to understand what the resident is trying to express (e.g., a resident who asks when he can go home may be reacting to unrelieved pain; a resident who asks for her small children may be reacting to a feeling of purposelessness in life; a resident who looks for her parents is looking for validation, security, and unconditional love). Truthfulness may hurt (e.g., telling the resident that this is his or her new home), and caregivers need to anticipate the resident's pain and take steps to relieve it.

Ultimately, being truthful is about honoring the resident's dignity. Therefore, respecting that dignity is each resident's right and our obligation. This is even more important for residents who are weakest (e.g., residents with severe dementia), as their dignity lies in our hands.

Ethical Dilemmas During End-of-Life Care

Ethical dilemmas are routinely encountered in LTC populations during end-of-life care. Examples include dilemmas around futile medical treatments, physician-assisted death, the discontinuation of a medical treatment that has a high burden, the discontinuation of artificial nutrition and hydration, and the use of life-prolonging treatments for residents with severe or terminal dementia. Futile treatment is a treatment or medical intervention that provides no meaningful possibility of extended life or an improved quality of life or other benefit for the resident. Medically futile situations can stimulate tremendous ethical conflicts, both within an individual and between individuals involved in the medical situation. For example, conflicts can arise when the family or surrogates demand treatment that the clinical staff views as excessively burdensome and futile for the resident.

Situations (e.g., terminal dementia) involving futile treatment commonly stimulate intense guilt in family members, who may go to great lengths to avoid actions that make them feel guilty. The prompt involvement of a physician (especially an experienced physician, and preferably one with expertise in geriatrics) is crucial to address ethical dilemmas in such situations and reduce the accompanying emotional suffering (in residents, their families, and clinical staff members). Health care providers with expertise in addressing such situations (e.g., psychiatrists) can often assist families and residents by helping them to bear their grief, guilt, and disappointment and to understand that physical helplessness does not automatically imply psychological helplessness. Medically futile situations may in fact promote the development of psychological mastery. Physicians, too, can experience psychological growth as they turn from action at any cost to empathetic care for the whole patient, including psychological care. Health care providers should address any family misunderstandings about suffering during end-of-life care and address the family's guilt and grief with patience and compassion. Listening to staff concerns and helping the staff understand the family's fears, guilt, and grief are helpful in reducing the staff's concerns and distress.

Determining the benefit of a particular treatment for a resident who has one or more terminal conditions is often difficult. In an LTC setting, the special relationships that are often established between the staff and residents may make the issue more ethically challenging. Sometimes members of the direct care staff feel that they understand a resident better than anyone else. In working through these issues with the staff, the clinician should distinguish between futile medical treatment and supportive care. Although a particular medical treatment may be considered to produce no benefit for the resident, staff members often need to be reassured that their caring is never futile or in vain. The decision to forgo a particular treatment must never be confused with abandoning the resident.

It is not uncommon for residents, or even some family members, to request physician-assisted death or euthanasia. Physician-assisted death can raise serious ethical conflicts, not only among professional caregivers but also with residents and their families. We strongly advocate palliative care (including palliative sedation) and hospice care in place of physician-assisted death. The preeminence of autonomy as an ethical principle in the United States can sometimes lead health care providers to disregard other moral considerations and common sense when making clinical decisions. An emphasis on individual autonomy reflects deeply held values in the United States: rugged individualism and self-sufficiency. Interdependence is not valued as much as autonomy in American society. We respect many individuals' beliefs and their wish to anticipate and overtake death by administering it themselves (i.e., we respect the person's wish for autonomy), but we strongly feel that the role of the medical profession is to understand but *not* to support such wishes. Every person's life is valuable, irrespective of one's physical and mental state, even when that person has ceased to deem life valuable. Yet all health care providers should also accept death as one of the conditions of human freedom. Valuing and promoting interdependence is crucial to providing dignity-conserving care to LTC populations and helping residents overcome the wish to end their lives.

Discontinuing medical intervention that poses a high burden often causes considerable ethical dilemmas, especially in caring for residents with severe dementia. For example, a decision regarding when to discontinue dialysis for a resident with severe dementia is difficult, especially if the resident does not appear to be suffering between dialysis sessions. Usually there is no guiding advance directive. The family or surrogates may be called on to decide whether it would be inappropriate to continue dialysis, based on their impressions of the resident's wishes or their estimate of the resident's best interest. If the resident's mental state leads him or her to interpret each dialysis as a threatening event that requires restraint or sedation or both, the decision to give up dialysis is clearly in the resident's best interest. We recommend an interdisciplinary team meeting, with the physician as the team leader and with the family present, to better understand the resident's values and make decisions that are in keeping with those values.

Withholding or withdrawing artificial nutrition and hydration also commonly raise ethical dilemmas. Because food and water are basic to human survival, and because feeding can be an expression of caring for and loving another person, caregivers may see the decision to withhold nutrition or to withdraw a feeding tube (e.g., for a resident in the terminal stage of dementia) not as the withholding of a medical treatment (e.g., not putting a patient on a ventilator) but as the denial of basic human care. Such situations often raise ethical issues, because of both the manner in which the decisions are made and the resident's capacity to make her or his wishes known. When residents are able to choose, the decision to withhold artificial nutrition and hydration may be more comfortable for the staff. In the absence of advance directives addressing artificial nutrition and hydration, some staff members may believe that there is a moral and legal obligation to do everything medically possible for the resident. Such ethical concerns of staff members should be addressed promptly with an interdisciplinary staff meeting and a sharing of recommendations from reputable organizations and journals (e.g., Mitchell 2007).

One area in which there is still controversy is whether antidementia drugs reduce mortality in LTC residents with dementia. There is preliminary evidence that they may indeed do so (Ott and Lapane 2002; Gasper, Ott, and Lapane 2005). Until further research clarifies this issue, we recommend including the modest potential benefits of antidementia drugs for some residents (e.g., a reduction in future agitation and the ability to maintain some current function [e.g., eating on one's own] for a few months longer than without the medications) in deciding between the risks and benefits of continuing antidementia drugs on an individual basis.

Restricting Autonomy in Different Cultures

In times of crisis and when facing one's own mortality, religious and familial or cultural values can be sources of strength and comfort. The traditional American emphasis on autonomy and full disclosure may not be respectful of dying residents from different cultural traditions. In Asian, Hispanic, and other traditions, autonomy must be balanced against such values as family and community support and compassion. For example, for a person from one of these cultural heritages, the family, rather than the resident, may make life support decisions. Many health care providers may have ethical issues related to restricting a resident's autonomy (e.g., the family's request to not tell the resident about a terminal prognosis). Full disclosure may be at variance with cultural beliefs about hope and wellness, and autonomous decision making may be counter to family-centered values (Gostin 1995). The resident's values should dictate whether it is beneficial or burdensome to be fully informed. The challenge to physicians is to understand and bridge the gulf between their own values and those of the resident. Although some differences may not be resolvable, residents and their families deserve a meaningful and dignified process of death and dying that is in keeping with their cultural and religious values.

Distributive Justice

The ethical dilemma of distributive justice arises when one has limited resources and multiple groups are trying to access those resources. How do you decide which resident should be given a single room if such rooms are scarce? How does one decide which person to admit when a bed becomes available? Such dilemmas are routine in LTC facilities. For example, a resident who was living in a private room (only one occupant) dies and different staff members want the room for various residents who are currently sharing a room with another resident. One staff member wishes the room to go to a resident who is a "yeller" and has disturbed every roommate he has had. Another staff member wants the room for a resident who is on hospice so that family members can stay with the resident during her last days. It is important to realize that both of these options (and many others) may be ethically right. There are often no wrong solutions. It is best to resolve such dilemmas as a group, rather than having one person on the leadership team make a unilateral decision.

Medicolegal Issues

Physicians and other health care providers should try to provide state-of-the-art care, although for medicolegal purposes, they are required to provide just the standard of care. The standard of care is defined as what a reasonable health care provider would have done in the same set of circumstances at the same time. Communication, the education of residents and their families, and the documentation of treatments are critical. Communication with the interdisciplinary team is important. Communicating with the resident and the family and educating them about the treatment should involve explaining the care plan and ensuring that they understand the resident's condition and the limitations of treatment. The clinician should document this conversation.

Medical directors have many more responsibilities to ensure that the standard of care is being provided to all residents. Medical directors are expected to have regular meetings with department heads at the facility, to be aware of trends or problems identified by facility personnel, and to be aware of the policies and procedures that need to be implemented about the problem (e.g., physical abuse of a resident by a staff member). Understanding proper reporting procedures can reduce the risk of government sanctions and criminal penalties for those working in LTC. It is incumbent on medical directors to familiarize themselves with criminal mistreatment laws in their state in order to ensure the residents' well-being, promote the staff members' integrity, and assist their facilities in managing the risk of criminal liability for abuse and neglect (MacLean 1999).

Conclusion

Abuse and neglect are prevalent in long-term care populations, they are underrecognized, and they are undertreated. Hence, during each encounter, the clinician should screen each resident for possible abuse. Addressing the abuse and neglect of residents includes prevention, reporting, and management of the negative health consequences. The most valuable intervention that a clinician can provide in cases of suspected abuse or neglect is in making an initial report to the appropriate agency. Health care providers must focus on the care of the resident and be an advocate for the resident. Clinicians who provide care for LTC populations are regularly challenged by ethical and legal issues. Ethical dilemmas are also commonly experienced by residents and their families. Most ethical issues can be resolved by guidance from an experienced physician. For complicated cases, we recommend a multidisciplinary approach.

Western civilization's concepts of personal autonomy and self-determination are at the core of health care decision making, but health care providers must be aware that other cultures do not always share that value system. Sensitivity to multicultural diversity in this context is imperative in maintaining individual self-esteem and respect for both the resident and the family (Zimring 2006). Attention to the medicolegal aspects of LTC practice (e.g., regular communication, and documentation of the risks and benefits of high-risk treatment interventions) is as important as high-quality clinical care.

CHAPTER 11

Palliative and End-of-Life Care

And in the end, it's not the years in your life that count—it's the
life in your years.

—*Abraham Lincoln*

Death and dying are central features of any practice in long-term
care. The most common causes of death in long-term care populations include terminal-stage dementia, congestive heart failure, cancer, and strokes.
In LTC populations that have underlying terminal conditions, pneumonia,
cachexia, dehydration, and hip fractures are the most common acute medical
events that precipitate death. Delirium and depression are the two most frequent psychiatric syndromes during the end of life for residents in LTC facilities. One in four Americans dies in a nursing home, and some 30 percent of
all nursing home residents die within one year of admission (Oliver, Porock,
and Zweig 2004). By the year 2020, it is projected that approximately 40
percent of Americans will die in a nursing home (Kapo, Morrison, and Liao
2007).

LTC residents often develop multiple chronic medical problems and endure
complicated medical courses with a variety of disease trajectories. Expertise in the diagnosis and management of diverse geriatric syndromes in LTC
settings (e.g., frailty, dementia, depression, delirium, agitation, pain, falls,
urinary incontinence, weight loss, pressure ulcers, dyspnea) is essential in
providing high-quality palliative care to LTC populations. End-of-life care for
residents has shifted from their families to health care providers, and much
of the cost of that care has shifted from families to the government. Deci-

sions about end-of-life care have moved from choices made by individuals to a negotiated plan of care among individuals, families, and health care providers and, in some situations, an ethics committee, the judicial system, and the government. Thus end-of-life care in LTC has become less of a medical problem and more of a problem for the community as a whole.

Much of the end-of-life care for LTC populations is for residents with dementia. These residents often die with inadequate pain control, with feeding tubes in place, and without the benefits of hospice care (Sachs, Shega, and Cox-Hayley 2004). Many family caregivers feel that their loved one did not experience a good death in the LTC facility (Bosek et al. 2003). End-of-life care in LTC settings may be inadequate because of chronic staff shortages, rapid staff turnover, poor staff training, poor reimbursement for palliative care, and limited participation by a physician (Miller, Teno, and Mor 2004). Last, but not least, prevailing societal attitudes and deeply ingrained prejudices against aging, frailty, and dementia are barriers to providing high-quality palliative care for all elderly people. The life of every human being is inherently valuable, and the end-of-life care needs of all residents should be reconceptualized to encourage more attention to the residents' quality of life and comfort and fewer active efforts to treat every medical exigency that arises.

Palliative Care

The World Heath Organization defines palliative care as an approach that improves the quality of life for patients and their families who are facing a life-threatening illness, through the prevention and relief of suffering by means of early identification, assessment, and the treatment of pain and other problems—physical, psychosocial, and spiritual. Thus the ultimate goal of palliative care is to help an individual make the best of every remaining day. The decision to intervene with active palliative care is based on an ability to meet stated goals (e.g., enhancing the person's quality of life, relief from distressing symptoms) rather than to affect the underlying terminal disease. All treatment options should be explored and evaluated in the context of the individual's values and symptoms. That person's choices and decisions regarding care are paramount and must be followed. The majority of LTC residents have one or more terminal illnesses (an illness from which there is little or no chance of recovery and that will most likely cause death in the near future). Thus palliative care should be offered to all LTC residents in custodial care and to many of the residents admitted for rehabilitation, regardless of their status as terminally ill or not. In many circumstances, health care providers may need to combine elements of palliative care with life-sustaining therapy to maximize the resident's quality and quantity of life, and no specific therapy should be excluded from consideration. This model abandons the either/or distinction between curative and palliative care and starts addressing quality-of-life and family issues once a diagnosis is made. In general, as curative treatment becomes less likely to be effective (and more burdensome), palliative care issues become greater.

The level and types of palliative care services that are provided vary among LTC facilities. Some nursing homes may have separate palliative care units or beds, some may be able to administer intravenous medications, and some may have access to physicians or other health care providers (nurse practitioners or physician assistants) who can assess an acute medical problem on site within four hours (thus avoiding a trip to the emergency room or hospitalization for many residents). Most assisted living facilities are still struggling to provide high-quality palliative care (Mitty 2004).

Palliative care is a popular term in LTC these days, but it is often misunderstood. Some facilities have a separate wing or unit for palliative care; others focus on pain management; and another approach is to train staff members in bereavement services. True palliative care has six components (table 11.1), and palliative care with all six components should be integrated into the routine care that is provided to all residents. All staff members, rather than only a separate palliative care team, should be involved in palliative care.

Palliative care preferably should start before admission, or at least at the time of admission. It starts with a review of the patient's and family's expectations of care and education about the philosophy and goals of palliative care. The next level of palliative care is implementing a formal palliative care

TABLE 11.1
Components of palliative care

Dignity-conserving care

Spiritual care

Encouragement of creative expression

Advance care planning: includes customized care that reflects the individual's preferences and respects that person's wishes, the thoughtful use of personal and family resources, and an ongoing discussion of the person's wishes regarding various medical emergencies

Relief of symptoms to ensure maximal comfort: includes physical (e.g., pain, dyspnea, incontinence, fatigue, cough, dry mouth, nausea), emotional (depression, anxiety, loneliness), and behavioral (agitation, aggression) symptoms

Care for the caregiver: includes caring for family and professional caregivers, and offering bereavement counseling, stress-reduction strategies, and staff empowerment program that involves six steps: (1) each resident is assessed for the six components described above, and one or more areas of focus (e.g., pain, agitation, caregiver grief) are identified; (2) measures to track outcomes (e.g., pain scale, depression scale, bereavement scale) are identified and preintervention measurements are taken; (3) evidence-based interventions are instituted; (4) postintervention outcomes are measured (e.g., a reduction in pain, a reduction in depression, a reduction in grief-related suffering); (5) results are shared with the staff and the family and their input is obtained; and (6) interventions are modified based on feedback and new research. Specific facility-wide goals can be set and outcomes tracked. For example, one goal may be an 80 percent reduction in moderate-to-severe pain symptoms within 72 hours of the initial assessment.

The ideal is in-house training in palliative care for as many staff members as possible (from housekeepers to physicians) by in-house palliative care leaders (e.g., the medical director, a consulting psychiatrist, or the director of nursing) who have themselves received advanced training in palliative care. Table 11.2 lists the topics for palliative care training. For example, housekeepers can be trained to watch for pain and other symptoms in residents, off-the-cuff grief remarks by family, and the like.

Dignity-Conserving Care

Upholding, protecting, and restoring the dignity of all patients is both the duty of every health care provider and the essence of medicine. Every resi-

TABLE 11.2
Topics for palliative care training

Basic principles of palliative care
Perceptions of death and dying
The concept of dignity-conserving care
Standardized tools for assessing pain
Prescription of appropriate pain medications
Bereavement counseling
Psychosocial-environmental interventions for managing challenging behaviors
Prescription of appropriate psychotropic medications
Stress-reduction strategies (e.g., mindfulness-based stress reduction, relaxation response)
Standardized tools for assessing depression
Advance care planning
Palliative sedation (and how it is different from assisted suicide and euthanasia)
Spirituality
Management of aggressive behaviors
Encouragement of creative expression

dent is worthy of honor, and there is meaning in the life of all residents, regardless of their cognitive, physical, and emotional conditions. Kindness, humanity, and respect—the core values of the medical profession, often overlooked in our time-pressed culture—can be reinstated by dignity-conserving care (Chochinov 2007). How residents perceive themselves to be seen is a powerful mediator for their dignity, and dignity is closely associated with a sense of being treated with respect. Factors that have been identified as fracturing a patient's sense of dignity include, but are not limited to, a loss of independence, fear of becoming a burden, no involvement in decision making, a lack of access to care (including palliative care), and some of the attitudes of health care providers, especially when patients feel vulnerable and lack power. Health care providers can uphold residents' dignity by seeing them for the people they were before dementia or a stroke, rather than for the illness they have. We recommend the A, B, C, D approach to dignity-conserving care (Chochinov 2007):

- Attitude: all health care providers should have utmost respect for all residents at all times (during life and after death).
- Behavior: all health care providers should show respect and kindness to all residents through their verbal and nonverbal behaviors at every interaction.
- Compassion: all health care providers should have compassion (a deep awareness of the suffering of another coupled with a wish to relieve it) for all residents at all times.
- Dialog: all health care providers should have an ongoing dialog with themselves (e.g., "Am I making ageist assumptions?"), with other health care providers (e.g., "Are we withholding life-sustaining treatment because of our assumption of a poor quality of life in a resident?"), with the resident ("What do you value?" or "What gives your life meaning?"; "What is your attitude toward suffering?"; "What is your identity?"), and with the resident's family ("What are the most important things in your loved one's life? Was there a hierarchy?") in order to know and value every resident.

Ensuring dignity thus involves spending more time with the resident and the family. These qualities of professionalism and connectedness also increases the likelihood that residents and their families will be forthright in disclosing personal information, which often has a bearing on ongoing care.

Every LTC facility should have a written policy of zero tolerance for a lack of dignity in the care of all residents.

Spiritual Care

There is a Sufi saying that two veils—health and security—separate us from the divine. The humbling circumstances of losing one or both may broaden us, in spite of ourselves. Similarly, to truly behold another is a spiritual act. Once we, as health care providers, take the trouble to know our residents, they will begin to feel seen, and in the course of feeling seen they will reveal more of themselves, because of a sense of safety in being known. Our giving and receiving will thus move into a sacred dimension (Lustbader 2000). Therefore, addressing residents' spiritual needs is vital to achieving the goals of palliative care (increased comfort and a timely, dignified, and peaceful death). For some residents, coming to peace with God, not being a burden to others, having funeral arrangements in place, and being mentally aware are important factors at the end of life. Chaplains or other appropriate spiritual providers can aid greatly in addressing residents' spiritual needs. Even residents with severe cognitive impairment can respond to religious rituals, intimate prayers, religious songs, and symbols. Although a person may be deep into the progression of dementia, continuities with the past usually exist amid the discontinuities.

The need for spiritual care varies greatly, not only from resident to resident, but also by race, gender, economic status, and ethnic heritage. Meaning-centered group therapy (offered to cognitively intact residents at the end of life) is a novel intervention that may successfully integrate themes of meaning and spirituality into end-of-life care. Professional caregivers need to realize that besides keeping the resident clean and comfortable, they should feel comfortable in helping residents transport themselves beyond their physical decline. This can be done in several ways, such as by reading them a favorite poem, singing a favorite song with them, or just spending time with them.

> **CLINICAL CASE** Mr. U, a 78-year-old man with severe dementia, developed acute bleeding from his rectum, and his wife was not sure if she should admit him to the hospital or opt for hospice care. The psychiatrist who had been involved in his treatment over the previous months helped Mrs. U understand the futility of hospitalization and that Mr. U would have wanted only comfort care at this point. Mrs. U agreed that her husband would have wanted comfort care only, but she wanted to be sure that

she was not giving up on him. Their daughter and son felt sure that their father would want comfort care only. After her children's input, Mrs. U decided on hospice care. Her dilemma was understandable, because just three months previously, Mr. U had been ambulatory and could feed himself with assistance, although he could not recognize family members by name (including his wife). He had developed pneumonia, and Mrs. U had admitted him to the hospital for treatment at that time.

Although the pneumonia was treated successfully, Mr. U had developed severe agitation and delirium during his hospital stay and needed large doses of antipsychotic medications to control the agitation. When he returned to the nursing home he could not walk, had lost the ability to feed himself, and was able to articulate only some words but not full sentences. After Mr. U began hospice care, the family and staff were surprised to learn that two different staff members on separate occasions had heard him clearly state, "I saw the heavenly gates" and "I was told to come back later." Mrs. U asked their pastor to come to the nursing home for spiritual support and to help her understand these statements. The pastor suggested that maybe Mr. U was waiting for his wife to say that it was okay for him to go. Mrs. U followed the pastor's advice, and three days later Mr. U died peacefully, with his wife holding his hand and his two children at his bedside.

TEACHING POINTS Even in the terminal stage of dementia, patients may be able to come up with complete sentences on rare occasions. Spiritual needs are more important than ever in the care of residents in the severe and terminal stages of dementia. The help of clergy during end-of-life care is crucial for the well-being of many residents and their families. Also, the family may need guidance to say goodbye to their loved one and to understand that allowing nature to takes its course (and thus allowing a natural dying process) is not giving up but letting go.

Creativity During the End of Life

Residents have enormous creativity that often remains untapped. Art is possible, and even enhanced, in a setting of disability and frailty. A small number of residents (e.g., some patients with early-stage frontotemporal dementia) may develop a new interest in art or express themselves more intensely through their artwork to cope with their emotional and/or physical suffering. Many residents, even if they have advanced dementia, have preserved their social function and their imagination, which allows them to participate in creative projects or programs such as "Memories in the Making" (a watercolor-painting activity) or "TimeSlips" (a group storytelling activity). The preserved strengths and abilities of all residents (irrespective of their frailty status or their level of cognitive impairment) need to be acknowledged, brought out, and maintained with innovative programs and creative activities. Finally, the majority of residents retain their capacity to appreciate and enjoy art, and this needs to be tapped into to improve their psychosocial well-being. Creating, looking at, and discussing art can be a spiritually rich and emotionally uplifting experience for residents who do not have full cognitive capacities. For some residents, engaging in creative activities can be a transforming experience. For residents who may wish to write about their memories or produce a poem, helping them jot it down may turn agony into peace.

Advance Care Planning

I will not relinquish old age, if it leaves my better part intact. But, if it begins to shake my mind, if it destroys its faculties one by one, if it leaves me not life but breath, I will depart from the putrid or tottering edifice. If I must suffer without hope or relief, I will depart, not through fear of the pain itself, but because it prevents all for which I would live.—Seneca, first century AD

Advance care planning documents ensure that a resident's wishes will be carried out when he or she is no longer capable of making care-related decisions. Advance directives should be conceptualized as an extension of the fully autonomous person. All states recognize advance directives as the reflection of a person's decisions regarding end-of-life care, and all health care providers have the responsibility of upholding advance directives in caring for residents. We recommend the "Five Wishes" document for planning advance care (available at www.agingwithdignity.org). This document addresses not only who would make decisions for the person when he or she cannot do so and what kind(s) of medical treatment the person would want during the end of life, but also how comfortable the person would want to be (e.g., pain control even at the cost of impaired cognition or consciousness), how the person would want others to treat him or her (e.g., to talk to the person periodically even if he or she is in a coma), and what the person would want loved ones to know (e.g., a wish for two family members who have grown apart to make amends to each other).

Medical decision making regarding residents with complex health problems requires a careful application of the best medical evidence combined with a clinical judgment that is balanced by resident-specific information based on the individual's life circumstances and personal values. Health care providers in any area of health care (nursing, social work, medicine, psychiatry, psychology) can take a leadership role in counseling residents and their families to discuss end-of-life wishes, what "quality of life" means, and the concept of substituted judgment versus a best-interest approach to making decisions.

Health care providers should encourage residents and their families to discuss the pros and cons of the following interventions on an ongoing basis and in the context of the resident's gradually increasing disabilities: do not resuscitate (DNR), do not intubate (DNI), do not hospitalize (DNH), do not call 911, do not insert a feeding tube, do not do laboratory tests, do not give antibiotics or intravenous fluids unless the reason is to improve comfort. Health care providers should discuss the risks and benefits of DNR with every resident or, more commonly, the surrogate decision maker. In general, because of severe and multiple comorbidities (especially dementia), the risks of resuscitation (further and severe cognitive impairment, rib fracture, the need for a ventilator) outweigh the benefits (successful resuscitation and discharge from the hospital) and the success rate of CPR for residents in LTC facilities is low (0.1%–5%). Hospitalization for a hip fracture may be appropriate for a resident with mild to moderate dementia and is otherwise healthy, but it may be inappropriate for a resident with severe dementia who has lost the ability to comprehend spoken language and is thus unable to participate in intensive rehabilitation after surgery. The family should be counseled that in situations in which surgery is forgone, the resident's pain can be adequately managed with medications and that the risks of hospitalization outweigh the benefits.

Communication about death and dying is vital, but the difficulties and stresses involved in bringing up the subject are so great that the discussion will usually be postponed for a "better opportunity," which seldom arrives. It is important for the clinician to remember that besides honoring the resident's wishes, an important goal of holding such a discussion is to ease the stress of both the resident and the family and to help them cope with the thought of impending death.

In anticipating a resident's potential loss of his or her decision-making capability, the health care provider should engage the resident early on in advance care planning, such as exploring the resident's values and goals and discussing advance care planning documents (e.g., a living will and a durable power of attorney for health care). The clinician should assure residents that such planning is a routine part of the admission process. With more intense communication occurring up front, the resident's and family's emotional and spiritual needs become a more integral part of the care.

The treatment team can trigger a dialog about end-of-life care by asking questions such as "Would we be surprised if this resident died in the next few months?" and "Is this resident sick enough to die?" and then using each episode of an acute illness, each visit to the emergency room, or each hospitalization as a rehearsal for end-of-life care discussions. Asking the resident and family if their goals of care would change "if this happens next time" is also helpful to clarify the types of end-of-life interventions desired.

Racial, ethnic, and gender groups may differ significantly in their end-of-life health care wishes. In some cultural groups (e.g., Asians, Arabs), families may be reluctant to tell the resident "bad news" and may avoid the use of words such as *death* and *cancer*. Health care providers need to be truthful with the resident but also sensitive to the wishes of the family, and they should communicate with the resident and the family in the least threatening manner possible. Also, health care providers should not generalize about all individuals in one group. It is important to respect the resident's preferences while considering the influences of race, ethnicity, and gender.

Health care providers need to understand the resident's religious/spiritual beliefs and financial circumstances, as well as the potential impact of any medical intervention on these concerns. Some residents and their families wish to participate actively in a discussion of treatment choices, whereas other residents and their families may defer most of the decisions to the physician after only a brief discussion. Health care providers need to communicate that the benefits and burdens may be uncertain for many end-of-life situations and interventions. They also need to help residents and their families emotionally negotiate this uncertainty.

Estimating Life Expectancy (Prognosis)

The terminal phase of life is difficult to predict for LTC residents who do not have cancer, but once the terminal phase is diagnosed, their survival time is usually short (one to two weeks). Estimating life expectancy typically involves LTC residents with severe or terminal-stage dementia, and a failure to recognize dementia as an incurable and progressive disease may result in inadequate end-of-life care, including late referral to a hospice. However, determining the prognosis in dementia is challenging. The time from diagnosis to death varies—from as little as three years if the resident is over 80 when diagnosed with dementia to 10 years or more if the resident is younger. A risk score based on 12 variables from the Minimum Data Set estimates the six-month mortality for nursing home residents with advanced dementia with greater accuracy than existing prognostic guidelines (Mitchell et al. 2004). The Mitchell et al. study also suggested that hypoactive delirium is a marker of a poor prognosis in dementia. Residents in this study who were "not awake most of the day" were likely to die in the nursing home within six months.

Estimating the life expectancy of LTC residents with terminal illnesses other than dementia (e.g., congestive heart failure, end-stage renal disease) is also challenging. Residents with end-stage renal disease tend to have a short life expectancy, multiple comorbidities, and a high symptom burden (e.g., itching, dry skin, fatigue, bone and muscle pain, muscle cramps). Many residents with end-stage renal disease may choose to stop dialysis (or the family may decide to stop it) when they feel that the burden of dialysis is high and the benefits, in terms of relief from daily symptoms, are low. Predictors of a poor prognosis for residents with congestive heart failure or end-stage renal disease include advanced age, reduced functional ability (e.g., dependence on staff for basic ADLs), poor nutritional status (e.g., a low serum albumin level), and the presence of comorbid illness.

Issues Pertaining to Hospitalization

Residents living in LTC facilities are at particular risk of admission to a hospital (Konetzka, Spector, and Limcangco 2008). More than 25 percent of long-stay nursing home residents are hospitalized in any given six-month period (Spector et al. 2007). Hospitalization and visits to the emergency room are extremely stressful for most LTC residents, especially frail, cognitively impaired residents. Poorly executed discharges from a hospital (e.g., poor coordination and communication among the hospital personnel, the patient, the family, and the LTC staff) may result in repeat hospitalizations of residents transferred from a hospital to an LTC facility. Hospitalization stemming from medical conditions thought to be largely avoidable or manageable with timely access to a physician and other medical support services has been termed *ambulatory care-sensitive hospitalization*.

Issues pertaining to hospitalization in relation to palliative care include reducing ambulatory care-sensitive hospitalization, preventing futile hospitalization, and recognizing the potential benefits of hospitalization for certain medical conditions and palliative care needs. Hospitalization for hip fracture surgery for a resident who is relatively cognitively intact may significantly improve that resident's quality of life. Hospitalization to an acute inpatient psychiatric unit (preferably a geriatric psychiatry unit) for the treatment of severe depression during a resident's end of life is also appropriate. Admission to a palliative care unit in a hospital for high-level and complex palliative care interventions (e.g., deep sedation for severe and refractory pain, deep sedation for end-of-life delirium with severe aggression and agitation), when available, may be necessary to relieve suffering for some residents during the last days of their life.

Among LTC residents, there is some evidence that low levels of RN staffing and poor quality-of-care practices significantly increase a resident's risk of experiencing ambulatory care-sensitive hospitalization (Carter 2003). Residents with dementia are at higher risk of ambulatory care-sensitive hospitalizations than residents who do not have dementia (Carter and Porell 2005). Increased RN staffing levels and on-site physicians and/or other health care providers (nurse practitioners, physician assistants) may reduce the risk of ambulatory care-sensitive hospitalizations in LTC populations (Konetzka, Spector, and Limcangco 2008). The availability of a highly trained nursing staff may improve timely identification of subtle changes in residents' symptoms (especially for residents with advanced dementia who may not be able to communicate their physical symptoms), allowing for prompt medical intervention. Other strategies to reduce hospitalization for LTC populations include improving the hospital-to-facility transition and aligning reimbursement policies such that providers do not have a financial incentive to hospitalize residents.

More than 50 percent of the people with advanced dementia who were admitted to a hospital with a diagnosis of a hip fracture or pneumonia died within six months of discharge, compared with only 12 percent of those who did not have dementia, suggesting that hip fractures and pneumonia are end-stage markers (Morrison and Siu 2000). Some 30 percent of hospital deaths occur within five days of transfer from a nursing home (Kapo, Morrison, and Liao 2007). Palliative care discussions based on a resident's wishes for expected medical emergencies (e.g., chest pain or acute neurological deficits in residents with unstable coronary artery disease, or acute neurological deficits in residents with a history of multiple strokes) may avoid unnecessary or accidental transfers to the emergency room for an evaluation of a possible myocardial infarction or stroke, since hospitalization for these problems has been deemed not to be in the best interest of the resident because of his or her end-of-life situation. Avoiding futile hospitalization, providing palliative care, and, if indicated, referring the person to a hospice may substantially reduce the suffering of many residents in LTC facilities. Do Not Hospitalize orders as part of their treatment plan should be discussed for all residents in the severe or terminal stages of dementia or other diseases.

Reviewing the Appropriateness of All Medications

A study found that 29 percent of the patients with advanced dementia who were enrolled in a palliative care program were taking medications that are never appropriate at that stage (Holmes et al. 2008). Determining the appropriate time to discontinue dementia-specific medications is a complicated decision. Ceasing to prescribe medication may result in a full spectrum of family responses, from significant psychological distress to great relief. In general, the clinician should discontinue prescribing antidementia medications when a resident reaches the terminal stage of dementia. Some residents with moderate to severe dementia may benefit from discontinuation without any adverse outcomes, whereas others may show increased cognitive impairments or behavioral symptoms and may need their antidementia medications reinstated.

The clinician should discuss the necessity of other medications for residents in palliative care (e.g., cholesterol-lowering agents, vitamins, medications for osteoporosis) and discontinue all medications that are deemed unnecessary (i.e., do not promote an improved quality of life). Certain drugs (e.g., warfarin) carry a significant risk of adverse effects and/or a frequent need for blood tests. Their prescription may pose a high burden for residents in the last phase of life and have few benefits. Hence the clinician should consider discontinuing these drugs.

LTC residents with advanced dementia frequently have an extensive exposure to antimicrobial drugs, often administered parenterally, and their use steadily increases toward the end of life (D'Agata and Mitchell 2008). The use of antibiotics imposes a considerable burden on residents (e.g., adverse effects, a prolongation of life that is not in keeping with the resident's wishes), especially for residents during the last stages of life. The clinician should consider prescribing antibiotics for a resident who is in the last stages of life only after a discussion about whether the resident's interests are being served (e.g., increased comfort by treating a urinary tract infection) despite the burdens imposed. For residents with terminal-stage dementia, we often do not recommend treating pneumonia with antibiotics, because such treatment may not prolong life and its adverse effects may affect the resident's quality of life.

Hospice

Hospice care focuses on the dying process and on helping individuals with a terminal illness (and their family and friends) go through this process more comfortably. Hospices also offer a 13-month bereavement benefit following the death of a resident. One of the key goals of palliative care is to identify those residents who would benefit from and qualify for hospice care. Within the context of Medicare benefits, hospice care is defined as an alternative to other Part A benefits, whereas Medicare and Medicaid do not recognize palliative care as a separate form of specialized care. To make a referral to a hospice, the physician must state that the resident's life expectancy is six months or less, due to a terminal (progressive and incurable) illness. Although many people with a terminal illness (including terminal-stage dementia) can benefit from hospice care, except for those with cancer, it is often difficult to determine when to refer someone to a hospice (Lunney et al. 2003). Eligibility for residents with a nonmalignant disease is based on clinical judgment.

The availability of hospice care in assisted living facilities has allowed many residents there to achieve a peaceful death without being transferred to a hospital or a nursing home. Although the use of hospice care with LTC populations is increasing rapidly, there is concern for both its underuse for many residents who may benefit from it and its overuse for many other residents (especially residents with dementia) (Casarett, Hirschman, and Henry 2001). Improving communication with the attending physician regarding a resident's goals for care and his or her treatment preferences is an appropriate way to improve when and for whom hospice referrals are made in LTC facilities. Residents and their families may benefit from the services that a hospice provides, such as better management of pain, dyspnea, and feeding tubes; increased satisfaction regarding the quality of a loved one's end-of-life care; and lower rates of hospitalization (Baer and Hanson 2000). After a resident is enrolled in a hospice, that person's care plan must document and designate which services the hospice will be responsible for and which services the LTC facility will provide.

Relief of Symptoms

Residents in their last days, weeks, or months of life may experience many distressing symptoms, such as delirium, agitation, dyspnea, pain, aggression, depression, and psychotic symptoms. Anxiety, fever, and gastrointestinal symptoms are also common. Intensive management of these symptoms is imperative, and rapidly worsening symptoms should be considered palliative care emergencies requiring immediate intervention. The terminal disease phase for most LTC residents is marked with distressing symptoms of low fluid and food intake, general weakness, and dyspnea. Direct causes of these conditions are diseases of the respiratory system (mainly pneumonia) and general disorders (e.g., cachexia). The two main underlying diseases in the terminal phase of life are dementia and diseases of the circulatory system. Cancer is the underlying disease in only 12 percent of LTC residents (Brandt et al. 2005), and residents with cancer show a different pattern of symptoms (e.g., a higher prevalence of pain) than those without cancer. The six most common symptoms or syndromes seen in the terminal phase of dementia (agitation and aggression; delirium; pain; dyspnea; nutritional problems; and depression, anxiety, and suicidal ideas) are discussed below.

Agitation and Aggression

> If no one turned around when we entered, answered when we spoke, or
> minded what we did, but if every person we met "cut us dead," and acted
> as if we were nonexisting things, a kind of rage and impotent despair would
> ere long well up in us, from which the cruelest bodily tortures would be a re-
> lief; for these would make us feel that, however bad might be our plight,
> we had not sunk to such a depth as to be unworthy of attention at all.
> —William James

Agitation and aggression are common near the end of life. The clinician should view them as a way for residents with a severe cognitive impairment to communicate their needs to their caregivers. The "difficult" residents may be fiercely protecting their dignity. They may demand, threaten, and rage until their requests are heeded. Often their assertiveness may be viewed as a problem that needs to be fixed or a symptom that needs to be controlled. The aim of person-centered care is to acknowledge the personhood of all residents (irrespective of their levels of frailty or cognitive impairments) in all aspects of care. It includes the recognition that the personality of someone with dementia is increasingly concealed rather than lost. Interpreting these behaviors from the viewpoint of the resident is thus the first step in helping residents who are agitated and aggressive feel comfort and peace. Occasionally aggression may be the only manifestation of delirium, depression, an undiagnosed acute medical condition (e.g., a urinary tract infection), medication toxicity, or a painful condition. Knowing the resident well is the key to a prompt and accurate diagnosis.

Often agitation and aggression are multifactorial (e.g., encompassing pain, depression, constipation, and a countertherapeutic caregiver approach). Successful treatment requires systematically evaluating residents for all causes of such behavior and then treating all identified causes. We recommend psychosocial-environmental interventions (e.g., aromatherapy, massage therapy, music therapy) as first-line options for treating the symptoms of agitation and aggression at the end of life. Pharmacological interventions may be needed for agitation and aggression that pose an imminent danger to oneself or to others or if the symptoms are severe and are not responding to psychosocial-environmental interventions. Atypical antipsychotics are the drugs of first choice unless the clinician suspects depression, in which case he or she should prescribe antidepressants first. We do not recommend prescribing benzodiazepines to treat agitation and aggression, due to the risk of worsening the person's cognitive impairment, but the clinician may add them if the resident's behavior is not responding to antipsychotic medications.

Delirium

Delirium is common during the last days, weeks, or months of life. Many residents may develop delirium as part of the syndrome of imminent death. Health care providers with expertise in palliative care should help manage not only hyperactive or agitated delirium, but also hypoactive delirium during the end of life, as both types of delirium are associated with similar levels of emotional distress (Ganzini 2007). Also, a resident's physical disability predicts family distress, and perceptual disturbances and severe delirium predict staff distress. Restlessness and mood lability are the most upsetting symptoms for family members. Health care providers with expertise in palliative care can educate the family and staff about delirium, thus reducing their distress.

Although delirium may be an inevitable part of dying, an LTC facility's efforts to minimize its impact are important. If delirium is associated with severe agitation, treating reversible causes of delirium (e.g., dehydration [with gentle intravenous fluids if necessary], urinary tract infections, untreated pain) may reduce the resident's agitation. Delirium-associated agitation and restlessness is often misinterpreted as a symptom of worsening pain. This interpretation may lead to excessive opiate use, which may worsen the delirium unnecessarily. Families must consider how aggressive and invasive they want health care providers to be in evaluating the causes of delirium, as burdens will accrue. Decreasing or stopping drugs that contribute to delirium may be easily facilitated. For opiate-induced delirium, we recommend rotating to an equipotent or slightly-less-than-equipotent dose of another opiate. Anticholinergic medications (e.g., tricyclic antidepressants) used to treat neuropathic pain, antisecretory agents (e.g., scopolamine) or antinausea drugs, benzodiazepines, and corticosteroids are among the medications most frequently implicated as being deliriogenic.

Delirium often progresses to a coma and then to death. It is frequently accompanied by anxiety, psychotic symptoms (delusions, hallucinations, illusions), and verbal and physical aggression. End-of-life delirium in LTC populations is typically multifactorial. Severe agitation associated with delirium may require the use of antipsychotics. During the last hours or days of life, the clinician may also treat the agitation associated with delirium by adding benzodiazepines to the antipsychotics. Despite the risk of increased confusion, benzodiazepines may be appropriate for treating agitation associated with delirium during this stage, especially for residents with myoclonus or seizures and for residents with severe dyspnea that is not responding to opiates. The goal for the treatment of end-of-life delirium is to relieve symptoms rather than to extend life. Psychosocial-environmental interventions—such as a calm, serene environment; adequate lighting; the correction of sensory impairments (e.g., addressing the need for appropriate eyeglasses or hearing aids) to correct misperceptions; frequent reassurance; and attention to safety (e.g., falls, wandering)—are also important.

Pain

Pain is a complex, pervasive, and difficult problem in LTC populations. Up to 83 percent of LTC residents experience pain daily. Pain in LTC populations is associated with high levels of functional disability and medical comorbidities (Ferrell 2004). The assessment and management of pain is a key aspect of palliative care. Pain in LTC residents can lead to depression, a lessened quality of life, decreased socialization, a diminished wish to live, insomnia, an unstable gait, and a loss of functional capacity. The frequency of untreated pain in LTC populations is as high as 30 percent (Bishop and Morrison 2007). LTC residents with severe cognitive impairments are particularly vulnerable to inadequate pain control (Husebo et al. 2008).

Musculoskeletal pain (e.g., due to osteoarthritis, chronic back pain) is the most common source of chronic pain in LTC residents. Residents who have a hip fracture, pressure ulcers, or cancer frequently experience excruciating pain (Teno et al. 2004). Other residents who experience excruciating pain often have been recently hospitalized (e.g., for surgery), have experienced weight loss, and/or have a terminal illness. Many residents may report pain during a pain assessment, but they may not report it spontaneously and they may not request pain medication. This may be because of a perception that persistent pain has little potential for change, stoicism, a belief that they are able to handle the pain, concerns about medications in general or pain medication in particular, and a concern about the staff's response to the request (e.g., fear of being labeled a "bad" resident) (K. Jones et al. 2005). For the assessment of pain in LTC residents, refer to chapter 2 on the assessment process.

Pain is eminently treatable with evidence-based pharmacological and psychosocial-environmental interventions. Standardized pain-management programs are critical in improving pain management in LTC settings (Keeney et al. 2008). Improvement in pain management can be obtained through a comprehensive program that involves staff education, changes in pain policies and procedures, and identifying pain management as an indicator of quality. The best way to relieve pain for residents with severe cognitive impairments is to have an attentive and consistent caregiver who notices that a resident is in pain and then observes that person's response to treatment. Nursing care, together with physical therapy and occupational therapy, can help to prevent contractures and increase mobility for residents with terminal-stage dementia.

The clinician may need to prescribe analgesics on a trial basis if he or she suspects pain. We recommend the American Geriatrics Society guidelines for the management of persistent pain in older persons as a basis for the selection of various analgesics (American Geriatrics Society Panel on Persistent Pain in Older Persons 2002). For residents who do not have hepatic dysfunction, acetaminophen is a reasonable first choice and is safer than nonsteroidal anti-inflammatory drugs (NSAIDs). The use of NSAIDs in LTC populations carries a significant risk of gastrointestinal bleeding and renal toxicity, especially if they are used on a chronic basis. The clinician may consider prescribing the short-term use of NSAIDs for residents with acute musculoskeletal pain and a low risk of gastrointestinal bleeding or renal toxicity. Antidepressants (preferably antidepressants with norepinephrine and serotonin reuptake inhibition activity, such as venlafaxine, duloxetine, and nortriptyline) may have a substantial beneficial effect on chronic pain, and the clinician should consider prescribing them for all residents with moderate to severe chronic pain, especially in the context of depression. The next group of medications in the analgesic ladder includes tramadol and codeine. We do not recommend the use of propoxyphene, because it has not been demonstrated to be more efficacious than acetaminophen and its use carries a higher risk of adverse effects (e.g., agitation, cognitive impairment).

The clinician may consider prescribing opiates that are more potent than codeine (e.g., hydrocodone, oxycodone, morphine) for moderate to severe pain. Their use carries a substantial risk of cognitive toxicity, constipation (and even delirium caused by constipation), fecal impaction, respiratory suppression, and death. Thus doses of these medications should be low and increased slowly, with close monitoring for any adverse effects. When used judiciously, opiates have the potential to dramatically reduce pain and thus improve the quality of life for residents with moderate to severe pain.

For residents with chronic moderate to severe pain, the clinician may consider prescribing long-acting opiates, such as a fentanyl patch (if an adequate subcutaneous fat reservoir is present) or methadone (available as a tablet and in liquid form and safer than morphine or oxycodone for residents with end-stage renal disease) if oral opiates have been shown to have significant benefits and have been well tolerated. Unlike acetaminophen and NSAIDs, opioids do not have a maximum dose, can be used for long periods of time without concern for organ damage, and can be administered through a variety of routes (oral, intravenous, subcutaneous, transdermal, rectal). For residents who cannot swallow pills, alternative routes of administration are useful and effective. For quick pain relief, transmucosal fentanyl can be as fast as intravenous administration. The clinician should avoid prescribing opiates that have anticholinergic properties (e.g., meperidine, pentazocine) because of their high risk of cognitive and cardiac toxicity. We strongly recommend the preventive use of laxatives (e.g., polyethylene glycol or sorbitol) whenever the clinician prescribes opioids, due to the high risk of constipation associated with their use.

For residents with severe renal disease or end-stage renal disease, we recommend avoiding codeine, meperidine, morphine, and propoxyphene, because their renally excreted active metabolites can accumulate and cause opioid neurotoxicity. Pain medications that are considered safe and effective for residents with severe or end-stage renal disease include fentanyl, methadone, hydromorphone, acetaminophen, gabapentin (at much lower dosages), and pregabalin. The clinician should use caution when prescribing hydrocodone, oxycodone, tramadol, desipramine, or nortriptyline for residents with severe or end-stage renal disease.

Dyspnea

Because most LTC residents die of noncancerous causes, dyspnea rather than pain may be the most prevalent symptom during their final 48 hours of life (Hall, Schroder, and Weaver 2002). It is important to elucidate its differential diagnosis, because palliative treatment interventions may differ considerably. Although many residents and their families may opt to forgo hospitalization for pneumonia in the terminal stage of an illness, a substantial reduction in the distress associated with dyspnea is achievable in an LTC facility. Opioids are effective in treating dyspnea by relieving feelings of suffocation. For acute exacerbations of dyspnea, a dose of as little as 25 percent of the typical analgesic dose of morphine every four hours may provide substantial relief. Supplemental oxygen can also have a beneficial effect, even when dyspnea is not related to hypoxia. Benzodiazepines also aid in the management of dyspnea, even for residents who do not have prominent anxiety symptoms or who have end-stage COPD. The clinician may also consider prescribing bronchodilators if he or she suspects dyspnea due to airway obstruction. For many residents, the onset of dyspnea may be a transition into the final stage of a disease. Clinicians should guide the staff in considering hospice care, monitoring for these conditions, and providing prompt treatment interventions with the goal of maximizing the resident's comfort.

Nutritional Problems

Severe nutritional problems, such as an unintentional weight loss associated with poor or absent food and/or fluid intake that results in cachexia and dehydration, are a common and fatal complication of many terminal diseases (e.g., dementia) in LTC populations. The clinician should first look for easily fixed causes of not eating: ill-fitting dentures, a sore in the mouth, a toothache. The clinician may consider prescribing dronabinol during palliative and end-of-life care to treat anorexia, as it may also improve nausea and one's general well-being and reduce pain (Morley and Thomas 2008). Residents with advanced dementia may reach a point when they are neurologically incapable of eating. In fact, at the end of any long and terminal illness, people often stop eating; this seems to be part of the wisdom of the body and is one of the most peaceful and comfortable ways of dying. Assisted feeding (including hand feeding) instead of a feeding tube is a better alternative for residents with advanced dementia who stop eating. Assisted feeding should be gentle and not overly aggressive.

Tube feeding is not usually beneficial for residents with advanced dementia, and it does not change the survival rate of residents with dementia who are unable to eat orally. Moreover, for residents with severe dementia, feeding tubes do not reduce aspiration or pressure ulcers or improve any malnutrition markers; rather, they lead to increased infections, more discomfort, increased oral secretions, and the use of physical restraints (Finucane, Christmas, and Leff 2007). One reason that many families and physicians continue to opt for artificial nutrition is that the case for feeding tubes is moral, not scientific (Gillick and Volandes 2008). What may be at issue for families is how best to demonstrate their caring. Health care providers should acknowledge the symbolic value of nutrition for residents in the terminal stage of dementia and seek an alternative means of satisfying the need to feed, such as hand feeding or giving the resident sips of water.

Depression, Anxiety, and Suicidal Ideas

Psychological distress is a source of substantial suffering at the end of life for many residents living in an LTC facility. Most residents experience at least some psychological distress (anxiety, fear, sadness, anger, agitation). Depression during the end of life is common not only among residents who do not have dementia (such as those with cancer, end-stage renal disease who choose to stop dialysis, and end-stage heart disease), but also among residents with terminal-stage dementia. These symptoms need comprehensive psychiatric assessment and treatment when they become pervasive. Occasional thoughts of suicide or a desire for death are fairly common among cognitively intact residents with a terminal illness (e.g., metastatic cancer), but preoccupation with a wish to die and/or a request for a hastened death is a psychiatric emergency. Cognitively intact residents and residents with mild to moderate dementia may make an explicit request or give hints for a hastened death. For example, a resident may say, "Doctor, I am ready to die. Will you help me?" Other expressions reflecting suicidal ideas and emotional suffering include, but are not limited to, "Just shoot me" [expressed verbally or by pointing to one's temple with a hand as if it were a gun]; "Just get Dr. Kevorkian"; or inquiring about the Hemlock Society (an organization that supports assisted suicide). Certain diagnoses (e.g., amyotrophic lateral sclerosis) are particularly associated with a request for assisted suicide.

Most frequently, such statements are an expression of the person's fears of suffering during the end of life rather than a fear of death. Such fears include the fear of pain, of loss of dignity, of loss of control, of dying alone, of being a burden to the family, and so forth. These expressions are often a way to elicit assurance from health care providers that the resident's suffering will be aggressively treated with a symptom-directed treatment plan using all available therapeutic strategies, including palliative sedation. The clinician can address the fear of pain by making it explicit to the resident and the family that a detailed pain management plan has been put in place, with multiple contingencies, in case pain becomes out of control. The clinician should consider a formal consultation with a psychiatrist for all residents with terminal illnesses who request a hastened death. To help the resident realize the potential harm of committing suicide and the potential benefit of being a role model for the next generation by going through the last days of life with dignity, the clinician may judiciously use information about stigmas and about putting first-degree relatives at greater risk of suicide if the resident commits suicide.

Many residents with a terminal illness meet the diagnostic criteria for major depression, which is a significant risk factor in a request for suicide. It is important for the clinician to clarify any request for death. Some residents and/or their families assume that by not accepting every possible treatment (e.g., antibiotics, dialysis), they are essentially committing suicide. The clinician should help the resident and the family differentiate between giving up and letting go: that by withholding certain treatments, the treatment team is allowing the natural process of dying to help the resident achieve a timely, dignified, and peaceful death. Health care providers can help alleviate the suffering of residents and/or their families by clarifying the difference between actively shortening the resident's life and not using medical treatments that aren't in keeping with the resident's preferences and values. Informing residents and their families that they can decline treatment interventions (including nutrition and hydration) and allow a natural death can relieve their stress.

Many of the somatic symptoms of depression—including fatigue, anorexia, a loss of energy, sleep disturbances, and cognitive impairments—are common in terminal illnesses. Hence psychological symptoms (e.g., hopelessness, worthlessness, guilt, helplessness, a loss of meaning, a preoccupation with death and suicide) are more useful in identifying major depression in these residents. When depression during the end of life is severe, different methods of diagnosing depression (e.g., replacing physical symptoms with psychologically oriented criteria) identify depression equally well (Chochinov et al. 1994). The presence of hopelessness correlates highly with suicidal ideation in these residents. Residents with terminal-stage dementia may also develop major depression, but its manifestations in this stage are mostly behavioral (e.g., a depressed affect, tearfulness, agitation, aggression, insomnia, poor oral intake, weight loss, social withdrawal, poverty of speech, an absence of smiles, an anxious or fearful affect).

An understanding of the potential impact of financial issues on the psychological well-being of residents and/or their families is a basic element in palliative care. Health care providers should inquire whether there are any financial matters that could be causing stress and creating barriers to the resident's receiving optimal palliative care that is in keeping with the resident's values and wishes.

Depression and anxiety symptoms are eminently treatable, even for residents in the last stages of life. Effectively controlling physical symptoms (e.g., pain) is the first step in treating depression. We recommend that the clinician conduct a thorough assessment to identify one or more triggers for depression (e.g., chronic pain) and look for general medical conditions that may masquerade as depression (e.g., hypothyroidism, hyperthyroidism, hypoadrenalism, hyperparathyroidism, medication-induced conditions), unless the resident has a short life expectancy (days to weeks). Residents with depression and chronic pain need simultaneous treatment of both the pain and their depression. A past history of major depression may indicate that current depressive symptoms may be a relapse of a depressive illness. Some residents (e.g., those with moderate dementia) may deny the presence of a terminal illness (e.g., metastatic cancer). Denial doesn't respond to reason, so it is best to honor the resident's psychological position and focus on providing comfort, rather than engage in an ongoing confrontation. Efforts to force residents to overcome their denial may do more harm than good. Denial is one of the stages of loss, so the clinician should anticipate it and respond with compassion. Residents who are in denial may nevertheless accept a comprehensive plan of care the family has agreed to without feeling stressed by medical decisions that they are not emotionally prepared to make.

Listening to the resident's wishes and emotional distress in a nonjudgmental manner can be tremendously therapeutic for the resident. Being mindful of the resident's situation and one's own emotional response to requests for assisted suicide, although difficult, can be profoundly healing to both the resident and the health care provider, because it can generate genuine compassion.

We recommend combining pharmacotherapy with psychological (e.g., meaning-centered psychotherapy, encouragement of creative expression), behavioral (pleasant activities), sensory (music, therapeutic touch [e.g., massage]), environmental (exposure to nature, sunlight), and spiritual interventions to treat end-of-life depression. Four simple statements—"Thank you," "I'm sorry," "I forgive you," and "I love you"—are powerful tools for easing the sufferings both of residents facing life's end and of their families. These four statements also help prepare the resident and/or the family to say goodbye. The key message the resident and the family need to hear from the treatment team is that dying does not have to be agonizing, physical suffering can always be alleviated, and the resident will not die alone. Also, it is important for the clinician to share information with the resident and the family indicating that this last stage of life holds remarkable possibilities for facilitating personal and spiritual growth, strengthening bonds with the people they love, repairing broken ties and making amends, and creating profound meaning in the final passage.

For residents with terminal-stage dementia, providing comfort through the use of all five senses (touch [soothing massage], smell [aromatherapy], taste [delicious food and fluids], sight [seeing natural surroundings, family], and hearing [listening to favorite soothing music]) and spiritual activities (e.g., saying prayers, listening to religious songs) may provide much-needed relief from emotional and physical distress. Life review and reminiscence therapy are also helpful in reducing depression and anxiety for residents with intact cognition or mild dementia. Life review is an important part of bringing one's life to a close. As life ends, many residents express a wish to know that they have truly been seen by someone in this world and that their life has had value and meaning. Reminiscence is common at the end of life, and many people find it helpful to reflect on their lives. This can be done in structured ways, to recall and sometimes document a life that is coming to an end. During this last phase of life, music often becomes a special form of support. It allows experiencing, sharing, and communicating feelings that otherwise would not be experienced, shared, or communicated.

We recommend referral to a mental health specialist (e.g., a geriatric psychiatrist) if the resident who has end-of-life depression is suicidal, the depression is accompanied by severe agitation or aggression, and/or the clinician is considering pharmacotherapy. The clinician should initiate a treatment of pain and/or other physical symptoms before or along with the initiation of a specific antidepressant treatment. The clinician should consider prescribing antidepressant medications for moderate to severe major depression and for residents with a past history of major depression and current mild major depression. Pharmacological treatment strategies involve stimulants (e.g., methylphenidate, dextroamphetamine) for a faster response (especially useful for resident with a short life expectancy [in weeks]), SSRIs (e.g., citalopram, sertraline, escitalopram), and other antidepressants (e.g., venlafaxine, duloxetine, mirtazapine, bupropion, nortriptyline). With the use of a psychostimulant, therapeutic benefits can be achieved within 24–48 hours of starting the medication. Psychostimulants may augment opioid analgesia and diminish opioid sedation. Psychostimulants may also reduce the feeling of fatigue in residents near the end of life. The clinician should consider prescribing ECT for residents with severe end-of-life depression when a quick response is needed (e.g., for residents who have suicidal ideas or have made a suicidal attempt). The clinician should also consider prescribing ECT to treat end-of-life depression with psychotic features and for residents with a past history of severe depression and a positive response to ECT.

Many residents who have mild anxiety symptoms during the end of life respond to psychosocial-environmental interventions. More severe anxiety symptoms or anxiety that does not respond to psychosocial-environmental interventions is usually best treated with an SSRI and/or benzodiazepines.

Caring for the Caregiver

The clinician should routinely address the emotional needs of family caregivers as part of the palliative and end-of-life care of all residents. Caregivers may not want to talk about death, but health care providers can help caregivers appreciate that talking and listening at this difficult time can help meet a dying person's spiritual, emotional, and physical needs. In addition, knowing that the caregiver did everything possible to follow the person's wishes may bring some peace. Caregiver stress and grief can be addressed through education, preparation for end-of-life care of the resident, and counseling. The bulk of suffering for the caregivers of residents with dementia occurs in the last years before the resident's death, and a majority of caregivers experience substantial relief after the loved one has died. Thus the clinician should institute caregiver grief- and stress-reduction interventions soon after the resident is admitted to the LTC facility, continue them throughout the resident's stay, and possibly intensify them during last few weeks or months of the resident's life. Family and friends should be allowed to visit as often and as long as they like without set visiting hours.

Most caregivers identify religious activities (e.g., going to church, reading sacred texts) as a major support for coping with difficulties in caregiving activities. Prayer is a particularly vital source of empowerment for many family caregivers. Praying often gives the family member a sense of peace, strength, and even answers to questions related to the loved one's end-of-life care. Struggling with and caring for a loved one who is frail and in an LTC facility may increase some caregivers' feelings of spiritual connectedness and emotional stability. Hence we strongly recommend identifying dimensions of religiosity to help the family develop effective and appropriate support systems. This, in turn, may make caregiving less stressful and more rewarding.

Support groups, bereavement groups, and mindfulness-based stress-reduction techniques are also useful in addressing caregiver stress and grief. Life review and reminiscence therapy can be helpful in relieving the caregivers' stress and grief. Some family caregivers (e.g., those with persistent depression, guilt, severe anxiety) may need referral to a mental health clinician for individual psychotherapy with or without psychotropic medications. It is also important for the clinician to address the grief and stress of professional caregivers who have grown emotionally close to the resident. Health care providers should not be afraid to show their compassion, respect, and sadness for the resident and the family.

Sending a sympathy card is helpful to the family, but a call from the physician inquiring about the family's well-being after the death of their loved one can have profound positive impact on the well-being of the family members and should be adopted as the standard of practice. If the clinician suspects complicated grief in a family member, encouraging the family to come for a formal office visit to address grief is an important aspect of palliative care for LTC populations.

Approximately 20 percent of bereaved caregivers will experience complicated grief after the death of their loved one (Schulz, Hebert, and Boerner 2008). Complicated grief is characterized by persistent grief symptoms (i.e., six months or more), such as an intense longing and yearning for the person who died and recurrent intrusive and distressing thoughts about the absence of the deceased, making it difficult to move beyond the acute stage of mourning. Psychosocial interventions designed to decrease caregiver burden and distress may prevent complicated grief after the death of the resident. We recommend early identification of complicated grief and aggressive psychiatric treatment with grief counseling, with or without the use of antidepressants.

Educating and Preparing the Resident and the Family for End-of-Life Care

Most families are faced with having to make all the decisions regarding end-of-life care because of their loved one's loss of his or her decision-making capacity, typically years before the end-of-life phase. Assessing the resident's and/or family's understanding of the prognosis and disease course is the clinician's first step in tailoring end-of-life education to their needs. Families often have a difficult time making end-of-life decisions because they are not emotionally prepared and/or informed. Also, family members may not reach a unanimous decision. The key strategies to prepare families for the end-of-life care of residents include promoting excellent communication with the family; encouraging appropriate advance care documents and decision making; demonstrating empathy for family emotions and relationships; and attending to the family's grief and bereavement. It is important to use simple, clear language that the resident and the family will understand, rather than clinical language. Health care providers should allow the resident and/or family to control the pace and flow of information whenever possible and let them indicate how much detail and how much information they are able to handle at any given time. The resident and the family may be more satisfied if they have a greater opportunity to speak while the physician listens. It is useful to provide residents and families with printed materials containing key points that will be covered during the discussion (e.g., the *Journal of the American Medical Association*'s patient page on "Hospice Care," dated February 8, 2006, available at www.jama.org).

The clinician should plan on repeat visits to readdress difficult issues, and he or she should view discussions of the prognosis as a spectrum from diagnosis to death, rather than as a one-time event. The clinician should reassure the resident and the family that it is normal to be confused and overwhelmed. Encouraging residents and/or their families to write down their questions as they arise, so that they can be discussed at a later meeting, is also a useful strategy. The task for families is to decide what their loved one would have wanted if that person was capable of making the decision (the concept of substituted judgment). If the family is not sure what their loved one would have wanted, then a decision based on what would be best for the resident's quality of life and in keeping with the resident's values (the concept of best interest) is an appropriate strategy. Some family members may need to be reminded that they have an ethical obligation to make decisions based on substituted judgment whether or not they themselves would do the same for their own end-of-life care.

The availability of health care providers with expertise in palliative care, and their accessibility, are key determinants of the quality of end-of-life care for LTC residents. Such health care providers can walk the family through the various stages of dementia or other terminal conditions and tell them what to expect, what interventions will replace aggressive medical interventions, how the resident's comfort will be maximized, the risks of interventions that promote comfort, and the differences among palliative sedation, assisted suicide, and euthanasia. Some families may need counseling on the appropriate amount of visits from friends and family. The physician and the LTC staff must strive to be on the same page before approaching the resident and the family, because the resident and/or the family may try to reverify what they heard, often for months after a meeting. The staff often know which family members to contact first, as well as a family's particular preferences for communication with the treatment team. It may also be useful to have the resident's social worker call each of the involved family members (e.g., the resident's children) with the same message. Although face-to-face meetings to discuss end-of-life care are ideal, a telephone conference call may also be arranged to include long-distance family members (Gwyther 2000).

Health care providers should understand the family's emotional distress, give information regarding steps to keep the loved one comfortable, and encourage the family to tell important things to the loved ones, as well as to treat the loved one in the same manner as when he or she was cognitively intact and healthy. Health care providers should never say "There's nothing more to be done" or ask "Do you want everything done?" Instead, health care providers should talk about the life yet to be lived and what can be done to make it better.

Addressing financial planning needs (e.g., inquiring about the adequacy of the resident's finances to meet the desired level of care for the remaining limited time, ensuring that the resident's finances are being used for the resident's care) is also part of comprehensive palliative care for LTC populations.

Educating and Training the Staff Regarding Palliative Care
Health care providers can lead the way in promoting a culture that normalizes death and dying in LTC facilities. Health care providers can conduct one-

to two-hour educational seminars for the staff on the topics listed in table 10.2. The goal of such seminars is to increase the staff's ability to discuss advance care issues, normalize the topic of dying for the staff, encourage discussion, and validate concerns. It can also model communication strategies and prompt shared experiences between older and younger staff. Such seminars can help the staff feel more confident in their ability to assess and manage pain, agitation, and family grief. They also may help staff members feel more competent to break bad news to a resident's family about that person's illness, to discuss the family's concerns regarding care, and to help in decision making (Zapka et al. 2006). Addressing grief not only in family members, but also in staff members who have grown close to the resident, is a crucial aspect of palliative care with LTC populations.

Conclusion

There is more to medicine than curing disease and/or defeating death. Life in the shadows of death can be immensely rewarding and fulfilling. End-of-life care is one of the most important components of high-quality care for all residents in long-term care facilities. Key factors to assure high-quality end-of-life care include facilitating choice (allowing the resident or proxy to retain as much control as possible within the limits of belonging to a community), respecting the choice (of the resident or proxy), providing evidence-based palliative care, securing the resident's network of significant relationships, and promoting sensitivity and respect for cultural diversity.

CHAPTER 12

Pharmacological Interventions

Pharmacological interventions are the primary treatments for many medical (e.g., moderate to severe pain) and psychiatric disorders (e.g., schizophrenia, bipolar disorder, recurrent MDD). Evidence-based pharmacological interventions, when used judiciously, have the potential to substantially improve the quality of life for many residents in long-term care facilities who are experiencing significant and persistent behavioral and psychological symptoms. Pharmacological interventions during psychiatric emergencies (e.g., physical aggression toward oneself and/or others) may be life saving not only for the resident, but also for others (e.g., staff members, other residents). Despite these benefits, pharmacological interventions need to be used judiciously in LTC populations, because their use is associated with a significant risk of increased morbidity and mortality.

LTC residents often do not tolerate medications well (prescription as well as over-the-counter ones), and even small doses may cause intolerable adverse effects. This is due to age and medical-illness-related changes in the disposition of a medication; altered sensitivity to the medication's adverse effects; complicated medication interactions because of polypharmacy; multiple comorbidities; and an impaired ability to physiologically compensate for even minor nuisance effects (e.g., mild sedation, nausea). The need to minimize risk and enhance outcomes in clinical practice entails taking into consideration all these age-related complications. There can be tremendous heterogeneity between residents in each of these areas, and there is often a lack of rigorous data on the efficacy and safety of many of the medications prescribed for LTC populations. Thus the task of managing medications for all residents, and particularly for residents who are frail, is complex and difficult. In addition, race and culture may irrationally influence prescribing patterns. For example, elderly African Americans are three times less likely to receive antidepressants than Caucasians, and atypical antipsychotics (compared with conventional antipsychotics) are more likely to be prescribed for middle-class Caucasians than for African Americans, perhaps because of their higher cost.

Pharmacological interventions for behavioral and psychological symptoms in LTC populations involve much more than the prescription of psychotropic medications. Table 12.1 lists pharmacological interventions for the prevention and treatment of behavioral and psychological symptoms in LTC residents.

Minimizing Medication Errors

A substantial number of daily medications are given in LTC facilities, and medication errors are common in LTC populations. The most common errors involve medications given at the wrong time (Young et al. 2008). Other common errors include a wrong dose given, a dose omitted, an extra dose given, an unauthorized drug given, or a wrong drug given. Medication errors carry the risk of adverse effects on cognition, behavior, and psychological well-being; they may also be fatal. Residents who are taking high-risk medications (e.g., warfarin) and residents with complex health problems are especially at risk of serious adverse consequences of medication errors. All LTC facilities should have policies and procedures in place to minimize medication errors. We recommend a systems-based approach to medication errors that

TABLE 12.1
Key pharmacological principles for the prevention and treatment of behavioral and psychological
symptoms in the long-term care population

Minimize medication errors (wrong drug, wrong dose, drug not given/taken)

Reduce the use of potentially inappropriate medications

Improve the prescribing of appropriate medications

Reduce and treat adverse drug events

Prevent and treat drug-drug interactions

Reduce the medication burden (i.e., reduce the number of medications and/or the amount of medication consumed)

Address psychiatric aspects/manifestations of medical problems (e.g., pain, constipation, falls, fractures, osteoporosis, seizures) commonly encountered in residents with behavioral and psychological symptoms

Consider pharmacological interventions for cognitive impairments in residents with dementia

Consider pharmacological interventions for persistent behavioral and psychological symptoms and for chronic and persistent mental illnesses assumes that individuals are doing their best. Such an approach should use proven protocols and processes that ensure effective communication, consistent knowledge and education, and a means of flagging errors and potential problems. We also recommend institutional safeguards to minimize medication errors.

> **CLINICAL CASE** Mrs. L, an 82-year-old married woman living in a nursing home, had chronic pain and chronic depression. She had been doing well on antidepressants (mirtazapine 15 mg at bedtime and duloxetine 30 mg daily) and a fentanyl pain patch (25 mcg/hour every three days) for more than six months, but she started showing drowsiness and unsteadiness over the last two days. The staff reported that Mrs. L had been shouting "Leave me alone, I don't feel like getting up" to various staff members, The staff called her psychiatrist, asking him either to request as-needed lorazepam to calm her or to reduce her "psych medications" due to her drowsiness. The psychiatrist recommended an urgent same-day assessment in his office, as this behavior was new, of sudden onset, and uncharacteristic. Mrs. L could not be brought in on the same day, but her husband brought Mrs. L in late the next day. Mrs. L was calm and pleasant during the visit. The psychiatrist asked Mr. L if he was aware of Mrs. L's drowsiness and aggressive behavior. Mr. L replied that he had figured out why Mrs. L's condition had changed. He had checked Mrs. L's pain patch (a fentanyl patch) and found that the staff had forgotten to remove the previous patch when they put on a new one two days previously.
>
> **TEACHING POINTS** Although psychiatric medications often may be responsible for sedation and an unsteady gait, we recommend that the clinician conduct a through assessment to identify other potential causes of any acute change in behavior. The clinician should always keep the possibility of a medication error in mind in the differential diagnosis, especially if the resident has been stable for some time. Also, an informed and astute caregiver (the husband, in this case) can often help quickly identify the cause of an acute change in behavior.

Reducing the Potentially Inappropriate Use of Medication

Despite long-standing guidelines listing drugs that expert panels consider unsuitable for older adults, inappropriate prescribing is still common both for community-dwelling older adults and residents living in LTC facilities (Fick et al. 2003). In fact, one out of two LTC residents may be taking at least one potentially inappropriate medication (Lau et al. 2004). This is almost 2.5 times the 21.3 percent frequency among community-dwelling elderly people. Some 17 percent of the potentially inappropriate medications were judged to have the potential for severe harm. Residents who receive a potentially inappropriate medication have a much higher chance of subsequent hospitalization or death (Lau et al. 2005). Even intermitted exposure to a potentially inappropriate medication may increase the short-term risk of death. The usual suspects are analgesics (e.g., propoxyphene), anticholinergics/antihistamines (e.g., diphenhydramine, hydroxyzine, cyproheptadine), antidepressants (e.g., amitriptyline), histamine (H-2) blockers (ranitidine), benzodiazepines (e.g., flurazepam), and medications for an overactive bladder (e.g., oxybutynin). Iron is often dosed beyond what can be absorbed, causing adverse gastrointestinal effects that may manifest as agitation in residents with severe cognitive impairment. Residents with COPD are often given sedatives that may worsen hypoxia and manifest as agitation if the resident has a severe cognitive impairment.

The use of drugs with moderate to high anticholinergic activity for residents who do or do not have dementia is common and rarely appropriate, because of the high risk of serious adverse events (e.g., accelerated cognitive decline and delirium, impaired vision, urinary retention, fecal impaction, intestinal obstruction) (Tune 2001). The clinician should replace these drugs with safer alternatives whenever feasible. Medications that have anticholinergic activity may also interfere with the beneficial effects of antidementia drugs (especially cholinesterase inhibitors, but also memantine). The combined effect of multiple drugs that have anticholinergic activity is referred to as anticholinergic load or anticholinergic burden. Among LTC residents, 21 to 32 percent take two or more anticholinergic agents; 10 to 17 percent take three or more; and 5 percent take five or more of these potentially impairing agents (Feinberg 1993). The clinician should closely monitor the cumulative anticholinergic burden of commonly prescribed drugs that have mild anticholinergic activity and try to replace some of these drugs with safer alternatives. We recommend that clinicians refer to a study that measured the anticholinergic activity of 107 medications commonly used by older adults, both when choosing among equally efficacious medications as well as in assessing the overall anticholinergic burden (Chew et al. 2008).

Many of the commonly used drugs having anticholinergic activity that are listed in this article are included in table 12.2, which displays anticholinergic drugs commonly used in LTC and some safer alternatives. Certain combinations of anticholinergic drugs (e.g., lomotil, used to treat diarrhea, is a combination of diphenoxylate and atropine) may carry an even higher risk of toxicity than individual drugs. Drugs for an overactive bladder, such as oxybutynin, carry a potential for higher cognitive adverse effects than tolterodine, as oxybutynin crosses the blood-brain barrier more readily and blocks the muscarinic receptors in the brain. Both oxybutynin and tolterodine may cause delirium, agitation, and hallucinations in frail elders. The clinician should consider discontinuing these medications and using scheduled toileting, prompted voiding, and other interventions for urinary incontinence. (For a comprehensive listing of drugs inappropriate for LTC residents and safer alternatives, refer to articles by Tune 2001; Fick et al. 2003; Desai 2004.)

Improving the Prescribing of Appropriate Medications

LTC residents often require complex medication regimens that substantially increase their risk of adverse events or of suboptimal pharmacotherapy. To

TABLE 12.2
*Anticholinergic drugs prescribed for long-term care residents, and safer alternatives
to consider*

Anticholinergic Drug	Safer Alternative(s)
Diphenhydramine (for insomnia)	Ramelteon
Hydroxyzine	None
Antidiarrheal agents (e.g., diphenoxylate sodium, dicyclomine, atropine, loperamide, belladonna, hyoscyamine, propantheline)	None
Tricyclic antidepressants for depression (e.g., amitriptyline, imipramine, doxepin, protriptyline, nortriptyline, desipramine)	Selective serotonin reuptake inhibitors (SSRIs), mirtazapine, venlafaxine, bupropion, duloxetine
Tricyclic antidepressants for neuropathic pain	Gabapentin, pregabalin, duloxetine
Thioridazine	Atypical antipsychotics
Mesoridazine	Atypical antipsychotics
Antinausea drugs (promethazine, prochlorperazine, trimethobenzamide, metoclopramide, tripelennamine)	Ondansetron
Metoclopramide (for gastroparesis)	None
H2 receptor antagonists (e.g., cimetidine, ranitidine)	Famotidine
Muscle relaxants (e.g., methocarbamol, carisoprodol, metaxalone, cyclobenzaprine)	Tizanidine
Antiallergy medications (e.g., chlorpheniramine, diphenhydramine, cyproheptadine)	Loratadine, fexofenadine
Analgesics (e.g., propoxyphene, codeine)	Acetaminophen
Analgesics (e.g., meperidine, pentazocine)	Tramadol, hydrocodone, oxycodone, morphine

improve appropriate prescribing, we recommend the Fleetwood Model, proposed by the American Society of Consultant Pharmacists. This model includes using consultant pharmacists with demonstrated expertise in geriatric pharmacotherapy, direct resident assessments by the pharmacist, increased interactions between the pharmacist and prescribing health professionals, evidence-based practices, and an explicit assessment of outcomes (Harjivan and Lyles 2002). Treatment algorithms have been developed for pharmacists to use when making clinical recommendations regarding safer alternatives to potentially inappropriate medications for the elderly population. One of the key principles of appropriate prescribing is the selection of drugs that have minimal or no anticholinergic activity.

When choosing an appropriate medication, the clinician should recognize the effects of nutritional status and lifestyle on drug metabolism. For example, impaired nutrition may be associated with decreased plasma protein (e.g., low albumin) and thus increased levels of some drugs that are highly protein bound (e.g., valproate); and alcohol misuse, associated with liver damage, requires the clinician to exercise extra caution when prescribing certain drugs (e.g., acetaminophen). The clinician should also recognize the effect of medical disorders on the pharmacokinetics of drugs. For example, bowel resection may increase the risk of drug-induced diarrhea (e.g., diarrhea induced by SSRIs), severe liver disease may decrease the rate of liver transformation/metabolism of most drugs, and renal failure or renal insufficiency may decrease the clearance of renally excreted drugs or their active metabolites (e.g., lithium, gabapentin, ramelteon).

Many drugs are continued much longer than necessary. This is especially true for drugs used to treat agitation and aggression in LTC populations. In many instances, the physician can safely discontinue psychotropic drugs (with a gradual withdrawal rather than an abrupt discontinuation) without any worsening of the resident's behavior or functional capacity (Cohen-Mansfield et al. 1999). In fact, the discontinuation of psychotropic medications may often result in some improvement in the resident's cognitive and functional status, indicating that subtle adverse effects of psychotropic agents were adding to that person's cognitive and functional impairment.

Principles of Pharmacological Prescription for Long-Term Care Populations

Prescribing medications for LTC populations is complex and should not be taken lightly. Table 12.3 lists several basic principles (Harjivan and Lyles

2002; Desai 2003; Lyketsos et al. 2006). Multiple factors affect the variability of a person's response to pharmacological interventions. For example, smokers clear olanzapine faster than nonsmokers or past smokers, men clear olanzapine faster than women, and African Americans clear olanzapine faster than other races (Bigos et al. 2008). African Americans usually require lower doses of lithium than do Caucasians, and a larger proportion of African Americans metabolize drugs more slowly. The FDA issued an alert that people of Asian ancestry (e.g., from China, India, Indonesia, Malaysia, the Philippines, Taiwan, Thailand) are at significantly increased risk of fatal skin reactions (e.g., Stevens-Johnson syndrome, toxic epidermal necrolysis) when treated with carbamazepine and should undergo genetic testing (for the presence of the human leukocyte antigen [HLA-B*1502]) to assess their risk before initiating therapy.

TABLE 12.3
Basic principles of pharmacological intervention for the long-term care population

Clearly document the reason(s) for prescribing medications (specific condition, target symptoms)

Involve a pharmacist with expertise in geriatrics to help select, initiate, and/or modify medication therapy; perform a comprehensive review of medications to identify, resolve, and prevent medication errors, adverse drug reactions, the use of potentially inappropriate medications, and drug-drug interactions; and help physicians and physician extenders follow the OBRA guidelines regarding the prescription of psychotropic medications

Ensure close collaboration between different prescribers

Avoid starting multiple medications concurrently

Start low, go slow

Use an adequate dose for an adequate time

Adjust the selection of medications and the dosage to accommodate a preexisting kidney or liver impairment

Periodically monitor renal function, as a substantial portion of the long-term care population have chronic kidney diseases that may advance over time

Adjust the selection based on available formulations (e.g., tablet, capsule, liquid, transdermal patch) and the resident's ability to swallow medications

Select an agent with the least likelihood of drug-drug interactions

Adjust the selection and the dose of drugs based on gender, lifestyle (e.g., smoker), and racial and ethnic differences in drug metabolism and tolerance

Use psychosocial-environmental interventions before pharmacological interventions, unless the resident is having a behavioral emergency

Monitor for drug response, drug toxicity, and drug interactions

Avoid prescribing more drugs simply to treat the side effects caused by other drugs

Discontinue the drug if there is a lack of or a marginal response

Consider periodic drug tapering and discontinuation (especially of antipsychotic medications) if the problem is under control for a sufficient period of time

Educate the staff to detect overt and subtle adverse effects of prescribed medications

Educate the staff and the family regarding realistic expectations from any pharmacological intervention

Consider cost / medication reimbursement

Genetically determined differences in drug metabolism may cause notable variations in a resident's blood levels for most psychotropic medications. For example, residents who are genetically slow or poor metabolizers via the 2D6 hepatic isoenzyme system may develop toxicity with low doses of drugs metabolized by this enzyme (e.g., codeine, paroxetine). For many residents (e.g., those who are frail, are age 85 or older, or have severe kidney and/or liver disease), microdoses (half the doses mentioned in the tables) may be sufficient for a therapeutic response. At the same time, the clinician may consider prescribing the usual doses of antidepressants even for residents who are in their 90s if they are tolerating low doses well but are not showing any benefit.

Drug-drug interactions are also a key factor in the selection of a drug. For example, hypertensive drugs may potentiate adverse effects of psychotropic medications (e.g., produce quetiapine-induced orthostatic hypotension), and anticonvulsants that have hepatic enzyme induction activity (e.g., phenytoin, carbamazepine) substantially lower the levels of psychotropic medications metabolized by the liver (e.g., antipsychotic medications). Many residents cannot swallow tablets or capsules and need to have the medication crushed. This may limit the use of certain psychotropic drugs (e.g., duloxetine is available as a capsule, and it cannot be crushed or have the capsule opened).

Given the complexities and risks involved in the pharmacologic management of behavioral and psychological symptoms in LTC populations, the principles of care require that the clinician seriously consider involving a specialist (such as a geriatric psychiatrist, geriatrician, or neurologist) who has specific expertise in the pharmacologic treatment of behavioral and psychological symptoms of dementia (Lyketsos et al. 2006).

Preventing and Treating Adverse Drug Reactions

Adverse drug reactions are prevalent in LTC populations, and more than half of the life-threatening adverse reactions are preventable (Gurwitz et al. 2005). Some 80 percent of preventable adverse reactions—many of them involving central nervous system agents—occur during ordering and monitoring; dispensing accounts for only 5 percent of such errors, and administration for 13 percent. The clinician should view adverse drug reactions (due to either the inappropriate or appropriate prescription of medications) as avoidable by altering existing medication regimens rather than assuming them to be an inevitable part of the aging process.

Adverse drug reactions are a serious safety concern and a key part of the larger quality-improvement picture in LTC. Adverse reactions can manifest as physical problems and functional decline, but often the only manifestation may be accelerated cognitive decline and/or behavioral and psychological symptoms, especially in residents with advanced dementia. Neuropsychiatric events such as oversedation, confusion, hallucination, and delirium are the most common adverse drug reactions, comprising 24 percent of the total and 29 percent of preventable events (Gurwitz et al. 2005). Hemorrhagic and gastrointestinal events follow closely behind. The medications most commonly implicated in producing adverse reactions in LTC populations include anticholinergics, warfarin, conventional and atypical antipsychotics, loop diuretics, benzodiazepines, opioids, insulin, digoxin, antiepileptics, and angiotensin-converting enzyme inhibitors. Adverse reactions are common because of a prescribing cascade that begins when a physicians misinterprets an adverse drug event as a new medical condition. Another drug is prescribed, and an adverse effect happens that is again mistaken for a new medical condition. Then a new drug is prescribed, and the resident is placed at risk of developing more adverse effects from the added medication.

Health care professionals need to do a better job of recognizing the impact that subtle medication-related adverse effects have on residents, as the residents themselves may not be able to recognize or communicate adverse effects of their medications. Therefore, health care providers should act preemptively to select medications with the best adverse effect profile and to avoid potentially toxic doses. Many drugs may cause or worsen preexisting vitamin deficiency. For example, the use of methotrexate, phenytoin, and trimethoprim is associated with folate deficiency, and the use of metformin, neomycin, and proton pump inhibitors with vitamin B_{12} deficiency (Sehl, Naeim, and Charette 2008). Anticholinergic drugs are often implicated in drug-induced delirium and drug-induced visual hallucinations. Antiparkinsonian drugs (dopamine agonists and anticholinergic agents) are frequently implicated in drug-induced psychoses. Dopamine agonists are implicated in sexually inappropriate behaviors. Benzodiazepines and opioids may cause depression. The use of steroids is associated with mania, psychosis, delirium, and depression. Beta-adrenergic agonists (often used to treat asthma) may cause anxiety symptoms. The FDA recently issued a warning regarding the risk of suicide, which has been linked with the use of all anticonvulsants, antidepressants (in younger populations), and varenicline (used in smoking cessation). The use of varenicline, interferon alpha (used to treat multiple sclerosis), singulair (used to treat asthma), or zanamivir inhalation powder (used to treat acute influenza symptoms) are all associated with a risk of depression. Hence the clinician should caution residents with a serious psychiatric illness (e.g., schizophrenia, bipolar disorder, major depressive disorder) regarding the use of varenicline in smoking cessation. For comprehensive information on the psychotropic adverse effects of commonly prescribed drugs in elderly people, see Desai (2004).

> **CLINICAL CASE** Mr. M, an 82-year-old widower with dementia, was transferred from the hospital to a nursing home for rehabilitation after being treated for syncope (due to severe bradycardia) with the implantation of a pacemaker and the initiation of 200 mg/day of amiodarone. A week after his discharge, he began developing mental status changes, including worsening disorientation, agitation, insomnia, aggressive behavior during personal care, and paranoia. The staff at the nursing home requested a psychiatric consultation, saying that he was "violent." After an emergency assessment, the consulting psychiatrist diagnosed amiodarone-induced delirium. After consulting with Mr. M's primary care physician and his cardiologist, the psychiatrist discontinued the amiodarone and prescribed risperidone (0.25 mg twice a day, increased the next day to 0.5 mg twice a day) for agitation and aggression. After two days the aggression improved dramatically, and after seven days it resolved completely. The risperidone was discontinued soon after.
>
> **TEACHING POINTS** Amiodarone (as well as many other prescription drugs) has the potential for significant cognitive adverse effects in older adults, especially those with dementia. Prompt short-term treatment of severe agitation in the context of delirium may prevent injury to oneself or others and may avoid hospitalization for severe aggression that cannot be managed in the LTC facility. We recommend that the clinician communicate and coordinate care with other health care providers before making any change in medications.

Preventing and Treating Drug-Drug Interactions

Drug-drug interactions that adversely affect a resident's health (physical, cognitive, and emotional) and functional status are prevalent in LTC populations because of the high prevalence of polypharmacy. For example, the addition of fluoxetine, which is a hepatic cytochrome P450 2D6 isoenzyme inhibitor, to nortriptyline, which is a 2D6 substrate, impairs the ability of 2D6 to metabolize nortriptyline, leading to an increase in the blood level of nortriptyline (in turn leading to nortriptyline toxicity [e.g., sedation, falls, urinary retention, hypotension]) (Armstrong, Cozza, and Sandson 2003). Another example of a clinically relevant drug-drug interaction is the addition of quetiapine to phenytoin. Quetiapine is primarily a 3A4 substrate, and phenytoin is an inducer of several cytochrome P450 enzymes, including 3A4. Thus when quetiapine is introduced and phenytoin is already present, there may be as much as a fivefold increase in the clearance of quetiapine (leading to lack of efficacy for quetiapine). If a resident is transitioned from taking phenytoin for seizure control to taking valproate (another effective anticonvulsant), which usually does not induce most liver enzymes, quetiapine may be more effective. Other examples of substituting a safer alternative (a drug with less risk of drug-drug interactions) for a drug that has a significant risk of drug-drug interactions include substituting omeprazole for lansoprazole and azithromycin for erythromycin. Pharmacy computer programs that alert health care providers to drug-drug interactions and maintain resident medication lists can assist in the prevention and treatment of many clinically significant drug-drug interactions. The clinician should maintain a high index of suspicion regarding clinically significant drug-drug interactions when prescribing any new drug for a resident who is already taking other medications.

Reducing the Medication Burden

Reducing the medication burden (i.e., reducing the number of medications consumed or the dose of current medications) may improve the resident's quality of life, and this goal can be achieved in several ways (table 12.4). Medication reduction is an important pharmacological intervention for all LTC residents in general, and specifically for residents who display behavioral and psychological symptoms, have difficulty swallowing, or are resistant to taking pills. Residents who experience subtle adverse effects from these medications may begin feeling and functioning better, and residents taking less medication will have a reduced risk of medication errors and drug-drug interactions. Staff time spent in dispensing medications may decrease, thus freeing up time for staff members to bond with residents.

Many LTC residents receive medications that are unnecessary, either because there is no clinical indication for such medicines and/or because the residents have a limited life expectancy (for example, the use of a statin for a resident with severe or terminal-stage dementia). A relatively high proportion of LTC residents taking antidementia drugs may not be benefiting enough from these medications to warrant continuing them (J. Lee et al.

TABLE 12.4
Strategies to reduce the number of medications consumed or the total dosage of consumed medications

Discontinue unnecessary medications
Discontinue medications that are not beneficial or that are only marginally beneficial
Discontinue medications that were effective before but are not expected to provide continued benefit
Discontinue medications that were given on a trial basis but were not found to be beneficial
Reduce the dose of a medication because of a significant change in the resident's health (e.g., increasing frailty, advancing dementia, a stroke, or a decline in liver or kidney function)
Use a combination of medications (e.g., acetaminophen with oxycodone)

2007). Discontinuing antidementia drugs by gradually tapering them off does not result in adverse outcomes for most residents. If there is a subsequent, clinically relevant decline that is temporally related to the discontinuation of the treatment, then the medication can be reintroduced. Withdrawal of antidepressants is successful for the majority of residents who do not have major depression or anxiety disorder and for residents who have been stable for more than one year and have current low scores on depression inventories (Ulfvarson et al. 2003; Lindstrom et al. 2007).

The application of a geriatric palliative methodology when dealing with disabled elderly people (e.g., there is an evidence-based consensus for using the drug for the indicated condition, the indication seems valid and relevant in a particular patient's age group and disability level, the benefits outweigh the risks for that particular resident, there are no significant adverse effects, there is not a safer alternative, and the dose can be reduced with no significant risk) may enable several medications to be discontinued simultaneously (Garfinkel, Zur-Gil, and Ben-Israel 2007). This, in turn, may improve the residents' quality of life, reduce mortality rates and referrals to acute care facilities, and lower costs and staff workloads. Residents with terminal-stage dementia are ideal candidates for a trial of discontinuing antidementia drugs.

Medications are often prescribed on a trial basis. Take, for example, a resident who is yelling and agitated, has severe cognitive impairment, and thus is unable to communicate the cause of the distress to caregivers and is, after a thorough evaluation, given a trial of an analgesic (e.g., acetaminophen) for suspected musculoskeletal pain or an antidepressant for suspected depression. It is important for the clinician to discontinue these agents if the target symptoms have not responded to treatment. This is frequently overlooked, with the result that the resident continues to receive an unnecessary medication.

Doses of medications that are beneficial may need to be reduced because of a decline in the resident's health. For example, the dose of gabapentin given for peripheral diabetic neuropathy should be reduced to avoid sedation if the resident's kidney function has declined due to worsening diabetic nephropathy. Strategies such as simplifying the drug regimen or using combination drugs, extended-release drugs, or other formulations may reduce the number of drug administrations and chances for errors (Dimant 2001). Some residents who are taking antiparkinson drugs and antipsychotics may not need the antiparkinson drugs once the antipsychotics are discontinued or switched for another antipsychotic with a low potential for extrapyramidal symptoms. For these residents, the clinician should discontinue the antiparkinson drugs or reduce the dosage as soon as possible, due to their high risk of cognitive, emotional, and behavioral adverse effects. Medication reviews and educational interventions are effective at reducing the prescription of psychotropic drugs (Nishtala et al. 2008).

Psychiatric Aspects of Medical Conditions Commonly Experienced by Long-Term Care Residents with Dementia

Medical conditions frequently manifest with behavioral and psychological symptoms. In this context, the treatment of the symptoms would involve identifying and treating the underlying medical condition(s). Common medical conditions associated with behavioral and psychological symptoms in LTC populations include urinary tract infections, constipation, pain, falls, fractures, osteoporosis, seizures, and dermatologic conditions. For many residents with dementia, treating these and other comorbid conditions may produce a greater improvement in their quality of life than focusing the treatment only on dementia.

Urinary Tract Infections

A urinary tract infection is one of the most common causes of an acute change in mental status and the acute onset of behavioral and psychological symptoms in LTC populations. Agitation may be the only manifestation of UTI in residents with advanced dementia. A high index of suspicion regarding and prompt treatment of the UTI quickly resolve agitation if a UTI is the cause. Trimethoprim, an antibiotic commonly used in combination with sulfamethoxazole to treat UTIs, may interfere with the elimination of memantine and thus has the potential for serious toxicity (e.g., myoclonus, delirium) (Moellentin, Picone, and Leadbetter 2008).

Constipation

Constipation may manifest as agitation in residents with advanced dementia, and fecal impaction may cause delirium. As a first step in treating constipation, the clinician should consider eliminating drugs that cause or exacerbate it (especially drugs that have anticholinergic activity, and opioid analgesics) and, if necessary, replacing them with safer alternatives. Bulking agents (bran, psyllium, methylcellulose) are typically used first in the treatment of constipation (Lacy and Cole 2004). The next group of agents are stool softeners (e.g., docusate). The clinician should be cautious in prescribing the third group of agents, osmotic agents (e.g., lactulose, sorbitol, and polyethylene glycol), for residents with diabetes mellitus, and he or she should monitor these residents for electrolyte disorders, especially with prolonged use. The next class of agents is stimulant laxatives (e.g., bisacodyl, senna). A combination of stimulant laxatives and bulking agents effectively treats most cases of severe constipation due to medications such as opioids. The clinician may consider prescribing a subcutaneous methylnaltrexone injection to treat refractory opioid-induced constipation for residents with an advanced disease who are receiving palliative care. The clinician may consider prescribing lubiprostone for residents with chronic idiopathic constipation.

Any pharmacological treatment for constipation must be part of a comprehensive strategy that involves efforts to increase physical activity, slowly increase fiber in the diet, and correct dehydration with increased fluid intake. Change in a pattern of chronic constipation should alert the clinician to look for serious medical conditions, such as bowel cancer, hypothyroidism, hypercalcemia, and the like. An enema (e.g., warm water, soapsuds) may be necessary in severe cases of constipation, when a rapid response is needed, or when medications are not effective. Manual disimpaction may be required if the clinician suspects impending impaction. Magnesium citrate may be useful in urgent situations. All medications used in the treatment of constipation may cause diarrhea, headaches, abdominal pain, abdominal distension, flatulence, and nausea. An excessive use of drugs to treat constipation may lead to fluid and electrolyte disturbances, including hypokalemia. The clinician should routinely look for these adverse effects in residents who are taking one or more medications for constipation.

Pain

Persistent pain is highly prevalent in nursing home residents (49% are in chronic pain), and diagnosing pain in cognitively impaired residents is challenging. Within LTC facilities, there is suboptimal compliance with geriatric prescribing recommendations, and acute pain may be an important contributing source of persistent pain (Won et al. 2004). Contrary to American Geriatrics Society recommendations (American Geriatrics Society Panel on Persistent Pain in Older Persons 2002), acetaminophen and opioids are typically given at low doses, and high-dose NSAIDs, which can cause toxicity, are given to one-third of LTC residents. Many residents (20%–25%) who are in pain receive no analgesic. Propoxyphene (a drug to be avoided in elderly people) is commonly used (18%) in LTC populations. Pain is a frequent cause of agitation, aggression, depression, and social withdrawal in LTC residents (American Medical Directors Association 1999). The use of analgesics (e.g., acetaminophen, opioid analgesics) has been associated with a reduction in agitation and inactivity and increased socialization in residents with dementia (Allen et al. 2003; Manfredi et al. 2003; Chibnall et al. 2005). The clinician may consider prescribing an empirical trial of analgesics for residents with severe agitation (e.g., persistent yelling). Before prescribing analgesics, the clinician should routinely consider discontinuing medications that may cause or exacerbate certain painful conditions (e.g., myalgia due to statins, headaches due to SSRIs). To maximize pain relief, the clinician should recommend psychosocial-environmental interventions (e.g., relaxation and breathing exercises, massage, music, exercise, tai chi, physical therapy) along with any pharmacological intervention. Adequate pain management is necessary for an adequate response to antidepressants in residents experiencing pain and depression, and vice versa.

For pain management in LTC populations, we recommend the American Geriatrics Society guidelines for the treatment of acute and chronic pain in older persons (American Geriatrics Society Panel on Persistent Pain in Older Persons 2002), as well as the American Medical Directors Association's *Clinical Practice Guidelines* for the treatment of pain in LTC (www.amda.com). The only update to these guidelines is a finding from several studies that the use of cyclooxygenase-2 (COX-2) inhibitors (e.g., celecoxib) may be associated with serious adverse cardiovascular events, and that the side-effects profile of these medications is not as benign as previously thought. One of the key principles of pain management with pharmacological interventions in LTC populations (especially for those with dementia) is using scheduled dosing rather than as-needed dosing, because residents with cognitive impairments may not be able to seek out staff when they have pain. Musculoskeletal disorders (e.g., osteoarthritis, chronic low back pain) are the most common cause of painful conditions in LTC populations.

Acetaminophen is probably the safest and most appropriate initial medication for residents with mild to moderate pain due to osteoarthritis or other musculoskeletal disorders. In LTC populations, acetaminophen can be dosed up to 3 grams/day. If the resident has mild liver disease, this dose should be reduced to no more than 2 grams/day to avoid hepatotoxicity. People with advanced liver diseases should not use acetaminophen, so the clinician should obtain liver function tests before prescribing acetaminophen or other analgesics.

For residents with moderate to severe musculoskeletal pain, NSAIDs may provide relief superior to that provided by acetaminophen. NSAIDs carry substantial risks (especially gastrointestinal and renal problems) when used by LTC populations, but the clinician may consider prescribing them to treat acute and chronic musculoskeletal pain for residents who do not have pre-existing medical conditions that would increase the risk associated with the use of NSAIDs (e.g., chronic kidney disease, recent coronary bypass surgery, peptic ulcer disease, recent gastrointestinal bleeding, residents taking warfarin). For residents subject to gastrointestinal risks, a proton pump inhibitor or misoprostol can be given as cotherapy with NSAIDs (e.g., naproxen) to reduce this risk, although the diarrhea associated with misoprostol may limit its use by LTC populations. Celecoxib (a COX-2 inhibitor) may be preferred over nonselective NSAIDs (e.g., naproxen, ibuprofen) for residents with minimal cerebrovascular risk but a history of gastric problems. Over-the-counter topical forms of analgesics (e.g., capsaicin and menthol combination creams, salicylate skin creams such as Bengay or Aspercreme) and prescription topical NSAIDs (e.g., diclofenac) may also help reduce pain associated with arthritis. Some residents may experience local burning or stinging when they first apply topical capsaicin, but that effect usually resolves after one week of continued use.

Tramadol is an analgesic medication that has a dual mechanism of action. It weakly binds with mu-opioid receptors and inhibits the reuptake of norepinephrine and serotonin. The clinician may consider prescribing tramadol to treat moderate to severe acute or chronic pain in LTC residents. The starting dose should be low (25 mg once or twice a day), with the dose gradually increased every three days to the lowest therapeutic dose. Adverse effects include dizziness, drowsiness, confusion, and a risk of serotonin syndrome and seizures when used along with SSRIs. The clinician should prescribe it cautiously for residents with significant kidney disease, because of their higher risk of toxicity. The clinician should avoid prescribing tramadol for residents with seizure disorders, as it can lower the threshold for seizures. The clinician may consider prescribing tramadol plus acetaminophen (available in a single pill under the brand name Ultracet) to treat moderate to severe musculoskeletal pain that is not responding to NSAIDs or when NSAIDs are not tolerated or are contraindicated.

Opioids are a mainstay for the management of acute and chronic, moderate to severe pain in LTC populations. They are indicated for both cancer and noncancer pain. Although tolerance and physical dependence may be unavoidable with opioids, psychological dependence or true addiction is extremely rare in current LTC populations. Unlike acetaminophen and NSAIDs, opioids do not have a maximum dose, can be used for long periods of time without concerns about organ damage, and can be administered through a variety of routes (oral, transdermal, rectal) (Bishop and Morrison 2007). Common adverse effects of opioids are nausea, constipation, and pruritus. In LTC populations, sedation, falls, fecal impaction, and urinary retention are also a concern. The clinician should expect constipation in all residents who are taking opioids, and we recommend a prophylactic bowel regimen (e.g., a combination of senna and polyethylene glycol) to prevent constipation. Common signs of opioid toxicity include severe sedation, myoclonic jerks, insomnia and nightmares ("bad dreams"), and delirium. If the resident is experiencing opioid toxicity, it may be useful to slowly administer one or two liters of fluid to flush out some of the drug and its metabolite. Methylphenidate or modafinil may be helpful in treating opioid-induced sedation. Opioids should not be abruptly discontinued, due to the high risk of serious withdrawal symptoms (e.g., dysphoria, agitation, insomnia, joint and back pain, muscle aches, lacrimation, rhinorrhea, yawning, fever, nausea).

Codeine or hydrocodone is the opioid of choice for the treatment of moderately severe acute and chronic pain, before using more potent opioids (e.g., oxycodone, morphine, hydromorphone). Both these opioids are metabolized by the hepatic cytochrome 2D6 isoenzyme system to active metabolites. Thus the use of other medications that inhibit 2D6 enzyme activity (e.g., paroxetine, fluoxetine) may reduce their analgesic effect. Long-acting formulations of opioids (e.g., transdermal fentanyl, long-acting morphine, methadone, long-acting oxycodone preparations) are effective in the treatment of persistent moderate to severe pain, but they require a great deal of care when titrating to a steady state. They may be started only after pain control is achieved with short-acting opioids, and they should not be administered to opioid-naïve residents.

All long-acting opioids must be prescribed on a fixed schedule for maximal efficacy. For breakthrough pain, usually a short-acting opioid (e.g., transbuccal fentanyl for residents on a fentanyl patch) is also necessary initially. Most residents respond to low starting doses and a slow titration upward. Long-acting morphine is a good choice for the long-term treatment of moderate to severe pain. Morphine has clinically active metabolites, which then undergo renal clearance. Thus the clinician should prescribe morphine cautiously for residents with kidney disease. Fentanyl patches work well, but they need a subcutaneous fat reservoir, so the clinician should avoid prescribing them for malnourished residents who require long-acting opioids. The starting dose for a fentanyl patch is 12 mcg/hour every 72 hours. Low-dose methadone (starting dose of 2.5 mg every 8–12 hours) is an appropriate long-acting opioid for the treatment of severe chronic pain. The advantages of methadone over other opioids include a lack of active metabolites and an analgesic effect by an opioid receptor agonist, as well as N-methyl-D-receptor antagonist activity (Ballantyne and Mao 2003). One key disadvantage of methadone over other long-acting opioids is that it is highly lipophilic and easily accumulates in tissues. This accumulation can lead to iatrogenic sedation, respiratory depression, delirium, and death. Long-acting opioids usually take three to five days to attain optimal analgesic effects, so the clinician should wait at least five days before considering an increase in the dosage.

Opioids are available in many forms besides pills (e.g., intensols of morphine, oxycodone; nebulized opioids), and the clinician may consider them for residents who need opioids to manage pain and are unable to swallow pills (but can swallow liquids). Other options for residents who have difficulty swallowing pills include a liquid preparation (e.g., liquid morphine [Roxanol]) to control acute pain and transdermal fentanyl to control chronic pain. A patient-controlled analgesia (PCA) pump (placed subcutaneously) is effective in controlling pain for residents with moderate to severe pain who are cognitively intact (e.g., a resident with metastatic cancer and bone pain), and therefore are reliably able to self-administer an opioid analgesic using the pump. A combination of acetaminophen and opioids for the treatment of moderate to severe pain improves analgesia and may require lower doses of opioids, thus reducing the incidence of adverse effects associated with these drugs. The clinician may also consider prescribing opioid rotation to reduce adverse effects linked with long-term opioid therapy. When a resident is rotating onto a new opioid, we recommend a dose reduction of 30 to 50 percent for the new opioid, due to incomplete cross-tolerance. We strongly recommend that the clinician avoid prescribing propoxyphene, meperidine, pentazocine, or buprenorphine to treat pain in LTC populations, due to their high risk-to-benefit ratio and the availability of safer opioids described above. Propoxyphene, a commonly used analgesic in LTC populations, has been shown to be not much more effective than acetaminophen, and it can cause sedation and dizziness, increasing the risk of falls and fractures.

Neuropathic pain (e.g., diabetic peripheral neuropathy, central poststroke pain, radiculopathy [e.g., sciatica], trigeminal neuralgia, postherpetic neuralgia) is a common but underrecognized cause of agitation and depression in LTC residents. We do not recommend amitriptyline and imipramine, although effective, for the treatment of neuropathic pain, due to the high risk of adverse effects (e.g., worsening cognition, cardiac toxicity). Carbamazepine is often used to treat neuropathic pain (e.g., trigeminal neuralgia). However, the use of carbamazepine is associated with significant neurotoxicity and a high risk of drug-drug interactions, because of its cytochrome P450 liver enzyme-induction properties.

Safer alternatives include gabapentin, pregabalin, duloxetine, and, for cognitively intact residents, nortriptyline. Common adverse effects of gabapentin are somnolence, peripheral edema, fatigue, confusion, depression, and ataxia. Gabapentin, if withdrawn abruptly, may cause a withdrawal syndrome that may present with anxiety, insomnia, nausea, pain, and sweating. The starting dose of gabapentin for the treatment of neuropathic pain in LTC populations should be 100 mg before bedtime, and the dose can be titrated up every three days to the lowest effective dose. One advantage of gabapentin is that it is primarily eliminated by the kidneys and thus has a low potential for drug-drug interactions; it can be safely used by LTC residents with hepatic dysfunction. Dose adjustments are necessary when gabapentin is used by residents with renal insufficiency. Pregabalin, as compared with gabapentin, has not been adequately studied in LTC populations, but the clinician may consider prescribing it for neuropathic pain and for fibromyalgia. Its adverse effects are similar to those of gabapentin. Duloxetine may be useful to treat fibromyalgia or diabetic neuropathy pain (it the only antidepressant approved for a painful condition). Local anesthetics (e.g., transdermal lidocaine [lidocaine patch 5%]) may be useful in the treatment of both neuropathic and localized pain. The patch should be applied for 12 hours and removed for 12 hours each day to avoid tachyphylaxis (Bishop and Morrison 2007). Up to three lidocaine patches per day may be used. Adverse effects from a lidocaine patch are uncommon, but they can include local skin reaction. Opioids may also be appropriate as adjuvants for neuropathic pain that does not respond to the usual pharmacological and psychosocial-environmental interventions.

We do not recommend prescribing opioids to treat pain due to fibromyalgia. Low-dose steroids may be necessary for the treatment of acute and chronic, moderate to severe pain due to rheumatoid arthritis or polymyalgia rheumatica. Although most muscle-relaxation medications are ineffective for chronic pain, tizanidine is effective both to relax muscle spasms and to reduce chronic pain symptoms. The clinician may prescribe it judiciously in LTC populations (starting at low doses, such as 1 mg before bedtime), with close monitoring for its sedating effects. For some residents with chronic pain, the clinician may consider referral to a pain clinic or a pain specialist for local pharmacological interventions (e.g., a PCA pump, epidural steroid injections [for spinal stenosis, a herniated disc, or single extremity pain], a facet block [for low back pain], trigger-point injections [for localized muscle pain], or a nerve block [for mononeuropathy, radiculopathy, or postherpetic neuralgia]), as well as more sophisticated procedures (e.g., radiofrequency neuroablation, vertebroplasty, spinal cord stimulation [TENS units]). The clinician may also consider neural blockade, neurolysis, or an implantable drug delivery system for selected cognitively intact residents with severe refractory cancer pain. Hospitalization in a palliative care unit may be necessary for residents with severe refractory pain who require highly complex pharmacological interventions for pain relief (e.g., severe postherpetic neuralgia, requiring intravenous lidocaine or oral mexilitene; a resident with metastatic bone cancer and excruciating pain, requiring palliative sedation).

Falls, Fractures, and Osteoporosis
LTC residents are more likely to fall or sustain a fracture than elderly persons in the community, because LTC residents often have problems with mobility, balance, cognition, and/or vision. Also, LTC residents take an average of seven to eight prescription medications, including many that increase the risk of falls and subsequent fractures. Approximately 6 percent of nursing home residents sustain a fracture during their nursing home stay (Spector et al. 2007). For the majority (85%), a fall causes the fracture (usually in the

hip or pelvis). Residents who are 85 or older and ambulatory, and residents who are agitated, are at a particularly high risk of falls and fractures. An estimated 70 to 85 percent of nursing home residents have osteoporosis (a loss of bone density), putting them at high risk of fractures (either after a fall or a spontaneous fracture), yet less than 1 in 10 newly admitted nursing home residents receives medications and/or calcium and vitamin D to treat osteoporosis (Wright 2007).

All psychotropic medications (including SSRIs) increase the risk of falls, so the clinician should prescribe them with extra caution for residents with osteoporosis (Cooper et al. 2007). A high percentage of hip fractures are related to the use of psychotropic medications (French et al. 2005). Besides psychotropic medications, anticonvulsants and analgesics also increase the risk of falls and fractures. The risk of a fracture may be reduced if residents with osteoporosis are treated with vitamin D and biphosphonates (e.g., alendronate, risedronate). The long-term use of high-potency antipsychotics (e.g., risperidone) in young adults is associated with hyperprolactinemia, although similar data are not available for the geriatric population. Until the effect of risperidone use on prolactin levels in the geriatric population is clarified, clinicians should be aware that long-term use of risperidone by elderly people may increase their risk of osteoporosis or worsen preexisting osteoporosis. All residents receiving psychotropic medications should be put on fall risk precautions. We recommend strength and balance training (e.g., tai chi) and physical therapy for all residents who have a recent history of falls or are at high risk of falls. The clinician should also consider other factors (e.g., improved ambient lighting, high staff-to-resident ratio) that reduce the risk of falls and fractures (Spector et al. 2007).

Seizures and Epilepsy

Residents in LTC facilities have a high prevalence of seizure disorder (due to a high degree of neurological disorders [e.g., stroke] and psychiatric disorders [e.g., dementia]) and a high risk of new-onset seizures. Cerebrovascular disease is the most common cause of new-onset seizures in LTC populations. The risk of epilepsy may be increased for more than a decade after a serious brain injury or a skull fracture. People with Alzheimer disease have an increased incidence of seizures that appears to be independent of the disease stage and highest in cases with early onset AD (onset before age 65) (Palop and Mucke 2009). Some cases of episodic wandering and disorientation in

AD are associated with epileptiform activity and can be prevented with antiepileptic drugs. Epilepsy in dementia has significant consequences; it can result in a worsening of cognitive performance, particularly in language, as well as a reduction in autonomy, a greater risk of injury, and a higher mortality rate (Hommet et al. 2008).

According to the Epilepsy Foundation (www.epilepsyfoundation.org), many residents who have dementia or have had a stroke may develop nonconvulsive or frontal lobe seizures that may present with agitation or behavioral and psychological symptoms (e.g., a sudden onset of anger or fear; unusual movements of the head, arms; aimless wandering; a trancelike appearance; periods of confusion that begin and end abruptly; sensory experiences [e.g., visual disturbances]) . These types of seizure are often not recognized or treated because the resident is unable to describe what he or she is experiencing, due to a preexisting cognitive impairment (e.g., a dementia-related cognitive impairment, stroke-related aphasia) (Mendez and Lim 2003). Manifestation of nonconvulsive seizures may also be mistaken for symptoms of underlying dementia. Clinicians may not routinely think of nonconvulsive seizures in the differential diagnosis of behavioral and psychological symptoms in LTC populations. Hence all residents showing behavioral and psychological symptoms that begin and end abruptly should be evaluated for possible seizure. The clinician should also first address easily reversible causes of seizure, such as dehydration, electrolyte imbalance, and a medication-induced seizure.

The clinician should prescribe antiepileptic drugs only after the diagnosis has been clearly established and when the risk of recurrence is high, and he or she should use monotherapy whenever possible. All antiepileptic drugs (especially topiramate and phenobarbital) have the potential to worsen cognition in residents with both seizures and dementia. The abrupt or rapid withdrawal of many psychotropic agents (e.g., benzodiazepines, sedative-hypnotics, mood stabilizers [e.g., valproate]) may precipitate one or more seizures. We recommend the use of anticonvulsants with low adverse effects on cognition (e.g., valproate, gabapentin, lamotrigine, and levetiracetam) whenever possible, along with using the lowest possible dosage and monitoring antiepileptic drug levels. Many residents with long-standing seizure disorders have comorbid depression and/or anxiety disorders that can often be adequately treated with appropriate psychotropic medications and psychosocial interventions. All antidepressants and antipsychotic drugs reduce the risk of seizures to varying degrees. The clinician should prescribe them cautiously for residents with seizure disorders and closely monitor these residents for the emergence of a new-onset seizure disorder.

Dermatologic Conditions

Dry skin (xerosis) is prevalent in LTC populations. Low humidity can greatly increase the risk of dry skin, especially during the winter months (Gilchrest 1996). Dry skin can cause itching (pruritus) and discomfort that may manifest as agitation in residents with cognitive impairments. Pruritus can lead to secondary lesions (e.g., eczema). Other signs and symptoms of dry skin include flaking, chapping, burning, erythema, pain, scaling, stinging, and tightness. If the skin splits and cracks deeply enough to disrupt dermal capillaries, bleeding fissures may occur. Dry skin occurs most often on the legs of elderly patients, but it may be present on the hands and trunk. Residents with generalized dry skin may complain of "itching all over." Clinicians may misdiagnose this as an allergic reaction and prescribe antihistaminic drugs (e.g., hydroxyzine or diphenhydramine) that have potentially serious adverse consequences (e.g., drug-induced delirium). Psychosocial-environmental interventions (e.g., turning down the heat, using a humidifier in the room, using soap sparingly, correcting dehydration), in combination with pharmacological interventions (e.g., discontinuing offending agents and using nonprescription moisturizing lotions, creams, or ointments on the hands and all other dry areas), usually improve dry skin problems. Repeated use of a moisturizing product over a period of time is needed before residents experience maximum benefits. A thorough application of a moisturizer once or twice daily is an appropriate regimen for most residents with dry skin. Keratolytics (e.g., 12% ammonium lactate lotion) may also be used for severe dry skin.

The treatment of comorbid depression and/or anxiety disorders may help improve the discomfort associated with xerosis, eczema, or psoriasis. For a successful outcome, the clinician needs to address nutritional deficiencies (e.g., zinc and essential fatty acids) and other conditions (e.g., thyroid disease, diuretic therapy, end-stage renal disease) that make the resident more susceptible to dry skin (Norman 2008). For complicated cases (e.g., a breakdown of skin due to excessive scratching; dry skin along with severe eczema or psoriasis), the clinician should consider referral to a dermatologist. The clinician should screen all residents for dry skin periodically (at least quarterly), as well as when they are complaining of itching and/or are agitated. The routine use of moisturizing products (especially during winter months) can help prevent dry skin in LTC populations.

Residents with eczema and psoriasis often see their symptoms flare up under dry winter conditions. Eczema and psoriasis are commonly associated with depression and anxiety disorders (Kimball et al. 2008). Many drugs (e.g., carbamazepine, lamotrigine, modafinil) may cause a serious and potentially fatal skin rash, especially in residents with a history of developing drug-induced skin rashes.

Pharmacological Interventions for Cognitive Impairment in Residents with Dementia

Cognitive decline confers the greatest burden of functional disability on LTC residents (Schultz et al. 2003). Antidementia drugs include ChEIs (donepezil, rivastigmine, and galantamine) and the NMDA receptor antagonist memantine. These drugs provide a modest but clinically relevant slowing of cognitive and functional decline in residents with Alzheimer disease, dementia with Lewy bodies, or Parkinson disease dementia (Desai and Grossberg 2005). For residents with AD, combination therapy (one of the ChEIs and memantine) may be better than monotherapy with a ChEI; the benefits of combination therapy increase with the amount of time a person spends on this treatment and are sustained for years (Atri et al. 2008). The use of antidementia drugs may delay the onset of behavioral disturbances in dementia and may defer a worsening of mild agitation (Cummings et al. 2004; Desai and Grossberg 2005).

Antidementia drugs may not reduce established moderate to severe agitation in persons with severe dementia (Howard et al. 2007). Hence antidementia drugs should not be the first-line or only treatment for residents with significant behavioral and psychological symptoms of dementia. Psychosocial-environmental interventions, with or without psychotropic drugs (e.g., antidepressants), should be the first line of treatment; once symptoms improve significantly, antidementia drugs may be added. Dual use of ChEIs and bladder anticholinergics (oxybutynin and tolterodine) in LTC populations may result in greater rates of functional decline than the use of ChEIs alone (Sink et al. 2008). Reducing the anticholinergic load of currently prescribed medications may improve the effectiveness of antidementia drugs. Memantine is primarily cleared through the kidneys and should be renally dosed. Drugs that interfere with the elimination of memantine—that is, other drugs using the organic cation transporter 2 in the renal tubule (e.g., trimethoprim, metformin, imipramine)—may lead to an accumulation of memantine and consequent toxicity (Moellentin, Picone, and Leadbettter 2008). For details on the use of antidementia drugs in LTC populations, see chapter 3 on dementia.

Pharmacological Interventions for Behavioral and Psychological Symptoms of Dementia and for Chronic Persistent Mental Illness

To date, the FDA has not approved any medication specifically to treat behavioral and psychological symptoms of dementia. After cognitive deficits are accounted for, behavioral dysregulation is also associated with significant functional disability in LTC residents. Thus interventions to ameliorate behavioral and psychological symptoms of dementia may also reduce functional disabilities. Pharmacologic interventions for these dementia symptoms in LTC residents are often effective in reducing the symptoms, enhancing the resident's quality of life, avoiding hospitalization, and avoiding chronicity. Nonetheless, the clinician must be prudent with psychopharmacologic interventions and recognize their complexity. It is also important to keep in mind that the focus of therapy may be not only the resident, but also the caregivers (family and professional) and other residents. Reducing harm to caregivers and residents from an aggressive resident is an important goal of psychopharmacologic intervention.

The clinician should carefully and frequently monitor such interventions for adverse effects, as well as for their effectiveness (using standardized rating scales when possible). The dose of psychotropic agents should be titrated slowly, and the final dosage should be in keeping with the physiological tolerance of the specific resident yet, whenever possible, ensuring that adequate therapeutic levels are achieved. Frail and oldest old (older than 85) residents are at greatest risk of pharmacodynamic sensitivity and polypharmacy-induced adverse effects. The clinician should review the duration of treatment and reduce drug dosages or discontinue drugs whenever appropriate. LTC residents are typically taking multiple other medications. These co-medications increase the risk of drug interactions, sensitivity to adverse effects, and the cumulative medication burden associated with any psychotropic medication. Adverse effects related to psychotropic medications (e.g., worsening cognition, a decline in function, unsteadiness) may not be recognized or may be attributed to other known problems (e.g., Alzheimer disease, cerebrovascular disease).

Antidepressants

We recommend antidepressants for the treatment of many depressive disorders and anxiety disorders in LTC residents (Pollock et al. 2007; see table 12.5). The clinician may also consider prescribing SSRIs for recurrent sexually inappropriate behaviors if psychosocial-environmental interventions have not helped. All antidepressants are equal in their efficacy and speed of response. The only exception to this are stimulants, which have a much faster onset of action (as fast as two to four days) and thus are the drugs of choice when a rapid improvement of depression is critical (e.g., for residents who have depression during the end of life). The choice of antidepressants is typically based on matching the adverse effect profile (e.g., the sedative properties and weight gain associated with mirtazapine) with clinical symptoms (e.g., the presence of insomnia and weight loss, thus making mirtazapine a preferred antidepressant), medical comorbidity (e.g., TCAs are more or less contraindicated for residents with cardiac conduction defects), and currently consumed medications (e.g., avoid prescribing SSRIs, which are linked with an increased risk of bleeding in residents also taking warfarin). If a person has a history of a good response to an antidepressant, the clinician should first consider that particular antidepressant. A family history of a positive response to a particular antidepressant may also move that agent further up the list of therapeutic options.

Drugs such as citalopram, sertraline, venlafaxine, mirtazapine, and bupropion are generic options. Escitalopram and duloxetine are nongeneric options. Any of these agents may be used as a first-line antidepressant. Second- and third-line options include any antidepressant in the first and second lines to replace the one that was tried and failed (due to intolerance or a lack of response). Desvenlafaxine has not been studied in LTC populations. We do not recommend fluoxetine or paroxetine except for patients who are already taking them and doing well, due to the higher risk of drug-drug interactions than with other SSRIs. Fluoxetine and paroxetine offer no advantages in efficacy over other antidepressants. Also, fluoxetine has a long half-life and paroxetine has dose-dependent anticholinergic activity. Residents who are stable taking an antidepressant (including the ones we do not recommend) should continue taking the same drug unless that antidepressant is causing serious adverse effects.

We recommend prescribing the newer antidepressant selegiline (in a patch form) only after all other treatment options have failed, both because of the

TABLE 12.5
Indications for antidepressant treatment

Depressive disorders
    Major depression (single episode or recurrent)
    Dysthymic disorder
    Poststroke depression and to prevent depression in a resident who had a stroke and is at high risk of
        depression (e.g., has a past history of depression)
    Severe depression in the context of dementia
    Depression in the context of chronic pain
    Medication (e.g., interferon)-induced depression when the offending medication cannot be
        discontinued
    Severe emotional lability / pseudobulbar affect
    Severe depression in a resident with schizophrenia
    Depression in a resident with schizoaffective disorder-unipolar type
Anxiety disorders
    Panic disorder (with or without agoraphobia)
    Post-traumatic stress disorder
    Severe social phobia
    Generalized anxiety disorder
    Severe chronic anxiety symptoms in the context of dementia
Other disorders
    Sexually inappropriate behaviors not responding to nonpharmacological intervention
    Agitation and/or aggression associated with dementia
    Persistent yelling when pain is ruled out as the cause or is adequately treated

risk of drug-drug interactions and dietary restrictions at higher dosages and because it has not been studied in LTC populations for its antidepressant effect. The only exception is for a resident with Parkinson disease. For such a resident, the clinician may consider prescribing a selegiline patch early in the treatment of depression. We do not recommend St. John's wort, due to the risk of drug-drug interactions with cardiovascular and other commonly prescribed medications. The clinician should avoid prescribing tertiary amine TCAs (e.g., imipramine, amitriptyline, doxepine) for LTC residents, due to the high risk of anticholinergic and cardiac toxicities.

For cognitively intact residents with severe depression, the clinician may consider prescribing secondary amine TCAs (e.g., nortriptyline, desipramine). For residents with a low albumin level, there is an increased risk of TCA toxicity due to decreased protein binding. The clinician should avoid prescribing TCAs for residents with preexisting bundle branch block. The use of TCAs (secondary and tertiary) is severely limited in LTC populations, because their adverse effects (e.g., cardiotoxicity, sedation, orthostasis, urinary retention, exacerbation of narrow-angle glaucoma) are much more frequent in this population.

The clinician may prescribe modafinil as a first-line agent for residents with depression who also have narcolepsy or excessive sleepiness in the daytime, along with OSA. The clinician may consider prescribing modafinil as an adjuvant for residents with refractory depression, depression with apathy, or depression with excessive daytime sleepiness. Mirtazapine is available as an orally disintegrating tablet; sertraline, escitalopram, and citalopram are available as liquid preparations. The clinician may consider prescribing these preparations for residents with depression who have trouble swallowing pills but not liquids.

Dosage

Table 12.6 displays recommended starting doses and usually effective doses of antidepressants for LTC residents. The starting dose can be increased over four to seven days to the usual effective dose. Residents with hepatic or renal disease and frail elderly people may start with a dose even lower than the recommended initial dose, and that dose may be increased after seven days.

Adverse Effects

Common adverse effects of SSRIs include insomnia, somnolence, nausea, diarrhea, headaches, the exacerbation of migraines, vomiting, anorexia, and weight loss, but most of these adverse effects diminish after the first week. For residents with preexisting nausea and/or diarrhea, the clinician should avoid prescribing antidepressants that may exacerbate these symptoms (e.g., SSRIs, venlafaxine, desvenlafaxine, duloxetine); antidepressants with the least risk of exacerbating these symptoms (e.g., mirtazapine, bupropion) are preferred. Combining SSRIs and ChEIs may increase the risk of anorexia, nausea, and diarrhea, especially if the resident starts taking the drugs within a short time of each other. SSRI-induced hyponatremia (due to central diabetes

TABLE 12.6
Recommended dosages of antidepressants for a long-term care resident

Antidepressant	Starting Dose (mg)	Usual Effective Dose (mg)	Maximal Dose (mg)
Citalopram	10	20–40	40
Sertraline	25	50–150	150
Escitalopram	5	5–10	20
Paroxetine	10	10–20	20
Fluoxetine	10	10–20	20
Venlafaxine	37.5	37.5–225	225
Bupropion	75	100–300	300
Mirtazapine	7.5	7.5–30	30
Duloxetine	20	20–60	60
Trazodone	25	25–100	150

insipidus) is rare, but clinicians need to monitor for this in residents who are taking diuretics. The clinician should avoid prescribing SSRIs or venlafaxine for residents who are at high risk of abnormal bleeding (e.g., residents taking warfarin), as their use carries an increased risk of bleeding, possibly due to their effect on platelet function. The clinician should instead consider prescribing an antidepressant with a low or no effect on serotonin (e.g., mirtazapine, bupropion) for these residents. For residents who are taking SSRIs, the clinician should avoid prescribing or minimize the use of NSAIDs and aspirin, because of the risk of bleeding. The use of SSRIs is also associated with an increased risk of perioperative blood transfusion. SSRIs should be tapered off over a one- to two-week period to avoid SSRI discontinuation syndrome, which includes dizziness, vertigo, headaches, nausea, and insomnia. For residents who are taking trazodone along with an SSRI and residents who are taking high-dose SSRIs, the clinician should monitor them for serotonin syndrome (flulike symptoms, myoclonic jerks, fever, agitation, hyperreflexia) and discontinue the offending agent promptly if this syndrome occurs, as it can develop into delirium and be life threatening. SSRIs may occasionally precipitate REM sleep behavior disorder and restless leg syndrome. SSRIs may also exacerbate parkinsonian symptoms (Chan, Cordato, and O'Rourke 2008). Finally, SSRIs may increase the risk of developing type-2 diabetes; hence the clinician should prescribe it cautiously for residents with diabetes (Brown, Majumdar, and Johnson 2008).

Venlafaxine and desvenlafaxine have adverse effects similar to those of SSRIs. In addition, high doses of venlafaxine are associated with increased diastolic blood pressure. Hence we recommend monitoring the resident's blood pressure when prescribing doses equal to or greater than 150 mg/day. The clinician should avoid prescribing duloxetine for residents with liver disease, because its use is linked with a transient small increase in liver enzymes, so it may worsen a preexisting liver disease. Mirtazapine is associated with sedation and weight gain, probably due to its antihistaminic effect. It may also cause constipation. Paradoxically, the sedating property of mirtazapine may decrease in some people as its dose is increased, because at a higher dose it also increases noradrenergic neurotransmission. Rarely, mirtazapine is associated with leucopenia. Bupropion may be associated with anxiety and insomnia. High doses of bupropion (greater than 300 mg/day) are linked with an increased risk of seizures, so the clinician should avoid prescribing it for residents with a seizure disorder (epilepsy) or an electrolyte imbalance (e.g., residents who exhibit vomiting, diarrhea).

Stimulants

Residents who have significant apathy associated with depressive symptoms and residents with depression at the end of life may benefit from a trial of stimulants (e.g., methylphenidate, dextroamphetamine). We recommend that the clinician consider prescribing methylphenidate to reduce fatigue and improve depression rapidly for some residents in a hospice. Start at 2.5–5 mg in the morning and the afternoon for three to four days and then double the dose. The therapeutic dose range for LTC residents is 5–20 mg/day in two divided doses. The clinician may consider prescribing stimulants to reduce depression more quickly in residents with poststroke depression if they are not participating in physical therapy because of severe depression, as other antidepressants may take a longer time to become effective. The clinician may consider prescribing stimulants to treat sedation due to opioids when reducing the dose of opioids is not a good option (because of increased pain with decreasing the dose of an opioid analgesic).

The use of stimulants may be associated with tachycardia, anorexia, insomnia, anxiety, blurred vision, increased blood pressure, restlessness, and agitation. Stimulants may exacerbate preexisting psychotic symptoms, and occasionally they may cause psychotic symptoms (e.g., paranoid delusions). Stimulants may increase the risk of cardiac arrythmias, especially for residents who have a preexisting cardiac disease along with a propensity toward tachyarrhythmias. The clinician should avoid prescribing stimulants for these residents and for residents with uncontrolled hypertension. Hence we recommend that the clinician collaborate with the resident's primary care provider and/or cardiologist and, if necessary, order cardiac tests (e.g., an EKG) before prescribing stimulants for LTC residents.

Drug Interactions

Residents typically are already taking several prescription medications, vitamins, and supplements. Paroxetine and fluoxetine decrease hepatic cytochrome P450 2D6 liver enzyme activity and P-glycoprotein activity in the gut. Hence paroxetine may increase drugs metabolized by 2D6 isoenzymes (e.g., desipramine, digoxin) to toxic levels (Yasui-Furukori and Kaneko 2006). Among all antidepressants, citalopram, sertraline, escitalopram, venlafaxine, and desvenlafaxine carry a low risk of drug-drug interaction.

Antipsychotic Medications

Antipsychotic drugs are indicated in the treatment of a variety of serious psychotic disorders (table 12.7). The primary use of antipsychotics for LTC residents is for dementia-related aggressive symptoms that pose an imminent danger to themselves and/or to others. Antipsychotics may be particularly effective for treating anger, aggression, and paranoid ideas in residents with dementia (Schneider et al. 2006; Sultzer et al. 2008). They do not appear to improve functioning, care needs, or the resident's quality of life (Sultzer et al. 2008). The clinician should first try psychosocial-environmental interventions to treat psychotic symptoms in residents with dementia, unless the resident poses an imminent danger to him- or herself or to others. After ruling out pain, depression, medical conditions, and medication-induced agitation, the clinician may consider prescribing the short-term use of antipsychotics to help reduce the severe agitation thought to be due to advanced dementia while psychosocial-environmental interventions are being implemented. In managing psychological symptoms of dementia with antipsychotic medication, a trial of drug reduction usually does not lead to a reactivation or a worsening of symptoms if they have been stable for three or more months.

Many states have laws that prohibit the involuntary administration (e.g., without consent, especially for intramuscular and intravenous use) of any psychotropic medication (including antipsychotics) to residents without a court order. Such laws, although well intentioned, may cause suffering in residents because of the need to involve law enforcement personnel in transferring the resident to an emergency room for hospitalization to an inpatient psychiatric unit and then waiting there until a court order to administer medications involuntarily has been received.

During the last decade, the newer atypical antipsychotic drugs (i.e., risperidone, olanzapine, quetiapine, and aripiprazole, in order of their introduction) have largely replaced the older conventional or first-generation antipsychotic drugs (e.g., haloperidol, thioridazine) and the former have been considered preferred treatments for behavioral disturbances associated with dementia (Alexopoulos et al. 1998, 2005). A standardized evaluation with an instrument such as the Neuropsychiatric Inventory (NPI) may be a clinical indicator of which people with dementia are likely to benefit from discontinuing antipsychotic treatment (Ballard et al. 2004). The selection of antipsychotic drugs is based on matching the adverse effects of the drug with clinical symp-

TABLE 12.7
Indications for prescribing antipsychotic medications for long-term care residents

Primary psychotic disorders
  Schizophrenia
  Schizoaffective disorder
  Bipolar disorder with or without psychotic symptoms
  Major depression with psychotic symptoms
  Other psychotic disorders (e.g., delusional disorder)
  Nonpsychotic disorders (e.g., pervasive developmental disorders with severe agitation or
    aggression)
Secondary psychotic disorders
  Psychotic symptoms and severe agitation or aggression in the context of dementia
  Drug-induced psychotic symptoms and agitation
  Severe agitation or aggression in the context of delirium
  Psychotic symptoms with agitation due to a general medical condition

toms, medical or neurologic comorbidity, and the risk of drug-drug interactions with existing drugs.

Antipsychotic drugs are currently overused in LTC populations. We strongly recommend that their use be short term (6–12 weeks) and restricted to residents with severe aggression who pose an imminent danger to themselves and/or others, and to residents with psychotic symptoms that do not respond to psychosocial-environmental interventions where the symptoms are linked with significant emotional suffering and/or aggression.

Serious Risks Associated with the Use of Antipsychotic Medications

The FDA has issued a "black box" warning regarding the risk of death associated with the use of atypical and conventional antipsychotics for people with dementia. Most of the deaths are thought to be due to an infection or a cardiovascular event (e.g., sudden cardiac death). Among patients with dementia, the use of atypical antipsychotics increases the risk of death from 2.3 to 3.5 percent. Thus for every nine to 14 individuals with dementia who take an antipsychotic and improve, one would expect one excess death (Schneider, Dagerman, and Insel 2005). This risk is highest earlier in the treatment (the first 10–12 weeks) and diminishes over time. Conventional antipsychotics are at least as likely as atypical antipsychotics to increase the risk of death among people with dementia (P. Wang et al. 2005; S. Gill et al. 2007; Schneeweiss et al. 2007). All antipsychotics are associated with an increased risk of strokes, and this risk may be higher in people taking atypical antipsychotics than in those taking typical ones (Douglas and Smeeth 2008). People with dementia may have a higher risk of strokes connected with the use of antipsychotics than those who do not have dementia. In light of these risks, clinicians considering the prescription of antipsychotic medications to treat the behavioral and psychological symptoms of dementia should discuss the potential risks and benefits of such treatment with the resident or surrogate decision maker and document this discussion in the resident's chart, especially for residents with risk factors for cerebrovascular disease. To reduce the risk of strokes, mental health care providers should consider prophylaxis for cerebrovascular events (e.g., the prescription of antiplatelet therapy) for residents with dementia who are taking atypical antipsychotics.

The use of both conventional and atypical antipsychotic medications is associated with an increased risk of hospitalization, falls, injuries, and an accelerated cognitive and/or functional decline, especially for residents with dementia (Rochon et al. 2008). These adverse effects (similar to the risks of death and strokes) are typically seen early on (in the first 30 days) after the initiation of antipsychotic therapy. Drug-induced extrapyramidal symptoms are a common complication of antipsychotic medications (especially high-potency antipsychotics, such as haloperidol or risperidone). Tardive dyskinesia is a serious complication from the long-term use of conventional antipsychotics (usually over several years), although it may be seen within one year of use in residents with dementia. Akathisia (motor restlessness and an uncontrollable urge to move [with or without inner tension], dysphoria, a feeling of jumping out of one's skin) may be an acute complication of antipsychotic medications (especially haloperidol, aripiprazole, or ziprasidone), as well as a complication due to many years of antipsychotic treatment (tardive akathisia). The clinician may mistake acute-onset akathisia for a worsening of agitation and further increase the antipsychotic, which in turn may worsen akathisia and precipitate a behavioral emergency. Thus the clinician should maintain a high index of suspicion regarding the early accurate diagnosis of akathisia. Careful assessment, communication (with the resident or surrogate decision maker), and documentation of potential risks and benefits from the use of antipsychotics are necessary before prescribing them for LTC residents.

The use of atypical antipsychotics (especially olanzapine, clozapine, quetiapine, and risperidone) is associated with hyperglycemia, weight gain, and hyperlipidemia. Thus prescribing them for residents with obesity, hyperlipidemia, diabetes mellitus, and metabolic syndromes carries extra risks that need appropriate monitoring. For residents with a limited life expectancy, these risks are usually not an issue. The clinician should consider all of these risks in the context of the medical need for the drugs, evidence of their efficacy, medical comorbidity, and the efficacy and safety of alternatives. In light of the many serious risks associated with the use of antipsychotic drugs by people with dementia, the clinician should prescribe these drugs only when there is an identifiable risk of harm to the resident and/or others, when the distress caused by the symptoms is significant, and/or when alternate therapies have failed and relief of symptoms would be beneficial (Lyketsos and Rabins 2005).

Conventional Antipsychotic Medications

Conventional antipsychotic medications include the phenothiazines (e.g., chlorpromazine, perphenazine, trifluoperazine, fluphenazine), the butyrophenones (e.g., haloperidol, droperidol), and others (e.g., thioridazine, mesoridazine, thiothixene, loxapine, molindone). In general, atypical antipsychotics are preferred over conventional antipsychotics to treat psychotic disorders in elderly people, because of the increased safety of the former and their possibly efficacious profile. Haloperidol is the drug of choice for residents with acute delirium and severe agitation or physical aggression. The advantages of haloperidol in this setting are its wide therapeutic margin of safety, its ease of administration by a variety of routes (oral, intramuscular, intravenous), and a relative lack of cardiopulmonary or anticholinergic effects at low doses. The major adverse effects of haloperidol use are drug-induced parkinsonism and akathisia. Drug-induced parkinsonism is associated with discomfort, choking, falls in ambulatory patients, and decreased bed mobility in nonambulatory patients. Drug-induced parkinsonism appears three to five days after the initiation of haloperidol, and in LTC residents it can develop even at low doses. Akathisia is a motor restlessness syndrome that can cause substantial discomfort and may be mistaken for worsened agitation. Akathisia can occur even with the first dose of haloperidol. Acute dystonias are rare in older adults, but even so, we do not recommend the long-term use of haloperidol because of its high risk of tardive dyskinesia and drug-induced parkinsonism.

The use of haloperidol by people with Parkinson disease or dementia with Lewy bodies is associated with high morbidity and mortality; thus it is more or less contraindicated for these patients. The clinician should also avoid the use of haloperidol for residents with a past history of drug-induced parkinsonism. The efficacy of conventional antipsychotics in treating agitation and aggression in people with dementia is low (average of 26%), and the adverse risks are high (averaging 25%) (Lanctot et al. 1998). Thioridazine and mesoridazine have been linked with a clinically relevant prolongation of QT intervals. The risk of tardive dyskinesia is high with the use of conventional antipsychotics for elderly people, especially LTC residents with dementia (Jeste et al. 1995).

All phenothiazines are metabolized by the hepatic cytochrome 1A2 isoenzyme system, and cigarette smoking (or otherwise using nicotine) causes induction of the 1A2 enzyme system, thus potentially lowering the levels of phenothiazine antipsychotic agents. Residents taking phenothiazepines may develop toxicity, due to elevated levels of the drug when they try to quit smoking. Many residents with a chronic persistent mental illness (e.g., schizophrenia, schizoaffective disorder) have been taking high doses of conventional antipsychotics for many years, and a sizeable portion of this group may have subtle or obvious drug-induced parkinsonism and/or tardive dyskinesia. The clinician should consider trying a gradual dose reduction for these residents if the psychotic disorder has been stable for a year or more, with close monitoring for any emergence of or increase in tardive dyskinesias or an exacerbation of the underlying psychotic disorder. Many residents with a chronic persistent mental illness are also taking more than one antipsychotic, and they may benefit from a gradual dose reduction and then discontinuation of one of the antipsychotic agents.

Atypical Antipsychotic Medications

Atypical antipsychotic medications include risperidone, olanzapine, quetiapine, aripiprazole, ziprasidone, clozapine, and paliperidone.

RISPERIDONE   Risperidone is a high-potency atypical antipsychotic agent, and it is one of the most rigorously studied antipsychotics in LTC populations. It is available in liquid concentrate and orally disintegrating forms. These may be useful if residents are unable to swallow pills. The clinician may consider prescribing liquid risperidone to treat behavioral emergencies, because its onset is quicker-acting than the tablet form. For residents who refuse to take oral antipsychotics despite the staff's best efforts, but still need antipsychotics to manage chronic psychotic symptoms (e.g., residents with schizophrenia who have a court order authorizing the involuntary administration of medications), the clinician may consider the use of injectable long-acting risperidone.

The use of risperidone is associated with a risk of sedation, dose-dependent parkinsonism (especially above 1.5 mg for residents with dementia), peripheral edema, and orthostasis (especially if the dose is rapidly increased or the starting dose is higher than 0.25 mg once or twice daily). The clinician should avoid prescribing risperidone for residents with a high risk of drug-induced parkinsonism (e.g., residents with Parkinson disease, dementia with Lewy bodies, or a past history of drug-induced parkinsonism). The use of risperidone is associated with an increase in prolactin levels, which may increase the risk of osteoporosis. Hence the long-term use of risperidone for residents with osteoporosis should be minimized. Risperidone is metabolized by the hepatic cytochrome P450 2D6 isoenzyme system and thus may interact with other drugs that affect the activity of this enzyme system (e.g., paroxetine, by inhibiting the 2D6 isoenzyme system, may increase levels of risperidone, resulting in risperidone toxicity [e.g., drug-induced parkinsonism]).

OLANZAPINE   Olanzapine has been rigorously studied in LTC populations. The clinician should monitor residents who are taking olanzapine for excessive sedation, falls, unsteadiness, weight gain, and hyperglycemia. For residents with anorexia, weight loss, or insomnia due to psychotic symptoms, some of these adverse effects may be beneficial. Olanzapine has mild anticholinergic activity in vitro, but this is usually not a problem if low doses (2.5–5 mg/day) are used. For residents who are taking other anticholinergic agents, the clinician should consider the potential for anticholinergic toxicity. The clinician should avoid prescribing olanzapine for residents with Parkinson disease, due to a high risk of falls. Residents who smoke may need higher doses of olanzapine, because chronic smoking causes the induction of cytochrome P450 1A2 isoenzymes, which in turn lowers the level of olanzapine. Conversely, residents who have been taking olanzapine and quit smoking may need to have their dosage of olanzapine reduced. The clinician should avoid prescribing olanzapine for residents with uncontrolled diabetes and/or morbid obesity. Optimal dosing of olanzapine in cognitively intact elderly people is 5–10 mg/day, and in elderly people with dementia, 2.5–5 mg/day. Olanzapine is available as a tablet, an instant-dissolve wafer, and an intramuscular injection.

QUETIAPINE   Quetiapine has a much lower risk of drug-induced parkinsonism than risperidone and olanzapine. It is the antipsychotic drug of choice to treat severe agitation due to psychotic symptoms for residents with Parkinson disease, dementia with Lewy bodies, or a past history of drug-induced parkinsonism. Its use is associated with sedation and orthostatic hypotension (which causes an increased risk of falls). Quetiapine is a short-acting drug that, in adults, needs to be given two to three times a day, but the clinician may consider prescribing it once a day at night for elderly, frail LTC residents. Quetiapine is also available in extended-release form, to be used once daily, usually at night. Quetiapine is available as a tablet and an oral solution.

ARIPIPRAZOLE   Aripiprazole is the only antipsychotic with the unique property of being a dopamine partial agonist and antagonist; thus it may be preferred over risperidone and olanzapine for the treatment of severe psychotic symptoms and agitation for residents with Parkinson disease or dementia with Lewy bodies who could not tolerate quetiapine. The clinician may also consider prescribing aripiprazole as an adjuvant for treatment-refractory depression. The use of aripiprazole is not associated with weight gain. Aripiprazole has a long half-life (75–146 hours), so adverse effects may take a longer time to clear, even after its discontinuation. Aripiprazole is available as a tablet, an intramuscular injection, an orally disintegrating tablet, and an oral solution.

ZIPRASIDONE   Ziprasidone has not been rigorously studied in LTC populations, but the clinician may consider it if risperidone, quetiapine, olanzapine, and aripiprazole have not been effective or could not be tolerated. We recommend obtaining an EKG before initiating this drug to check for a corrected QT interval, as the use of ziprasidone has been associated with dose-related prolongation of QT intervals. Hence it is more or less contraindicated in persons with a known prolongation of the QT interval, a recent myocardial infarction, or uncompensated heart failure, and it should not be given with QT interval-prolonging medications. The use of ziprasidone has not been linked with weight gain. It may be preferable to risperidone and olanzapine for residents with Parkinson disease who are experiencing psychotic symptoms and could not tolerate quetiapine, clozapine, and aripiprazole. It is available in tablet, rapid-dissolve wafer, liquid concentrate, and intramuscular injection forms.

CLOZAPINE   Clozapine substantially lowers the seizure threshold, which can be problematic for residents who have had a stroke or have advanced dementia. Clozapine also has anticholinergic properties that can further impair cognitive function in this population, and it may provoke delirium. The use of clozapine has been associated with orthostasis, tachycardia, cardiomyopathy, and myocarditis. The clinician may consider prescribing it for residents who have Parkinson disease without dementia and are experiencing severe psychotic symptoms. Residents with a chronic persistent mental illness who are stable taking clozapine and tolerate it well should continue taking this drug, but the clinician should closely monitor them for adverse effects. Many residents with a chronic persistent mental illness may benefit from a gradual dose reduction, especially if they are experiencing subtle adverse effects. LTC residents may tolerate low doses of clozapine (12.5–50 mg/day) because low doses may avoid most of the adverse effects, but the need to monitor for agranulocytosis is a major liability. The clinician may consider prescribing low-dose clozapine for treatment-resistant severe aggressive behavior in residents with dementia (H. Lee et al. 2007).

PALIPERIDONE   Paliperidone has not been studied in LTC populations, but the clinician may consider prescribing it either if a resident has not tolerated the usual antipsychotics or if the usual antipsychotics have not been effective. As with risperidone, the clinician should avoid prescribing paliperidone for residents with preexisting extrapyramidal symptoms, Parkinson disease, or dementia with Lewy bodies, due to the high risk of worsening these symptoms and increased mortality. Paliperidone may be a safer choice than other antipsychotics (all of which require hepatic metabolism) for residents with liver disease and a psychotic disorder, because it is primarily excreted unchanged via the kidneys. For residents with chronic kidney disease, paliperidone may cause toxicity even at low doses (3 mg/day). The starting dose and dose range of paliperidone in LTC populations are unclear. It may be started at 3 mg/day and the therapeutic dose range may be 3–6 mg/day.

Dosages of Atypical Antipsychotic Medications
Table 12.8 displays dosages and common adverse effects of atypical antipsychotic medications. In general, the doses of antipsychotics are much higher for residents with severe persistent mental illnesses (schizophrenia, schizoaffective disorder, bipolar disorder) than for residents with dementia and severe psychotic symptoms who are naïve to antipsychotics. Table 12.9 lists antipsychotics available in formulations other than pills.

TABLE 12.8
Recommended dosages of atypical antipsychotic medications for residents with dementia

A. *Standard Dosages*

Antipsychotic	Starting Dose (mg/day)	Average Therapeutic Dose Range (mg/day)
Risperidone	0.125–0.5	0.25–1.0
Quetiapine	12.5–50	25–200
Olanzapine	2.5–5	2.5–5
Aripiprazole	2–5	2–10
Ziprasidone	20–40	40–120
Clozapine	12.5–25	12.5–50

B. *For Behavioral Emergencies*

Antipsychotic	Dose (mg)	Route
Haloperidol	0.5–1	Oral, intramuscular, intravenous
Risperidone	0.25–0.5	Oral (liquid, rapidly dissolving tablet)
Olanzapine	5–10	Rapidly dissolving tablet, intramuscular
Aripiprazole	5–10	Rapidly dissolving tablet, intramuscular, liquid concentrate
Ziprasidone	10–20	Intramuscular

TABLE 12.9
Some commonly used antipsychotic medications in special formulations

Risperidone: rapidly dissolving tablet, liquid concentrate, and long-acting intramuscular injection typically given every two weeks

Olanzapine: rapidly dissolving tablet and intramuscular preparation

Aripiprazole: rapidly dissolving tablet, liquid concentrate, and intramuscular preparation

Ziprasidone: intramuscular preparation

Haloperidol: liquid, intramuscular preparation, intravenous, intramuscular depot preparation typically given once every four weeks

Fluphenazine: intramuscular depot preparation typically given every three to four weeks

Hypnotic Medications

Numerous prescription and nonprescription agents have been used to treat insomnia. Hypnotics are drugs approved by the FDA for the treatment of insomnia. Hypnotics recommended for use in LTC populations include zolpidem, zaleplon, eszopiclone, temazepam, and ramelteon. The clinician may also consider prescribing hypnotics for the short-term treatment of insomnia in residents with depression, as antidepressants usually take several weeks to be effective. The use of hypnotics for LTC residents carries a high risk-to-benefit ratio (for details, refer to chapter 8). The clinician may consider the lowest effective doses of zolpidem and zaleplon for short-term use (e.g., the resident is anxious and has insomnia a few days before scheduled surgery). Zaleplon has a short half-life of one hour and is not associated with tolerance or rebound insomnia. Zolpidem is available in both short-acting and long-acting preparations. Unlike zaleplon, zolpidem is associated with dependence and the potential for abuse (Messinger-Rapport et al. 2007). Eszopiclone works by binding the GABA-A receptor and may be considered to be a second-line treatment for insomnia because of its higher cost than zolpidem and zaleplon. Temazepam is a third-line treatment because of its higher toxicity than zolpidem, zaleplon, and eszopiclone. Ramelteon (a melatonin receptor agonist) has not been studied in LTC populations, but the clinician may consider prescribing it for a resident who is experiencing chronic insomnia characterized by difficulty with sleep onset. Ramelteon is not a sedating medication, and residents may experience the maximal therapeutic effects over a period of several nights or weeks. Ramelteon lacks abuse liability, although this is not a concern in the majority of LTC residents who need sedative-hypnotics. The typical recommendation is to take hypnotics 30 minutes before bedtime.

Alternatives to hypnotics for the treatment of insomnia include mirtazapine and trazodone. Mirtazapine promotes sleep and thus may be preferred over other antidepressants for residents with depression and insomnia. The clinician should prescribe trazodone sparingly for insomnia in LTC residents because of the risk of daytime sedation, dizziness, psychomotor impairment, falls, and orthostatic hypotension even at low (25–50 mg) doses in this population (Mendelson 2005). For residents with insomnia in the context of depression or nighttime agitation, the clinician may consider prescribing low-dose trazodone. Alcohol and sedating antihistamines (e.g., diphenhydramine) are the most commonly used self-treatments for insomnia. The clinician should inquire into their use and discontinue them, while taking appropriate precautions (e.g., monitoring for alcohol withdrawal symptoms) (Buysse 2008). Diphenhydramine is a potent anticholinergic available over the counter (e.g., as Tylenol PM), and it may cause delirium in older people. The clinician should avoid prescribing it. Drinking a nightcap (a drink containing alcohol taken at bedtime) is a poor choice for addressing insomnia because alcohol can impair the quality of sleep, resulting in daytime somnolence. Alcohol is also associated with the rapid development of tolerance. We do not recommend the use of sedating antipsychotics (e.g., quetiapine, olanzapine) to treat insomnia.

Table 12.10 displays recommended doses of hypnotics for LTC populations. We do not recommend the use of flurazepam, triazolam, estazolam, quazepam, doxepin, amitriptyline, trimipramine, diphenhydramine, doxylam-

TABLE 12.10
Recommended doses of drugs used to treat insomnia
in the long-term care population

Drug	Dose Range (mg)
Benzodiazepine receptor agonists	
Zolpidem	5–10
Zaleplon	5–20
Eszopiclone	1–2
Benzodiazepines	
Temazepam	7.5–15
Melatonin-receptor agonist	
Ramelteon	8
Other agents	
Trazodone	25–50
Mirtazapine	7.5–15
Melatonin	1–6

ine, hydroxyzine, chloral hydrate, or ethclorvynol to treat insomnia in LTC residents, due to the high risk of adverse effects (e.g., cognitive toxicity, falls) that are linked with their use. All hypnotics (except ramelteon) are associated with an increased risk of postural instability, falls, injuries, anterograde amnesia, the induction or exacerbation of delirium, daytime sleepiness (especially in the early morning), and the potential to worsen preexisting pulmonary conditions, such as obstructive sleep apnea. Hence the chronic use of hypnotics (except ramelteon) should be minimized. Residents who have been taking hypnotics for a long time and appear stable may continue taking these medications with close monitoring for adverse effects and, if possible, a slow gradual tapering off of the hypnotic agent. We do not recommend abrupt discontinuation of sedative-hypnotics, due to the risk of rebound insomnia and other withdrawal symptoms that may manifest as agitation, especially for residents with dementia. The long-term use of hypnotics is associated with tolerance and dependence. Although the majority of hypnotics have a potential for abuse, this is not usually an issue for LTC populations. Melatonin works best for jet lag, which is not a typical insomnia seen in elderly populations, and its use may be linked with depression. Valerian may be useful for mild insomnia.

Antianxiety Medications (Anxiolytics)

Antianxiety medications include antidepressants (already discussed), benzodiazepines, buspirone, propranolol, and pregabalin.

Benzodiazepines

Benzodiazepines (BZs) have excellent anxiolytic properties and work quickly. Hence they are the drugs of choice to treat an acute episode of severe anxiety in LTC residents. BZs are also the drugs of choice for alcohol withdrawal (as well as to treat serious withdrawal symptoms resulting from the long-term use of BZs) and for agitation, myoclonus, and/or seizure during the last days of life (including for a resident with end-stage COPD). BZs in this setting can facilitate calm, sedation, and anxiolysis, but they may worsen confusion and hasten death. The clinician should counsel family members regarding these benefits and risks. In some severe cases of anxiety associated with dementia, the short-term use of low doses of short-acting BZ (lorazepam, oxazepam) may be necessary until the antidepressants become therapeutic. The clinician may consider prescribing low-dose clonazepam for REM sleep behavior disorder associated with DLB and for Parkinson disease.

The use of BZs by older adults is linked with cognitive impairment (attentional and memory problems, slowed psychomotor performance), a worsening of preexisting cognitive impairments, daytime sedation, dysphoria, ataxia, falls, hip fractures, delirium, and a paradoxical increase in agitation and disinhibition. LTC residents are even more susceptible to these adverse effects than community-dwelling older adults. Some BZs with longer half-lives (e.g., diazepam, flurazepam) are on the Beer's list of medications not appropriate for older adults. The concomitant use of BZs and alcohol greatly increases the risk of adverse events. Moreover, the long-term use of BZs is associated with tolerance and dependence and the risk of serious withdrawal symptoms (e.g., insomnia, anxiety, visual hallucinations, shocklike sensations, delirium, seizures, and death). Thus the clinician should first consider safer alternatives and minimize the use of BZs.

BZs still have a significant role in the treatment of acute severe anxiety symptoms in LTC residents. The clinician may consider periodic, careful, and gradual discontinuation of BZs for residents who have been taking BZs for decades for underlying chronic anxiety disorders. A subgroup of residents with disabling chronic anxiety disorders who need long-term BZs (at a gradually lower dose as age or disability increases) may be identified with such a discontinuation trial. For residents (or surrogate decision makers) who do not want to try a reduction of BZs, we recommend close monitoring for adverse effects. Tapering off and discontinuing BZs should be at a dose-reduction rate of no more than a quarter of the usual daily dose per one to two weeks, resulting in a taper time from full dosage to discontinuation of four to eight weeks. Some residents may need an even slower taper over three to six months.

The clinician should avoid prescribing BZs for residents with COPD, as they decrease respiratory drive, compromise lung function, and worsen exercise tolerance. BZs may also suppress respiratory drive, so the clinician should avoid prescribing them for residents with OSA. Lastly, the clinician should avoid prescribing BZs for residents with delirium, because they worsen cognitive impairments.

Some BZs are available in other forms besides pills (e.g., orally disintegrating alprazolam [Niravam] and clonazepam [Klonopin wafers]; intensols [alprazolam, lorazepam]), and the clinician may consider prescribing them for residents who have difficulty swallowing pills but not liquids.

Buspirone

The clinician may consider prescribing buspirone for residents with a long-standing generalized anxiety disorder (GAD) and GAD-like symptoms in the context of dementia (Desai and Grossberg 2003a). Persistent anxiety in residents with dementia may manifest as persistent agitation, irritability, and verbal or even physical aggression. The clinician should exercise caution with the concomitant use of buspirone with verapamil, diltiazem, erythromycin, or itraconazole, because competitive enzyme inhibition will substantially increase the plasma concentration of buspirone. Buspirone may also interact with fluoxetine, fluvoxamine, paroxetine, and bupropion, producing adverse consequences such as agitation (Ramadan, Werder, and Preskorn 2006).

Propranolol

The clinician may consider prescribing propranolol for the management of drug-induced akathisia, for agitation and aggression in residents with brain injuries, for severe essential tremors, and for some residents with severe post-traumatic stress disorder, which is associated with autonomic symptoms (palpitations, tachycardia). Its use carries a significant risk of hypotension, bradycardia, tiredness, and occasionally depression.

Pregabalin

Preliminary evidence and clinical experience indicate that pregabalin may have an anxiolytic effect. It is a good choice for treating anxiety symptoms in residents with fibromyalgia, epilepsy, or pain associated with neuropathy. Adverse effects include dizziness, sedation, and falls.

Mood Stabilizers

Mood stabilizers include lithium, valproate, carbamazepine, oxcarbazepine, and lamotrigine.

Lithium

There is a 10 to 15 percent decrease in total body water from young adulthood to old age. This leads to a slower rate of elimination and an increased concentration of water-soluble drugs, such as lithium, in body fluids. Aging-associated changes in distribution patterns may make plasma levels of the drug unreliable; for example, lithium may remain clinically active long after plasma levels decline. Residents with bipolar disorder who are stable and tolerating lithium well should continue taking lithium, albeit with close monitoring for adverse effects. Residents with bipolar disorder who are taking lithium and whose symptoms are partially controlled should also continue taking lithium, as there is a significant risk that their symptoms may worsen considerably if lithium is discontinued. Lithium is preferred over other agents for people with bipolar disorder who have a high risk of suicide. For residents with bipolar disorder who are experiencing adverse effects with lithium, lowering the dose (and thus the plasma levels) may resolve these adverse effects and yet have some therapeutic value, even if their levels are below the therapeutic range. The use of lithium in LTC populations carries a high risk of delirium, falls, the exacerbation of a preexisting cognitive impairment, psychomotor slowing, tremors, diarrhea, leukocytosis, renal toxicity, cardiac conduction defects, and hypothyroidism. Residents taking NSAIDs and/or diuretics are at a higher risk of lithium toxicity. Hyponatremia (low serum sodium levels) due to any cause may result in lithium toxicity, even for residents who are taking a previously stable dose of lithium, because sodium is needed for lithium to be cleared by the kidney. Residents with a preexisting kidney disease are also at high risk of lithium toxicity.

Valproate

Valproate may be an appropriate choice for residents with bipolar disorder and hypomanic or manic symptoms, or mixed symptoms. Although rigorous data do not support the use of valproate for residents with dementia, expert consensus guidelines and clinical experience suggest that the clinician consider prescribing a trial of low-dose valproate for some residents with chronic moderate to severe agitation and/or impulsive aggression without psychotic symptoms if psychosocial interventions have not helped (Rabins et al. 2007). For residents with migraines or seizure disorders who are experiencing chronic agitation, valproate may be a good choice. Its use is associated with ataxia, falls, daytime sedation, thrombocytopenia, gastric distress, tremors, weight gain, and a decline in one's ability to carry out ADLs. The risk of sedation and falls is particularly high when valproate is used with other sedating psychotropic medications (e.g., antipsychotics, benzodiazepines). Valproate is highly protein bound, so the protein binding of valproate may be low in residents with low albumin levels, resulting in increased free valproate levels and an increased risk of toxicity, although such toxicity will not be apparent from the total serum valproate levels. Drugs that induce hepatic enzymes (e.g., phenytoin, carbamazepine, phenobarbital) can double the clearance of valproate, requiring an increased dose of valproate to produce therapeutic benefits. Valproate may double the levels of lamotrigine. In addition, valproate and other anticonvulsants have been linked to an increased risk of suicide.

Carbamazepine

The clinician may consider prescribing carbamazepine (CBZ) for residents who have bipolar disorder with mixed mood symptoms or residents who have hypomanic or manic symptoms and cannot tolerate valproate. The clinician may also consider it for residents who have bipolar disorder along with alcohol abuse, have been advised to abstain from alcohol, and are undergoing alcohol withdrawal symptoms (anxiety, insomnia, tremors, etc.). For residents experiencing alcohol withdrawal, CBZ may be a reasonable alternative to benzodiazepines. CBZ appears to be modestly efficacious for the management of agitation and aggression in residents with dementia, although side effects and concerns about drug-drug interactions limit its use (Herrmann and Lanctot 2007). The clinician may consider prescribing CBZ for the management of severe and persistent agitation refractory to psychosocial-environmental interventions and other pharmacological interventions (e.g., antidepressants, antipsychotics, valproate, analgesics).

Although classically used for trigeminal neuralgia, CBZ is not used as firstline agent for this indication in LTC populations, because of the high risk of adverse effects and drug-drug interactions. Residents who are taking CBZ for trigeminal neuralgia, are doing well, and have minimal adverse effects may continue taking it. Its use carries a significant risk of drug-drug interactions, induction of many cytochrome P450 liver enzymes (including autoinduction of its own metabolism, requiring a dose adjustment after a few weeks), osteoporosis with long-term use, and, rarely, aplastic anemia and leucopenia. Other adverse effects of CBZ include daytime sedation, ataxia, falls, dizziness, and delirium. A long-acting preparation of CBZ (Equetro) is available and can be given as a single nighttime dose. Many residents have difficulty tolerating CBZ levels at or above 8–10 mcg/ml, but they may show therapeutic benefits at lower levels (4–8 mcg/ml). Fluoxetine, propoxyphene, and cimetidine are some of the many commonly used drugs that can significantly increase CBZ levels. Routine adverse effects associated with the use of CBZ, such as unsteadiness, tremor, and sedation, may be underreported in LTC residents. Hyponatremia produced by CBZ, due to a syndrome of inappropriate antidiuretic hormone secretion, is more common in LTC residents, especially those taking diuretics.

CBZ is short acting, and the total daily dose is given in two or three divided doses for adults. For frail, elderly LTC populations, the clinician may consider once-a-day dosing (usually at night). CBZ is highly protein bound and, like valproate, may cause toxicity for residents with low albumin levels despite having normal serum levels (because the free or unbound fraction is increased). CBZ and other anticonvulsants (e.g., valproate, oxcarbazepine) have been linked to an increased risk of suicide.

Oxcarbazepine

The clinician may consider prescribing oxcarbazepine (OXC) as an adjuvant for the treatment of hypomanic or manic symptoms when other drug interventions have not been successful or tolerated. The clinician may consider prescribing OXC in place of valproate to treat chronic agitation and/or aggression in the absence of psychotic symptoms for residents with dementia. The use of OXC is associated with hyponatremia, sedation, and an increased risk of falls. OXC is usually better tolerated and has less risk of enzyme induction than CBZ. Oxcarbazepine is also available in a liquid formulation.

Lamotrigine

Lamotrigine may be useful to prevent depressive episodes for residents with bipolar depression. The titration needs to be done slowly to achieve a therapeutic dosage, and its primary adverse effect is the risk of a serious skin rash, which may be fatal, especially if the dose is increased rapidly. Residents who have history of skin sensitivity to drugs or preexisting dermatologic conditions may need extra precautions during the initiation of lamotrigine therapy. Valproate doubles lamotrigine levels, so lamotrigine should be started at half the usual dose for residents who are already taking valproate.

Dosages of Mood Stabilizer and Anticonvulsant Medications

Table 12.11 displays doses of mood stabilizers for LTC residents.

Vitamins, Herbals, and Supplements

Older adults commonly take dietary supplements (including vitamins, herbal remedies, and synthetic supplements), and an estimated one out of five patients takes such substances in an effort to maintain or promote health (Ashar and Rowland-Seymour 2008). Clinicians should routinely ask residents about their use of supplements, because of potential toxicity and drug-drug interactions associated with the use of supplements.

Many LTC residents have a vitamin B_{12} and/or vitamin D deficiency and would benefit from vitamin replacement therapy. Vitamin B_{12} deficiency is prevalent in LTC populations and may contribute to cognitive impairments, depressed moods, and fatigue (due to macrocytic anemia). In severe cases, B_{12} deficiency may cause dementia, peripheral neuropathy, and subacute combined degeneration of the spinal cord. The most common cause of B_{12} deficiency is reduced absorption, due to atrophic gastritis. A high oral dose (1,000 mcg) of B_{12} daily is sufficient to treat B_{12} deficiency, except for residents with pernicious anemia, who may require monthly injections of B_{12} (100 mcg). For residents with depression, even levels that are normal (but at the lower end of the normal range) may indicate a B_{12} deficiency and should be treated with oral B_{12} supplements.

LTC residents are prone to vitamin D deficiency, due to their limited exposure to sunlight (a major source of vitamin D, which is formed when ultraviolet light catalyzes its synthesis from 7-dehydrocholesterol in the skin)

TABLE 12.11
Recommended doses of mood stabilizers for long-term care residents

Drug	Usual Daily Starting Dose (mg)	Usual Daily Therapeutic Dose/Level
Lithium	75–300	Therapeutic levels 0.4–0.9 (level)
Valproate	125–500	Therapeutic levels 40–100 (level)
Carbamazepine	100–200	Therapeutic levels 4–8 (level)
Lamotrigine	12.5–25	25–150 mg
Oxcarbazepine	150–300	300–600 mg

as well as their limited intake of dairy products, which are usually fortified with vitamin D (A. Thomas and Gambert 2008). Vitamin D is useful for bone health (reducing the risk of fracture), and it also may have beneficial effects on heart health, chronic pain, fall risk, cognitive health, and moods (reducing depression) (Messinger-Rapport et al. 2007). Hence we recommend that the clinician routinely test vitamin B_{12} and vitamin D_3 levels in LTC populations unless a resident is in the terminal stage of dementia or has another terminal condition (Morley 2007). Vitamin D deficiency may be treated with vitamin D_2 50,000 units once or twice weekly for eight to 12 weeks. Following that loading regimen, vitamin D_3 800 to 1,000 units daily can be initiated. For residents with renal failure, we recommend calcitriol, as the kidneys cannot convert the 25-hydroxxy vitamin D into 1.25 dihydroxy vitamin D in end-stage renal disease. Hypervitaminosis D is rare, but it has severe adverse health effects (e.g., irreversible renal and cardiovascular damage, adverse effects of hypercalcemia), and clinicians prescribing vitamin D should keep this in mind.

In the past, many clinicians recommended that people with dementia take vitamin E to slow the progression of their dementia, but due to recent reports of a small increase in all-cause mortality and the potential to increase the risk of bleeding (especially if vitamin E is taken with warfarin), we recommend against the use of vitamin E (especially daily doses above 400 international units [IU]) for residents with dementia (Bjelakovic et al. 2007). If a resident wishes to take vitamin E because of its antioxidant properties, the clinician should recommend taking less than 400 IU and closely monitor that person for adverse effects.

Multivitamin and mineral supplementation does not have a significant effect on the incidence of infection in the majority of LTC populations, although a subgroup of residents who do not have dementia may benefit from supplementation (Liu et al. 2007). In contrast, nutritional supplements fortified with higher levels of antioxidants (vitamin E, vitamin C, and beta carotene), B vitamins, selenium, and zinc than the traditional supplements (e.g., Ensure Plus) may have benefits for the immune system, as well as a clinical benefit (e.g., less fever, fewer prescribed antibiotics), for frail LTC residents (Langkamp-Henken et al. 2006).

Older adults commonly use herbals and supplements (Desai and Grossberg 2003b). Many elderly residents may be self-medicating (or a family member may be medicating the resident) with over-the-counter herbals and/or supplements for a variety of problems (e.g., memory impairment, depression, insomnia), typically before admission to an LTC facility and occasionally while they are in the facility. The clinician should routinely inquire about such use and evaluate its risks and benefits, preferably in collaboration with a pharmacist. Clinicians who are knowledgeable about the use of over-the-counter herbals and supplements may consider recommending them, although there is little research to guide the use of herbals and supplements for LTC populations.

The clinician may consider prescribing valerian (400–900 mg) for residents with mild insomnia, although it often requires one to two weeks of nightly use for best results. Valerian carries a small increased risk of oversedation with the concomitant use of hypnotics, and symptoms similar to BZ withdrawal may be seen if it is abruptly discontinued after several weeks. The clinician may consider recommending chamomile tea for enhancing sleep, but the resident should not take it if he or she is allergic to ragweed. It carries a small risk of oversedation with the concomitant use of sedative-hypnotics and a risk of excessive bleeding with the concomitant use of anticoagulants. The clinician may consider prescribing melatonin (3 mg before bedtime) to treat insomnia in some residents (e.g., residents with delayed sleep phase syndrome or who are blind and have insomnia) (Doghramji 2006).

The use of melatonin may worsen depression; for residents with depression or who develop depressive symptoms after taking melatonin, this problem may be avoided or treated with exposure to 10,000 lux bright light in the daytime (from 9 a.m. to 6 p.m.) (Riemersma-van der Lek et al. 2008). We do not recommend prescribing ginkgo biloba to treat mild to moderate dementia because of its lack of efficacy (McCarney et al. 2008). Many residents (with or without dementia) may wish to take ginkgo to enhance their cognitive functions and cerebral circulation. The clinician should monitor these residents for the risks associated with the use of ginkgo (e.g., excessive bleeding if used concomitantly with anticoagulants). Many elderly people take ginseng to improve their energy levels. Ginseng carries increased risks of tachycardia, excessive bleeding with the concomitant use of anticoagulants, mania and headaches with the concomitant use of monoamine oxidase inhibitors, and insomnia and nervousness with the concomitant use of stimulants. Some elderly people take St. John's wort to treat low-grade depression. The use of St. John's wort is linked with an increased risk of lowering the blood levels of many prescription drugs, due to its enzyme induction properties and the risk of serotonin syndrome if it is taken with SSRIs and trazodone. SAM-e is often taken to treat low-grade depression, but its use is associated with gastrointes-tinal distress, insomnia, dry mouth, and restlessness.

Residents who are cognitively intact or have a mild cognitive impairment may wish to take omega-3 supplements for their potential cardiovascular ben-efits (e.g., reducing the risk of sudden death in people with coronary artery disease), potential benefits for rheumatological disorders (e.g., rheumatoid arthritis), and potential cognitive and emotional benefits. Omega-3 supple-ments, though usually safe, carry a small risk of increased bleeding time, are difficult to swallow because of the large size of the capsules, and may cause mild gastrointestinal distress. Some residents may wish to take glucosamine plus chondroitin for osteoarthritis. Its benefits for pain relief are modest and are usually seen within three months (Ashar and Rowland-Seymour 2008).

Although many herbal remedies are marketed as "natural," it is impor-tant for clinicians to know that *natural* does not necessarily mean *safe*. For a comprehensive listing of herb-drug interactions and supplement-drug in-teractions, readers can use Epocrates (www.epocrates.com) and the book *The Essential Herb-Drug-Vitamin Interaction Guide* (Grossberg and Fox 2007). Epocrates has a database of more than 400 herbals and more than 3,000 prescription medications, accessible through a handheld device or online. Ep-ocrates provides custom-tailored information, including appropriate dosage recommendations and typical uses of commonly reported herbs. Physicians can also receive regular health care updates on herbal preparations, as well as other alternative and traditional medicine matters, through Epocrates. Herbals and supplements are not well regulated by the FDA; we recommend checking them at www.consumerlab.com.

Pharmacological Interventions for the Management of Behavioral Emergencies

Although psychosocial-environmental interventions (especially by a veteran staff member) may be sufficient to manage many behavioral emergencies (e.g., acute verbal and physical aggression, agitation), pharmacological in-terventions are often necessary and, if used appropriately and promptly, may prevent serious injury to the resident or to others (staff, other residents) and avert transfer to an emergency room. The clinician should suspect and inves-tigate delirium and its various causes, as well as acute pain, for any resident with a behavioral emergency. Often, the cause of the behavioral emergency is known and is being treated (e.g., delirium due to a UTI in a resident with dementia). In such situations, the clinician may consider prescribing atypical antipsychotics (e.g., liquid or orally dissolvable risperidone) with or without BZs (e.g., orally dissolvable alprazolam). The staff may consider asking the resident's family to help administer medications (e.g., antibiotics, psychotropics) if the resident is refusing to take them. Many state laws forbid controlling the resident's behavior with the parenteral administration of psychotropic medications (e.g., intramuscular haloperidol with or without intramuscular lorazepam) at an LTC facility, so the facility may have to seek a court order approving the use of medications against the resident's will. This usually requires hospitalizing the resident in an acute psychiatric unit before obtaining the court order. Residents who have an acute exacerbation of a chronic mental illness (e.g., schizophrenia, bipolar disorder) may require the court-ordered involuntary administration of medication for stabilization. We recommend keeping the psychotropic medications needed to treat behavioral emergencies (on an immediate-use basis) in a contingency box or a behavioral emergency management kit similar to a crash cart for medical emergencies. The as-needed use of antipsychotics and BZs should be restricted to the management of behavioral emergencies. The clinician should closely monitored such use for its effectiveness, the appropriateness of its use by the staff, and adverse effects. We strongly recommend setting a start date and an end date for the use of as-needed psychotropic medication.

OBRA Guidelines for the Use of Psychotropic Medications in the Nursing Home Population

In nursing homes, the use of all psychotropic medications (excluding antidementia drugs, as they are not considered psychotropic medications) requires careful documentation of the targeted behavior as well as any adverse effects from the medications, plus an adjustment of the dosing to the lowest effective dose possible. These dosing adjustments are outlined in the Centers for Medicare and Medicaid Services's *State Operations Manual* for nursing homes. These regulations were first authorized by the Omnibus Budget Reconciliation Act of 1987, which took effect in October 1990 and, as revised and amended, is still in effect.

The specific regulation regarding psychotropic medications, F329, states that the resident has the right to be free from unnecessary drugs. To be considered a necessary drug, the medication must have a supporting diagnosis or reason listed in the medical record, be adequately monitored, be given in an age-appropriate dose and for an appropriate duration, not be duplicative therapy, and be free of significant adverse effects or adverse consequences. If a medication fails to meet any of these conditions (e.g., depressive symptoms have been completely resolved with antidepressant treatment), the prescriber must document that the benefit of continuing the medication outweighs the risk (e.g., a high risk of a relapse of the depression and an increased risk of suicide if the antidepressant dose is reduced or discontinued).

Also, psychotropic medications need to go through a periodic gradual dose reduction, unless this is medically contraindicated. If so, the reason for medical contraindication needs to be documented. The schedule for a gradual dose reduction is as follows: within the first year (either after admission [if the resident is already on psychopharmacologic therapy] or after initiation), taper the dose in two separate quarters, with at least one month between attempts; after the first year, taper annually. Tapering is clinically contraindicated if the resident's target symptoms returned or worsened after the most recent tapering attempt within the facility and the prescriber has documented the clinical rationale. OBRA guidelines specify that a gradual dose reduction should be done at least twice a year after psychotropic therapy has begun, unless the dose has already been reduced to the lowest possible dose that will control the symptoms. Residents undergoing dose reduction should be monitored closely for breakthrough symptoms or withdrawal reactions.

The guideline gives maximal daily doses of many psychotropic drugs for residents with dementia (e.g., the maximal doses of olanzapine are 10 mg/day, of quetiapine are 200 mg/day, of risperidone are 2 mg/day). These figures are not an absolute maximum, but rather indicate which higher levels must be specifically explained. Some other examples of F329 guidelines include the following: the use of drugs for sleep induction is to be for less than 10 consecutive days, unless an attempt at gradual dose reduction is being made and the dose is equal to or less than the dose listed; the (daily) use of benzodiazepines should be for less than four consecutive months unless an attempt at gradual dose reduction is unsuccessful. The OBRA regulations have had an effect on the prescribing of psychotropic medications in U.S. nursing homes, but it is unclear if this has translated into better outcomes for residents (Hughes et al. 2000).

Conclusion

Many serious psychiatric disorders in long-term care populations are amenable to pharmacologic interventions, provided that these interventions are evidence-based and individualized. Pharmacologic interventions that may prevent and treat many behavioral and psychological symptoms in LTC populations involve discontinuing offending, inappropriate, and/or unnecessary drugs and avoiding drug-drug interactions. The risks and benefits of all drugs prescribed for LTC residents should be reviewed collaboratively by the prescriber, the pharmacist, the resident's nurse, the resident, and the family. Appropriate and judicious use of psychotropic drugs has the potential to dramatically improve the quality of life of both many LTC residents with psychiatric disorders and their caregivers. We recommend controlling the use of as-needed medications with education, clear dosing instructions, and monitoring of their use. The prescription of all psychotropic medications in nursing homes should to be in keeping with OBRA regulations.

CHAPTER 13

Psychosocial and Environmental Interventions

As you ought not to attempt to cure the eyes without the head,
or the head without the body, so neither ought you to attempt to
cure the body without the soul . . . For the part will never be well
unless the whole is well.

—*Plato*

Psychosocial and environmental interventions are the primary mode of treatment for behavioral and psychological symptoms in the majority of long-term care populations (Morley 2008). Not only are psychosocial-environmental interventions effective for treating behavioral and psychological symptoms, but pharmacological interventions are associated with significant adverse effects and are often ineffective because they do not address the most common underlying reasons for agitation, such as loneliness and boredom. Even in situations in which pharmacological interventions are the primary mode of treatment (e.g., for schizophrenia, bipolar disorder, behavioral emergencies, severe psychosis, severe depression, or pain), psychosocial interventions are needed to maximize the effects of pharmacological interventions. A systematic algorithm for providing individualized psychosocial-environmental interventions involves searching for the underlying causes of agitation (alternatively labeled *problem behaviors* or *disruptive behaviors*) (Cohen-Mansfield, Libin, and Marx 2007). Multiple factors typically cause agitation, so a combination of interventions may be needed for successful outcomes. Psychosocial-environmental interventions are sometimes termed *nonphar-*

macological interventions or *nondrug interventions*. We prefer the term *psycho-social-environmental interventions*, as it is more person-centered.

Person-Centered Care

Person-centered care is a process where the goal is improving the residents' quality of life (Kitwood 1997). The adoption of person-centered care may prevent many problem behaviors. For example, if a resident is looking for his or her home and this behavior is addressed with efforts to make the resident's room look and feel more like home, such actions may reduce the need for physical or chemical restraints and may provide an effective alternative to psychotropic medication, including antipsychotics (Andrews 2006; Fossey et al. 2006). Psychosocial-environmental interventions implemented in the context of person-centered care, along with ongoing staff training, staff education, and adequate staffing, may not only improve the residents' quality of life, but also improve staff satisfaction, reduce staff turnover, and decrease the necessity of prescribing psychotropic medications. The concept of person-centered care involves several key components (table 13.1).

A person-centered LTC community fosters a culture that supports autonomy, diversity, and individual choice. Leadership and community involvement cultivate relationships among residents, families, support systems, and personnel. The community itself fosters responsiveness, spontaneity, and continuous learning and growth. Residents and staff celebrate the cycles of life and connect to the local community, continuing relationships that nurture the quality of everyday life. In such a community, the residents are the experts regarding life in their home. They participate in decisions about the rhythm of their days, the services provided, and the issues that are important to them. Their families and support systems are welcomed. A person-centered LTC community is a place where the residents want to live, where the staff members want to work, and where both choose to stay. The challenge is to transform the LTC institutional culture of efficiency into a home environment that focuses on the individual.

A person-centered model of care encompasses transformational practices and procedures in three domains: workplace practice, care practice, and the surrounding environment. Strategic changes in these domains assist an LTC facility in moving from a traditional institutional model to a homelike model.

For the residents, their relationship with the staff is the most important measure of quality. The second most important measure is choice: in food, in routine, in decorating one's room. Well-planned activities that create mean-

TABLE 13.1
Components of person-centered care

Knowing the resident
Maintaining the dignity and selfhood of every resident
Recognizing purpose in every resident's life
Facilitating inner exploration
Facilitating spirituality
Facilitating creativity
Facilitating adjustment to a "new home"
Facilitating preserved strengths
Providing a therapeutic physical environment
Facilitating sensitivity to and expression of the residents' cultures
Making the relationship central to all aspects of caregiving
Strengthening existing healthy relationships and facilitating healthy new relationships
Caring for the family caregiver
Caring for the professional caregiver

ing and purpose in the lives of the residents are the next significant measure. Although the residents may need the physical support offered in an LTC facility, they have established their own rhythms of daily life. Person-centered care means that the resident is at home, and the staff—not the residents— have to change their schedule.

Key Factors in Person-Centered Care
Knowing the Resident

The hand that holds the fork that feeds the resident must belong to someone who has a feeling for who that resident is. All of us caring for the residents must remember what we learn about the resident, and our awareness must grow from one encounter to another. One of the ways to start knowing a person is to read a one-page biography (perhaps created by family), written as if the resident wrote it. Another way is to review a life-history book created by the family that chronicles the life of the resident, including passions, travels, achievements, love of life, and many other aspects that reflect the richness and resilience of the resident throughout life and up to this moment. Health care providers should encourage and guide the family in creating such a biographical page or life-history book and take an active role in ensuring that the staff caring for the resident read it, so that they know who the resident is and that he or she is loved. We recommend a facility-wide directive for all staff members (including physicians) to truly know the residents.

Maintaining the Dignity and Selfhood of Every Resident

The "difficult" people in LTC facilities are those who refuse to be diminished! They demand, threaten, and rage until their needs are heeded. Their dignity causes trouble in care systems that are designed for efficiency. Such residents insist on the prickly assertion of self in places where assertiveness is inconvenient. These are the people who will not let the staff forget what makes them different from the others. "You'd better open Martha's drapes the way she likes them or you'll hear about it." Thus Martha's spirit survives in the ways she makes sure her preferences are respected. In the predicament we currently call LTC, outrage remains one of the best ways for people to preserve themselves. The residents express their selfhood in their preferences, in the way they like to arrange things in their rooms, and in the importance they give to wanting a bed near a window so that they can find peace by looking at the sky through the branches of a tree. Everyday actions such as eating when a resident wants to (or is used to) and sleeping when he or she wants to (or is used to) are to be ensured in order to maintain selfhood and give the resident some control over his or her life. By sharing our own lives (e.g., by telling the resident about our spouse and children, our own quirks), by laughing together, we may even help the resident temporarily forget the reality of frailty. We can have a relationship rather than a "clinical encounter" and the staff can have a relationship rather than a "feeding time."

One major problem in achieving this is the impersonal culture of medicine. Caring for the residents in an LTC facility is different from caring for a young adult in an office. Holding the resident's hand, rubbing his or her shoulder or back, or hugging the person, if done with concern and respect, can be immensely healing, yet this is not routinely taught in medical school. Dementia and disability obscure personhood like a mask. When a physician speaks to the person pushing a wheelchair rather than to its occupant, negation occurs. "How is she feeling today?" The one who has been negated can always shout "I'm fine, doctor," thereby declaring her continued status as a person, but the harm has already been done. To be overlooked, to be discounted even for a moment, wounds even after apologies have been extracted or hasty recognition has been won (Lustbader 2000). To have to fight to be seen is what causes the damage.

Recognizing Purpose in Every Resident's Life

Helplessness is the pain one feels when one receives care but is unable to give care (Mitty 2005). Many LTC residents experience this. Finding out what gave a resident purpose in life may relieve that person's loneliness and shed light on the cause of his or her agitation. Mrs. W's purpose in life was to take care of her family (her spouse just after marriage, her children until they were grown, and her spouse since then), so her current behavior of looking for her small children (when she now has grandchildren and great-grandchildren) may be an expression of her need to take care of someone, to be needed, to be useful. Helping the residents find meaningful activities every day is one of the fundamental goals of person-centered care.

Facilitating Inner Exploration

Inner exploration is one of the chief benefits of slowing down in later life (Lustbader 2000). Keeping the residents physically active in their later years is important, but movement inward may prove even more important. Although cognitive impairments make inner exploration difficult for residents, they are nevertheless doing so, and we can facilitate this journey. Many residents faced with long stretches of silence turn inward. When they then express some finding from this inner exploration, person-centered care recognizes and encourages these moments, which happen spontaneously and often out of the blue. Caregivers (professional and family) should respond to such moments with deep awareness that something tender is being shared. Just being with the resident (e.g., squeezing his or her hand to communicate that you heard) during these moments is sufficient. Such moments may also deepen the caregiver's own connection with life.

Facilitating Spirituality

Spirituality refers to meaningful connectedness within oneself, with other people, with the environment, and with the sacred. The Sufis say that two veils separate us from the divine: health and security. When we loose these attributes, we may find ourselves dealing with questions that belong to the spiritual realm. Thus humbling circumstances may enlarge us, in spite of ourselves (Lustbader 2000). For the majority of residents, spirituality has played an important role in their life. Spirituality can be an enormous source of comfort, providing hope, meaning, and purpose (Koenig 1999). It may ward off depression, speed up recovery from depression, and increase one's quality of life. Better mental health, in turn, may increase the motivation for self-care activities and even help the residents view their problems as less disabling.

As we take care of residents, we can help them be in touch with their spirituality. We can share the times when they experience and express spiritual moments, such as their commenting on the sunbeam lighting up a crystal saltshaker in colors and sparkles. Many residents are religious and depend on religion as a major way of coping with health problems and other adversities. They should be given as much opportunity as possible to express their faith and participate in the religious rituals they were practicing before coming to the LTC facility.

The spiritual experiences of those with dementia are often most profound at the end of life. Residents with cognitive impairments need help expressing and then finding these meaningful connections. Rituals, prayers, and sacred liturgy from childhood often stay firmly rooted in memory long after dementia takes its toll. Hence spiritual activities, such as saying prayers for the well-being of other residents or family or even unrelated people (e.g., people suffering in another country), can make the residents feel satisfied that they have reached out beyond themselves to support someone else. Residents may sleep and eat better if they say a prayer before bedtime or grace before a meal. Having a ritual of grieving, such as gathering for prayers when a resident passes away, can also provide spiritual satisfaction. Religious formats may vary over time, so the clinician might consider using an earlier edition of a devotional book or hymnal or asking older relatives what the standards were when they were growing up. People with dementia, or who have suffered a stroke and have been mute for months, have been observed to spontaneously sing the words of a religious hymn or otherwise participate in a religious service. Clergy should design religious services as multisensory experiences that emphasize noncognitive pathways (e.g., visual symbols). A visit from a spiritual counselor may help fill the void left by a resident's inability to attend a familiar place of worship due to frailty.

Spiritual distress may be indicated by the residents' statements, such as "God has forsaken me!" or "Is there life after death?" We recommend that a member of the clergy who is familiar with the resident intervene to address spiritual distress. The LTC facility should offer religious book study (either one-on-one or in a group) for residents who are more cognitively intact. *A Guide to the Spiritual Dimension of Care for People with Alzheimer's Disease and*

Related Dementias: More than Body, Brain, and Breath, by Eileen Shamy, has suggestions for offering spiritual care to people with dementia.

Hope is the subjective sense of having a meaningful future despite obstacles, and the preservation of hope can maximize a person's psychological adjustment to a progressive disability. Clergy can encourage hope despite the future perils of terminal cancer, advancing dementia, or another disability. Hope can address secular matters, such as future plans and relationships, or religious matters, such as one's ultimate destiny (Post and Whitehouse 1999).

Facilitating Creativity

Creativity can be any behavioral or psychological activity that is new and benefits the soul. By this description, creative activities can cover a spectrum, from artistic expression (e.g., painting, writing poetry) and performance (e.g., dancing, music) to daily activities (e.g., dressing, cooking) to problem solving (e.g., a resident with dementia negotiating barriers to going outdoors). For residents with cognitive impairments, creative activities can offer ways to express one's feelings (which may reduce anxiety and depression), experience the joys of using cognitive and motor skills (which may help maintain and even improve cognition, mood, and motor skills), experience delight in solving a problem (which can bolster a sense of mastery, control, and self-esteem), and enhance personal growth. Thus facilitating creative expression, which is already occurring spontaneously almost daily in every resident's life, through structured activities (e.g., group storytelling, painting, song writing) and during the activities of daily living (e.g., during caregiving) is a key component of person-centered care.

Facilitating the Adjustment to a "New Home"

For most individuals moving into an LTC facility, the new room will become their new home. "Being at home" often means an existence that offers possibilities (i.e., choices), whereas "not feeling at home" may reflect an inability to find meaning and connectedness (Hammer 1999). Moving the resident's clothes, a chair, photographs, and other belongings into the room and otherwise making the room ready are activities that should be done before the resident moves into the new home. Many residents may become agitated after the move and try to leave the facility. Such behavior is a normal expression of the loss of one's home and therefore is to be expected. Residents often take two to six weeks to settle into their new home, and a few may take several months. Many residents ask to be taken home. For residents with advanced dementia, this often means their childhood home rather than the home where they were living just before moving to the LTC facility. Many residents may show significant disturbed behavior and disorientation for up to three months after a move. Relocation has the greatest effects on mortality among people with moderate cognitive impairments, which suggests that a certain degree of cognitive awareness is necessary for a negative outcome to occur. For people with dementia, a sudden or unplanned relocation can increase their depressive symptoms and mortality. Conversely, a positive change in their environment, such as a planned relocation from home (and loneliness) to a vibrant LTC facility, can result in improvements in mood, motor function, and even cognition.

Several strategies can ease the new resident's adjustment to LTC. These strategies, however, are guidelines rather than firm recommendations. They may not apply to everyone (e.g., a resident with severe or terminal-stage dementia), and they should be individualized (e.g., using only a few appropriate selections from the strategies).

The person moving into an LTC facility should be as involved as possible in all aspects of moving. If the person has dementia, the possibility of a move should be discussed soon after the diagnosis of dementia is made (e.g., several years before the move needs to occur). He or she should again be told two to three months before the move, with periodic reminders about the reason for the move. We recommend telling a person who does not want to move that it is the physician's recommendation (rather than the family's decision) that he or she move into an LTC facility, due to that person's medical conditions and medical needs.

Have the resident make several visits to the LTC facility before moving to become familiar with the place and the people and even to take part in activities before moving in. People may be encouraged to volunteer at the LTC facility for months to years before moving in. In fact, all of us should try to volunteer in an LTC facility to make helping frail elders a routine part of our lives. This may also help change the part of our culture that tries to deny the existence of frail elders, in order to deny our own future of dependency and frailty.

A high level of social support and the involvement of family and friends is also beneficial. This includes allowing opportunities for the new resident to vent, expressing grief and anger. The involvement of younger children, if done judiciously, may be helpful, as they may be fun and creative and perhaps help the resident cope with the multiple losses involved in moving into an LTC facility. Sometimes, the use of the terms *almost home* or *retirement community*, rather than *nursing home* or *assisted living facility*, is preferable.

The family could bring a one- to two-page life story or a life-history book for the staff to read and get to know the resident better. The family could also bring a list of favorite activities, favorite foods and drinks, favorite topics of conversation, favorite music, favorite movies, favorite family members, favorite animals, spiritual preferences, and cultural preferences. Other very helpful information would be for the family to give the staff a list of the resident's daily routines (sleep time, wake-up time, mealtime, bathing rituals), as well as a list of that person's unique personality characteristics (e.g., likes to be touched, likes to be left alone, easygoing, easy to please, assertive, particular about cleanliness), family role (e.g., has always been the decision maker, a patriarch), and relevant past experiences (e.g., poverty during childhood resulted in the person's being frugal; experiences in World War II resulted in the person's being sensitive to news regarding wars and terrorist attacks).

The family could make a list of the resident's strengths (e.g., can play a musical instrument, can sing, is good at card games) to share with the LTC staff. The family could also make a list of the psychosocial-environmental interventions that they found useful before the resident moved to the LTC facility (e.g., responds well to humor, is easily distracted by favorite music, does better if left alone and reapproached later, calms down easily after talking to a particular family member), in addition to a list of the resident's common triggers for agitation (e.g., dislikes someone telling him or her what to do or not to do instead of offering options, likes bed sheets and other things in the room arranged in a particular manner).

To help create a homelike environment, a room filled with memorabilia, personal furnishings, pictures, and perfume or other scents that person is familiar with are helpful. The facility may offer a welcome gift or welcome bag for a new resident from the residents already living at the facility. This may help the new resident feel accepted and more comfortable in a strange place.

Prior experience in an adult day center often helps persons with dementia emotionally make the transition from the community to an institutional residence. It may also reduce the cognitive decline seen in many residents soon after admission to an LTC facility (Wilson et al. 2007), which may reflect difficulty in adapting to an unfamiliar environment. Adult day programs also help the family become accustomed to the idea of their loved one's admission to LTC. Ideally, the adult day program should be in the LTC facility into which the person with dementia is moving.

The family could request staff from the Alzheimer's Association to attend one or two family meetings to offer suggestions and resources (e.g., books, pamphlets, videos from the association's own library) to ease the transition. Such meetings should be held weeks to months before the transition date. Family members could also consider seeking professional help from the local Alzheimer center and from memory clinics for individual therapy for the resident, family therapy, and, if necessary, medications (e.g., antidepressants, as-needed benzodiazepines for a few days around the transition period) to emotionally prepare both the new resident and the caregivers for the stress involved in the transition and to reduce the anxiety, depression, and agitation surrounding issues of moving into an LTC facility.

We recommend that the family spend a lot of time with the person in the first few days to weeks after admission, so that he or she does not feel abandoned. Family members can gradually reduce their visits as the person becomes adjusted. The family should try to continue as many family rituals and activities as possible after the transition, albeit with necessary modifications (e.g., smaller and shorter gatherings during birthdays, celebrating at the facility rather than at a family member's home).

Family members themselves may benefit from attending support groups and learning creative tips from other family caregivers who have "been there, done that." Alternatively, the staff at the LTC facility may ask other residents' family members to talk to and help the new resident's family cope with this difficult time. Family and staff members need to have patience, as it usually takes several weeks for a new resident to adjust to a new living situation. Transition to an LTC facility is hard on almost everyone. It is important to recognize and accept that this stress is normal and to avoid denial or attempts to fix the stress with drugs. Family members need to realize that they are not alone, and that many other residents and families have also experienced difficulty transitioning. Last, but not least, family members need to tap into the power of humor and spirituality to help themselves and the resident negotiate this difficult time.

Facilitating Preserved Strengths

Each resident has a unique repertoire of strengths that help him or her cope with challenges and enjoy the good things life offers. Our current care culture focuses too much on the problems and too little on the assessment and preservation of existing strengths and skills. Person-centered care seeks to correct this imbalance. Skill-appropriate activities facilitate engagement, maintain skills, and enhance the enjoyment a resident can gain from them (Manepalli, Desai, and Sharma 2009). Helping to preserve strengths may also be considered restorative care that focuses on helping the residents do, rather than doing for them, as well as abilities-centered care that focuses on maintaining and strengthening the residents' specific abilities during daily personal care.

Providing a Therapeutic Physical Environment

The design of an LTC facility can have a tremendous impact on the residents' physical and psychosocial well-being, especially for residents with dementia (Day, Carreon, and Stump 2000; Zeisel et al. 2003). Therapeutic design may also reduce the residents' aggressive behaviors toward others. For example, overcrowding and the frequent intrusion of others in one's personal space is a risk factor for physical aggression, so increased personal space and private rooms may reduce the risk of aggressive behavior (Rueve and Welton 2008). An LTC facility should be a place that supports healthy aging, active engagement in life, spirituality, and the peaceful last years of a resident's life.

A recent trend is to diverge from the traditional medical model (large facilities with a focus on providing medical care) to a social model (small, homelike environments with terraces, landscaping, windows that make the outdoor relevant). Such social models involve well-designed facilities (e.g., large facilities housing two or more "neighborhoods" [each neighborhood having two to four houses and each house having 10–12 residents], as well as small-scale homes caring for 9–10 people with dementia) that not only are esthetically pleasing, but also may be spiritually uplifting (e.g., more contact with nature) and give the residents reasons to get out of bed and socialize, enjoy the outdoors, or just wander safely. Across the country, many small LTC facilities (e.g., Corrine Dolan Center near Cleveland, Ohio, and the Dolan Centers in St. Louis, Missouri) as well as large LTC facilities (e.g., Brewster Village in Appleton, Wisconsin; Evergreen Retirement Community in Oshkosh, Wisconsin) have adopted a social model in their design.

Table 13.2 lists some examples of environmental designs for an LTC facility that may promote the physical, cognitive, emotional, and spiritual well-being of the residents. Well-designed facilities may also reduce the prevalence of depression and agitation in residents, reduce the need for psychotropic medications, reduce family caregiver stress, and reduce staff burden (e.g., reduce

TABLE 13.2
Examples of environmental designs that may help or hinder the overall well-being of long-term care residents

Designs that may help well-being
Small, homelike environment
Adequate personal space
All rooms private, not shared
Large windows or skylights that allow plenty of natural light to come in and offer beautiful views of nature outside
Indoor (continuous, well-defined) pathways and secure outdoor walking paths and a sheltered garden to encourage the enjoyment of nature outdoors, casual strolling, and exercise in a safe environment
Therapeutic garden with nontoxic plants for horticulture programming
Craft studio
Privacy room where residents can go when they want to meditate, spend time alone, or be sexually intimate with a spouse or other loved one
Family room with a fireplace where residents can spend time with family or have family functions and holiday celebrations
A room for staff to "chill," which may have a treadmill, soothing music, comfortable chairs, and the like to help the staff "de-stress"
Fitness center and temperature-controlled indoor and/or outdoor swimming pool (especially in large LTC facilities) with wheelchair ramps and walking rails
Dutch doors for each bedroom (closed doors may agitate residents with dementia; and with the top half open, the closed bottom prevents wanderers from meddling in someone else's room)
A toilet situated in view of the bed so that the resident has fewer incidents of incontinence or of toileting in inappropriate places
Traditional nurses' station replaced by nourishment centers that provide opportunities for social interaction in addition to the enjoyment of ice cream or other delicious food or beverage items
Photos, shadow boxes, or curio cueing cabinets outside resident bedrooms, holding meaningful mementos to trigger long-term memories and help the resident identify his or her room
Glass-sided refrigerator door showing residents the food (residents are free to open the refrigerator and eat the food inside)
Food prepared in the facility kitchen and served restaurant style, with second helpings encouraged
Designs that may hinder well-being
Long corridors
Food delivered on trays
Glare from lighting or insufficient lighting
Limited amounts of natural light
Dark-colored floors or parts of the floor (which may be mistaken for a hole by a resident with a cognitive impairment)
Glass walls, which residents may inadvertently walk into
Audible intercoms, which may be distracting and cause irritability

the incidence of cleaning residents who soiled their clothes by having a toilet the resident is able to see from the bed, encouraging that person to toilet in an appropriate place).

Unless a facility is not-for-profit and accepts a portion of its residents based on financial need, the only option for someone receiving Medicaid is a nursing home. Some states are creating small, homelike assisted living facilities (e.g., community-based residential facilities in the state of Wisconsin) as less-costly alternatives to nursing homes for older adults with dementia who have limited financial resources. Most assisted living facilities that have adopted the social model do not have medical services on site (e.g., a physician and/ or a physician extender coming to the facility to provide medical care, the round-the-clock presence of a registered nurse, supervision or administration of medications by a nurse). Many large LTC facilities (including nursing homes) have begun modifying their architecture to adopt the social model. We recommend a hybrid: LTC facilities based on a social model which also incorporates the positive aspects of the traditional medical model, such as the availability of high-quality medical, psychiatric, and nursing care on site.

Technological solutions to enhance and maintain the residents' independence and freedom are being studied, and in the future such solutions may become affordable and a routine part of living in an LTC facility. For example, if a resident gets out of bed in the middle of the night, a light would turn on; if a resident is detected exiting through a main door at an inappropriate time, a prompt would encourage him or her to go back; should the resident continue to exit, the staff are alerted.

Proper lighting in LTC facilities is important, especially in areas such as hallways and bathrooms, where the residents are at increased risk of falls, and during cloudy days, at dusk, and after dark. For LTC residents, appropriate lighting should be considered a primary line of prevention against depression, sleep disorders, a loss of independence, and falls (Noell-Waggoner 2004; Riemersma-van der Lek et al. 2008). Light levels should be increased without creating glare. In addition, all lighting fixtures, with the exception of those in day-use-only activity spaces, should be able to be dimmed to evenly lower the overall lighting during the evening and nighttime hours.

The integration of cognitively intact and cognitively impaired residents may result in worsened agitation for the residents with dementia as well as irritation for the residents whose cognition is intact. A separate LTC facility, or a specific unit or wing within a facility solely for people with dementia, may help address this problem. Such a specialized facility may help the residents function better in ADLs, decrease their anxiety/fear, and increase their interest in activities, because there would be a high likelihood that the facility's staff is better trained in understanding dementia and in caring for residents with dementia. Such a facility may also have adopted therapeutic environmental designs. Decorating some areas with scenes of nature or home life, including recorded sounds and smells, has been associated both with the residents spending more time in these areas and with an increase in their level of pleasure. Using contrasting colors and textures on the walls, doors, and furniture, as well as signs on the doors, may help the residents be more independent.

Facilitating Sensitivity to and an Expression of Residents' Cultures

As our communities become more diversified, so too will our LTC resident populations. In large metropolitan areas, this has already started to happen. Respecting the beliefs and traditions of the residents and the staff (who often are from a different culture) is a fundamental component of person-centered care. Some beliefs may provide emotional relief in dealing with incurable and progressive conditions such as dementia. For example, many Asian cultures accept many hardships of life, including dementia, as destiny and do not resist or fight, whereas Western culture often reacts initially (and frequently in later stages) with resistance and a wish to fight the condition. The Japanese martial art aikido teaches us to go with the force that threatens us, rather than oppose it. Without resistance, there can be no collision. Instead, there is fluid motion, more like rushing water than the intransigence of stone (Lustbader 2000). This philosophy can apply to dealing with dementia, especially by family caregivers and by interested residents with mild dementia.

Making the Relationship Central to All Aspects of Caregiving

As we come to know a resident and develop a bond over time, a unique relationship often follows, giving purpose to both our lives. Once we take the trouble to know a resident, at some level that resident begins to feel seen, heard, valued, and respected. In the course of such an interaction, positive things can happen. A person who has not spoken for a long time may blurt out "I love you" or "Thank you." A caregiver may come to realize that he or she is receiving as much of a blessing as being the person who is giving one. These brief moments of intimacy may make both the resident and the caregiver less fearful of the future.

Strengthening Existing Healthy Relationships and Facilitating Healthy New Relationships

It is important for the residents to connect in a meaningful way with other residents and with caregivers besides the family. A compassionate, nurturing, and loving relationship can protect the residents from the stress of their declining health and functional abilities. Facilitating relationships may not only prevent emotional distress due to loneliness, but it can also help calm a resident who is agitated. Unexpected embraces, uncharacteristic expressions of feeling—these are some of the many ways that relationships can grow despite the demands of dementia and frailty. To accept help, to depend, and to embrace attention may satisfy yearnings long suppressed. When the loved one's plight is relieved even for a brief moment, both the giver and the receiver learn a lesson in hope.

Facilitating intergenerational connections is also important. The presence of children often brings a smile, a laugh, or a caress. Even residents with advanced dementia who are usually silent may initiate a conversation in the presence of children. Families with small children are encouraged to visit their loved ones in an LTC facility with these children, who can color with the resident (or the children can color on their own), play with toys, watch television (cartoons, educational programs) or movies with the resident, or just bring some laughter and joyfulness by their playful presence. Sharing stories and activities with children from a local school may also help. The children do not have to interact with the resident (especially if that person has advanced dementia and has lost the ability to converse); their mere presence in the room may be sufficient to provide the sense of peace that comes from knowing that loved ones are around. Facilitating visitors and companionship may also enhance the residents' quality of life in unexpected ways. Most residents love having visitors. Indeed, any visitor generates excitement among the residents. Even when residents have lost the ability to comprehend speech and express themselves, they can still savor the physical presence of someone who sits and listens to their incoherent speech, makes eye contact, and responds with facial gestures or a touch.

Facilitating a sense of being a part of the greater community is an integral part of person-centered care. Attending a concert at a local theater, going fishing with friends or family, participating in a community service project, going to local museums, or playing with local children through an intergenerational program can be fun and can give the residents a sense of being part of the greater community.

Relationship-building care involves the following:

- securing a network of the residents' families and friends to participate in enhancing the residents' quality of life
- facilitating relationships between residents
- facilitating relationships between the residents and their health care providers
- facilitating relationships between the residents and the staff

- helping the residents cope with relationships that are unhealthy (e.g., frequently hostile, overinvolved, critical, and/or insensitive interactions)
- if necessary, protecting a resident from obviously harmful relationships (e.g., abusive relationships [physically, sexually, verbally, emotionally, financially])

CLINICAL CASE Mr. T, an LTC resident for 12 months, became increasingly depressed because his wife had reduced the frequency of her visits to once a week and would visit for only a few minutes. His wife reported that visiting him was depressing, as he was not the active and intelligent person she married. Over time, Mr. T lost weight and stopped going to group activity programs he previously attended. The physician was about to prescribe an antidepressant when Mr. T's mood began to improve. He started eating better, started taking part in activities, and seemed to be happy. This was because Mr. T had developed a friendship with a female resident and they would spend several hours together, watching television or sharing stories. When asked what Mr. T liked about this new friend, he replied, "I like the way she laughs."

TEACHING POINTS This case illustrates the power of friendship, attachment, and intimacy in healing emotional pain. It also illustrates the resiliency of Mr. T (and many other residents) in the face of adversity.

Caring for the Family Caregiver

Enhancing the family caregiver's health is as important as improving a resident's psychosocial well-being, and it is an integral part of person-centered care. The transition to institutional care is particularly difficult for spouses, almost half of whom visit the resident daily and continue to provide help with physical care during their visits (Schulz et al. 2004). We recommend interventions to prepare the caregivers for the transition and to treat their depression and anxiety following the admission of a loved one to LTC. Such interventions can include efforts by staff members to improve the quality of family members' visits, support groups within the facility, individual counseling (including stress-management techniques [e.g., mindfulness-based stress reduction, relaxation training, breathing exercises]; addressing grief, loss, guilt, and resentment; coping strategies), encouragement to caregivers to build a social support network, encouragement to caregivers keep their own physical and mental health a priority (regular visits to their primary care pro-

vider, regular exercise and healthy diet, etc.), and, in some cases, psychotropic agents to treat severe anxiety and depression (Selwood et al. 2007). When
staff members become more involved with the residents' families and help
make their visits more meaningful, the families feel more satisfied with the
visits (Volicer et al. 2008).

Spouses often have difficulty asking for help from their children because of
concerns that they are a burden to their children. Counseling spouses regarding the benefits of asking for help from one's children (e.g., reduced stress and
improved physical health of the caregiving spouse, which in turn will help
the spouse meet the needs of the resident better and for a longer time) may
help not only the resident and the caregiving spouse, but also the children,
who are often struggling with how best to help both parents. Counseling family caregivers can also help address the caregivers' conflicts with siblings or
stepchildren, their frustrations with feeling unappreciated, and their confusion over ambivalent feelings, as well as optimizing the caregivers' attitudes
and helping them deal positively with inherent sacrifices. Counseling for the
family and the resident by a health care provider, several months before the
resident's move into an LTC facility, may prevent caregiver depression and
ease the resident's transition into his or her new home. The resident's children may also benefit from these interventions, although psychological issues
experienced by children are somewhat different from those experienced by
spouses. Caregivers need to be informed that research has shown that caregiving may have important positive effects: a new sense of purpose or meaning in life, fulfillment of a lifelong commitment to a spouse, an opportunity
to give back to a parent some of what the parent has given to them, renewal
of religious faith, and closer ties with people through new relationships or
stronger existing relationships (Sorrell 2007).

Many family caregivers stop visiting their loved one, or only visit for a short
time, because they feel that the dementia is so advanced (e.g., the loved one
cannot recognize the family member) that it makes no difference whether
they visit or not. Some family members (especially some children and, less often, some spouses) may not visit because it is too painful for them to see their
loved one in such a diminished state. Health care providers can play a crucial
role in counseling families that all visits have meaning for the resident (even
one in the advanced stages of dementia) in ways that may not be obvious, as
well as in addressing their grief so that visits can continue and future feelings
of guilt can be prevented.

Health care providers need to address not only the physical and emotional losses experienced by the family caregiver, but also the sheer physical fatigue resulting from grief and caregiving. Grieving while caregiving is hard work, is tiring, and drains the caregiver's vitality. Ira J. Tanner, in his book *Healing the Pain of Everyday Loss*, offers helpful advice: loss is natural to life; people and objects do not have permanence, feelings of grief are normal, grief offers opportunities to help establish or reestablish values and goals. Spouses of residents may be referred to the Well Spouse Association (www.wellspouse .org), a national nonprofit organization that offers support to people caring for husbands, wives, and partners with various forms of chronic disability, including dementia. If possible, LTC facilities should offer support groups for family caregivers. Support groups can provide social support, a place to share and learn creative ways of coping with the loved one's illness and behavior and to express one's grief and frustration. Spirituality is equally important for caregivers, as a way to cope with the immense stress of seeing their loved one decline due to dementia or another terminal illness.

Families are increasingly multigenerational and dispersed, and many residents' significant others may not be blood relations but can still be considered family. Many families find it difficult to understand complex and abstract information in today's fast-paced world and fear making a wrong decision. Many children may not understand their parents (who are residents) in the context of their parents' culture. The traditional generation gap has been widened by the technology gap. In addition, many adult children do not understand their parents' need to mourn what has been lost to them and to reminisce. Convening family meetings to address these issues may improve not only the emotional well-being of the family members, but also the quality and frequency of interactions between the family members and the resident. The latter, in turn, can have a positive impact on the resident's psychosocial well-being.

Often, the seeds of dissension between siblings were sown when they were children. Health care providers can help adult children focus on the resident's well-being by encouraging them to help each other in a polite manner and to avoid trying to resolve long-standing differences. The clinician should encourage family members to keep any criticism of each other to a minimum while in the presence of the resident. "I want to go home" is one of the most common complaints of residents in an LTC facility. Family members often may be split in their opinions regarding this issue and may give mixed messages to the resident, further worsening the resident's emotional distress. Deciding whether a loved one should be taken home after rehabilitation versus staying in the nursing home can be facilitated by input from all team members. A realistic appraisal of the resident's needs and coming to a compromise that would best meet the resident's needs in the long run is essential. Avoiding short-term fixes is vital, despite the strong emotions and wishes of the resident and some family members. The clinician should encourage families to approach the resident together when informing him or her that the family has agreed that the resident needs to stay in the LTC facility on the physician's recommendations (instead of having one family member become the "bad guy").

Health care providers can also recommend that the siblings not expect other siblings to view the parent as they do, as the experiences and relationship of each child with his or her parents are unique and influenced by a multitude of factors that are different in each relationship (e.g., birth order, stressful events during birth and later, etc.). The primary sibling caregiver should keep other siblings up to date on the loved one's condition. Other siblings should provide support and frequent verbal and nonverbal appreciation, and minimize any criticism or demands, in order to enhance the primary caregiver's emotional well-being and reduce that person's stress. Each sibling should evaluate what he or she can reasonably and honestly do to help the loved one who is living in an LTC facility.

> **CLINICAL CASE** Mr. L, the 90-year-old husband of Mrs. L, an 85-year-old woman with advanced dementia, commented during an interview with her psychiatrist that "my wife is there, but she isn't there. She needs a wheelchair now and her speech is largely gone. She recognizes me by face at times but calls me 'Dad' when she says a few words that I can make sense of. She is starting to be combative. This is so unlike her. I find myself getting angry even though I know that it's her disease that makes her behave so. Then I get depressed." The psychiatrist treating Mrs. L provided emotional support to Mr. L and suggested that Mr. L see a social worker who specialized in helping spouses adjust to dementia in their loved one and to their loved one's admission to an LTC facility. Mr. L was reluctant, but he agreed after his daughter promised to accompany him during the first visit to the social worker. After several weekly meetings with the social worker, Mr. L gradually felt less guilty, was able to express his grief and loss, and learned ways to make his visits with his wife meaningful and even fun at times. Mr. L also started attending spousal support groups run by the local chapter of the Alzheimer's Association. Mr. L resumed his

regular exercise program at a health club after the psychiatrist indicated to Mr. L that if he keeps himself healthy, the treatment team could focus better on improving Mrs. L's emotional well-being. Mr. L also became more mindful of the little gifts from his wife, such as her breaking into a big smile when she would see him approach.

TEACHING POINTS Addressing family caregiver grief and stress is an integral part of addressing the emotional well-being of LTC residents.

Caring for the Professional Caregiver

A professional caregiver who has not been adequately trained (in person-centered care, in psychosocial-environmental interventions, and in understanding dementia and the behavioral disturbances associated with dementia), or has not been given adequate resources (e.g., adequate staffing) and emotional support and appreciation, cannot be expected to manage challenging and complex behavioral problems in a systematic, calm, and evidence-based manner. In fact, caregiver stress can often lead to untherapeutic or countertherapeutic approaches and, not uncommonly, even verbal and/or physical abuse or neglect. Growing research calls for LTC facilities to make every effort to find managers (e.g., administrators, directors of nursing, supervisors) who know that the well-being of the resident is inseparable from the welfare of the professional caregivers and that professional caregivers' needs transcend mere bread-and-butter considerations. Such managers fashion a workplace that recognizes the individual persons behind their roles on the front-line staff (e.g., CNAs, nurses), challenges and supports them, and helps them achieve, grow in, and enjoy their work. The engagement of the front-line staff deepens when managers care about them as people, appreciate their work, evaluate them fairly, and communicate with them on important matters. In fact, managers play a critical role in the satisfaction, loyalty, and commitment of staff (Tellis-Nayak 2007). The front-line staff members usually perceive of their managers as exerting a pervasive influence in their work lives.

Another important area for managers to address is workplace safety. Staff members (especially CNAs, but also nurses and other staff) are frequently pushed, grabbed, or shoved by a resident or are verbally abused. Staff members are often asked to handle residents (e.g., transfers, lifting) with inadequate assist devices, putting them at risk of serious injury and even persisting disabilities.

Caring for the professional caregiver is a key component of person-centered care. The first step in caring for professional caregivers is providing high-quality education and training so that they can not only deliver high-quality care, but also enjoy their work and feel proud of their contributions to the well-being of the residents and their families. Caring for professional caregivers may also involve having a "room to chill" for the staff (see table 13.2). In addition, caring for professional caregivers involves helping them mature; maintaining their motivation to care for frail and vulnerable but challenging LTC populations; helping them be mindful that for some residents, the professional caregivers may be the only people the residents have a chance to touch and to engage with in conversation; helping them adjust to the realities of working in an LTC facility (e.g., limited resources); helping them balance their personal and professional lives; encouraging them to have a self-care plan (physical, emotional, and spiritual); and helping them find and cultivate hidden strengths and successes. Offering on-site services for professional caregivers—such as yoga, mindfulness-based stress reduction, breathing and other relaxation-training exercises, tai chi, day care for their children, healthy and delicious food and drink from an in-house café, and other amenities—goes a long way in improving professional caregivers' well-being.

Models for Understanding the Behaviors of Residents with Dementia

Various models have been described to help understand the meaning and causes of the behaviors of LTC residents with dementia. Training caregivers (family and professional) regarding these models can improve the residents' quality of life and may reduce the caregivers' stress and improve their confidence in dealing with the behaviors (Volicer and Hurley 2003).

The Need-Driven, Dementia-Compromised Behavior Model

The need-driven, dementia-compromised behavior model views behaviors as stemming from a need or goal of the individual with dementia. This model recognizes that it is difficult to influence background factors (e.g., the pathological processes causing dementia), but proximal factors (e.g., assistance with performing ADLs) are more amenable to modification. These modifications are then customized according to individual needs and goals. This model is used by recreational therapists.

The Progressively Lowered Stress Threshold Model

The progressively lowered stress threshold model is based on the assumption that one's stress threshold is progressively lowered with the progression of dementia and that behaviors are thus response to stress (Smith et al. 2004). This model identifies five stressors: fatigue; a change in environment, routine, or caregiver; misleading stimuli or an inappropriate stimulus level (over- or understimulation); demands that exceed the person's functional ability; and physical stressors (pain, discomfort, acute illness, depression, psychotic symptoms). For example, a resident may be agitated because he or she is tired, and a short nap may be what is needed. Or the resident is stressed and anxious before a dental procedure and may be less resistive during the procedure if he or she has had a period of relaxation (with soothing music, hand massage with a lotion) before the procedure.

The Antecedent-Behavior-Consequence Model

The antecedent-behavior-consequence model instructs caregivers to identify the antecedents of a specific behavior as well as to clearly define the behavior's consequences. For example, a male resident with dementia is sitting in one corner and there is an activity group in another corner involving a group of female residents. The male resident becomes agitated and restless and, after some time, starts masturbating. A staff member reprimands the male resident for inappropriate behavior and the resident starts crying and becomes more agitated. Here the antecedent could be boredom and a wish to join the group, the behavior is masturbation, and the consequence is being reprimanded, resulting in more behavioral disturbances. By altering the antecedent (a staff member gently approaches the male resident when he begins to grow agitated and restless and involves him in the group activity), the behavior is changed (no masturbation), and the consequence is changed (the resident is calm and happy in the group instead of agitated and tearful).

For most residents with advanced dementia, a behavioral plan may not be appropriate, due to their inability to recall the antecedents (i.e., the positively reinforcing events). For residents whose cognition is intact and for residents with mental retardation (or low borderline intelligence) but no dementia, the antecedent-behavior-consequence approach may help some specific behavioral problems. Examples of situations in which the antecedent-behavior-consequence approach (including a written outline of a behavioral agreement [behavioral contracting]) may be beneficial include issues surrounding cigarette smoking, the need for water restrictions for polydipsic residents, residents frequently making financial requests to staff members, and the necessity of rationing soda or candy for residents who dwell on the availability of these items.

The Habilitation Approach

The habilitation approach aims at maximizing the functional independence and morale of residents with dementia, a stroke, or another disabling condition. It is a caregiver-controlled environmental therapy that addresses six domains in which positive emotions can be created and maintained: physical environment (e.g., providing limited choices of clothing to facilitate dressing); communication (increasing the use of body language, a calm soothing voice, eye contact, pictures); functional assistance (prompting to void, to snack); social (e.g., encouraging a resident who can read to read aloud to others); perceptual (e.g., putting a large stop sign on the door); and behavioral (changing the caregiver's behavior or approach, or approaching the resident later for the same task). This approach eliminates attempts at reasoning and replaces the word "No" with distraction and the elimination of triggering events.

The Psychosocial-Environmental Model

The psychosocial-environmental model postulates that, for each resident with behavioral or psychological symptoms, modifiable and unmodifiable biological (includes medical causes and dementia-related neurochemical changes), psychosocial (includes spiritual and cultural issues), and environmental factors are predisposing, precipitating, and perpetuating the symptoms, as well as being factors that are protecting the resident from symptoms. Evaluating each resident with behavioral and psychological symptoms for modifiable factors and intervening appropriately and comprehensively improves the success rates of managing the symptoms.

Research has highlighted a whole array of psychosocial-environmental approaches and strategies that, if applied appropriately (e.g., in an individualized, systematic fashion in the context of person-centered care), have the potential not only to improve behavioral and psychological symptoms, but also to dramatically improve every resident's quality of life. To help residents with behavioral disturbances, caregivers must try to understand the meaning implied by the behavior (Norberg 1996). For example, a resident with advanced dementia who starts disrobing during an activity program may be feeling hot rather than acting in a sexually inappropriate manner. If health care providers overcome the barriers associated with cognitive impairment, and if they decipher the subtle messages in the resident's actions, they may be able to realize that much of what is considered challenging behavior is not meaningless, unpredictable, and manageable only with psychotropic medications and/or restraints.

The residents' psychosocial needs include the needs for unconditional love, comfort, trust and attachment, safety, autonomy and control, initiative and inclusion, pleasure, industry and occupation, a meaningful social role and identity, intimacy, legacy and generativity, and integrity (wholeness and meaning). Often most of these needs are not adequately met. We recommend that caregivers learn to replace the words "difficult behavior" with words that indicate some understanding of the meaning of that behavior. For example, instead of saying that the resident "resisted personal care," say that the resident "seemed anxious and did not allow me to clean her properly." In addition, continuous activity programming can provide several opportunities throughout the day for the residents to participate in meaningful activities. A facility can institute continuous activity programming without staffing changes, but the benefit is increased if additional staffing is available (Volicer et al. 2006).

Table 13.3 lists some basic Dos and Don'ts of interacting with an agitated resident.

Boredom and loneliness are pervasive in the lives of LTC residents, and they manifest as excessive time spent sleeping during the day, down time, and times when the residents are not actively engaged in meaningful activity (Ballard et al. 2001). Boredom and loneliness have a tremendous negative impact on the residents' quality of life. The first step in bringing back fun and joy for LTC residents is to correct the negative attitude that pervades our society—even among health care providers—that life in an LTC facility

TABLE 13.3
Dos and Don'ts for interactions with an agitated resident

Do—take the resident's complaints seriously

Do—empathize, sympathize, and be compassionate and understanding

Do—try to redirect or change the subject if the resident believes you are trying to harm or hurt him or her

Do—allow the resident to vent

Do—show patience

Do—let go of any negative or accusatory statement that the resident makes to you

Do—say "I'm sorry that you are feeling this way"

Don't—argue or try to "make the resident understand"

Don't—ignore the resident's complaints

Don't—try to defend yourself

Don't—overreact to any false claim the resident makes against you is merely a lamentable stage of life and that boredom and loneliness are an inevitable last stage of life. Person-centered care, along with a variety of specific psychosocial-environmental interventions and innovative programs, are needed to optimally address boredom and loneliness for all residents (table 13.4). Although not all residents respond to these interventions, and their effects may be short lived, for many residents these interventions not only provide relief from suffering, but also avoid the use of psychotropic medication and prevent complications, such as an escalation from agitation to physical aggression. These interventions may also improve the milieu for other residents by calming the agitated resident.

Caregiver-Oriented Strategies

Caregiver-oriented strategies are some of the most important psychosocial-environmental strategies to improve the psychosocial well-being of LTC residents (Livingston et al. 2005). The success of any psychosocial-environmental intervention relies on the quality of caregiving. A resident's behavior (e.g., pacing, wandering) is often disturbing to the caregivers (professional and family) but not to that resident. In such cases, the treatment of these behaviors involves educating caregivers rather than treating the resident. In fact,

TABLE 13.4
Key psychosocial-environmental strategies that may help reduce behavioral and psychological symptoms in long-term care residents

Caregiver-oriented strategies
    Changes in the way the family interacts with the resident
    Changes in the way the staff interacts with the resident
    Improvement in staff-family relationships
    Enhancement of communication skills

Resident-oriented strategies
    Meaningful structured (e.g., bingo) and unstructured activities (e.g., folding napkins)
    One-on-one strategies
    Massage and other approaches involving therapeutic touch
    Exercise or another physical activity
    Music
    Nutrition
    Humor
    Simulated presence therapy
    Bright light therapy
    Animal-assisted therapy (Pet therapy)
    High-tech interventions
    Cognitive rehabilitation
    Individual psychotherapy
    Reminiscence therapy
    Aromatherapy
    Validation therapy
    Dance or movement therapy

educating and training caregivers so that they can change their approach with a resident who has behavioral disturbances is one of the key caregiver-oriented psychosocial-environmental interventions to treat LTC residents' agitation. Also, a caregiver's stress can, at times, result in an inappropriate interaction with a resident, which in turn may cause behavioral disturbances in that resident. Addressing caregiver stress may thus prevent or decrease the residents' agitation. Last, but not least, a caregiver's emotional distress (sadness, anger, anxiety) may spill over to the resident, in turn causing the resident to become emotionally distressed. Residents (especially those with cognitive impairments) may misinterpret the caregiver's emotional distress as having something to do with them and therefore react with agitation.

Educating Family Members

Family caregivers may unwittingly act as precipitating and/or perpetuating factors in behavioral disturbances by their loved ones when they visit them in an LTC facility (Lawlor 1996). Family caregiver distress and poor interpersonal interactions between the resident and the family caregiver(s) can exacerbate depression and anxiety. For example, when one or more family members place excessive demands on the resident, catastrophic reactions may occur. When the resident and the family caregiver have had a poor premorbid relationship, the caregiver may misinterpret agitated behavior as being purposefully provocative and thus worsen the situation with an angry reaction. Because of burden-induced intolerance, caregivers often underestimate the resident's functional abilities, which can contribute to or aggravate behavioral disturbances. Furthermore, family members under stress may perceive behavioral disturbances when they are not present or describe depression in a resident when they themselves are the ones who are depressed.

Educating the family about dementia, the importance of not arguing, and other supportive interactions should be a routine psychosocial-environmental intervention for all family members. Health care providers should also make efforts to improve the quality of visits by family members, because visiting provides LTC residents with a link to their families and communities and promotes the residents' quality of life. This improvement can be made by educating the family regarding factors that may agitate the resident (e.g., directing too many questions to a cognitively impaired resident), helping them decide the best times to visit the resident, and offering specific suggestions (e.g., walking with the resident for five to ten minutes, arranging flowers together, reminiscing, listening to music together, reading a chapter of a religious book to the resident). The family needs to understand that the resident's behavioral and psychological symptoms are often part of dementia or a stroke, and this does not mean that the resident's feelings toward the family member(s) have changed. Involving the resident in activities can be enhanced by the family's involvement in their care and by staff encouragement.

Educating and Training Staff Members

Staff training programs and environmental modifications appear to be the most effective strategies for managing aggressive behavior (Landreville et al. 2006). Interactive training has been demonstrated to be an effective approach to shaping more appropriate staff reactions to aggressive resident behavior. This training can be delivered effectively on the Internet, where it is led by health care providers with geriatric expertise (Irvine et al. 2007). Staff and physician education regarding psychosocial-environmental interventions and the risks of pharmacological interventions (especially antipsychotics) and restraints has been found to dramatically reduce the use of antipsychotic medications and restraints without worsening behaviors (Avorn et al. 1992; Ray et al. 1993; Doody et al. 2001).

The staff needs to be taught that tasks are secondary to relationships, and supervisors should be trained to not supervise the staff in a regimented manner that precludes the staff responsiveness that every resident needs. Staff members who provide personal care need to be given more power and a greater say in decision making and to be seen as doing the most valuable work in the facility. The staff need to be taught that their relationship with the residents is the hub of life in an LTC facility. Staff members should be rewarded for spontaneous, innovative approaches (e.g., a new staff member who decides to read a resident's favorite poem aloud to lessen that resident's unease with the staff member and even to help transport that resident beyond his or her cognitive and physical diminishment).

Whether caregivers are skilled at coping with behavioral disturbances can affect the quality of care a resident receives. The staff should be trained in person-centered care to improve their knowledge of and skill in caring for residents with dementia, their knowledge of and skill in meeting the psychosocial needs of residents who need psychosocial-environmental and pharmacological interventions, and their knowledge of and skill in mentoring other staff members. Many local chapters of the Alzheimer's Association (e.g., the Education Institute at the St. Louis Chapter of the Alzheimer's Association) have affordable programs that provide excellent staff education and training in all of these areas. Residents in LTC facilities in which the staff receive intensive training to understand and manage behaviors experience fewer behavioral symptoms related to dementia. Such person-centered care and intensive training may also reduce staff turnover and increase the staff's satisfaction with their jobs.

Staff training should involve direct, systematic clinical supervision and supervised implementation of individually planned care. Such training can lead to a more positive perception of the residents, less burnout, increased creativity, increased job satisfaction, and improved resident-caregiver interactions (Hallberg et al. 1995). Staff training should include the understanding that although there is a significant neurochemical basis for many behavioral disturbances, this does not mean that there was not a previous experience behind the behavior or that the behavior cannot be affected by human interaction (Kirby and Lawlor 1995). Kihlgren et al. (1992) encouraged caregivers to promote an integrative experience (wholeness and meaning) during all care activities for patients with moderate or severe dementia. The authors interpreted integrity in accordance with Erikson's "eight stages of man" theory, thus presupposing an experience of trust, autonomy, initiative, industry, identity, intimacy, generativity, and integrity.

Caregivers must make an effort to find meaning in the attempted communications by residents with severe dementia, which is a prerequisite for these caregivers experiencing the care they perform for these residents as worthwhile and for them being able to help the residents lead a meaningful life despite severe dementia. Caregivers need to train themselves not to personalize any unkind statements voiced by the resident, not to argue with the resident, not to misinterpret the resident's agitated behavior as purposefully provocative, and to avoid responding with anger. One of the goals of staff training is to reduce ineffective approaches, such as arguing or appealing to logical thinking, when the resident is unable to think logically because of advanced dementia. Staff members who are educated to understand dementia, its expected progression, and its resulting behavioral and psychological symptoms are likely to be less judgmental and more caring. In utilizing a person-centered approach, staff members need to be trained in the towel bath technique to reduce behavioral and psychological symptoms during bathing. The staff members also need to be trained in the hand-under-hand technique, in which the caregiver's hand is under the hand of the person with dementia. This technique is an effective way of helping residents with dementia participate in their daily care (e.g., feeding, bathing, changing clothes), even if they are not doing the task on their own, and it can reduce the residents' resistance to care. Training caregivers to help the residents balance activity with quiet time is also important.

During personal care activities such as feeding, many caregivers may act in a task-oriented way, saying "Open your mouth" and "Swallow," and not address the resident as a person. This may occur even though the caregivers understand that the resident's behaviors are expressions of that person's feelings of anxiety, abandonment, or dissolution. The reason for the discrepancy is that caregivers may feel ineffective, helpless, and powerless. By avoiding the residents, they try to avoid these feelings.

Caregivers should watch for agitation triggers and do their best to avoid them. Both family and professional caregivers need to learn to compromise, and to simplify things in the resident's life. Some residents may be helped by establishing set routines (eating meals at the same time each day, going to bed and waking up at the same time).

Improving Relationships between the Family and the Staff

A resident's psychosocial well-being depends to a considerable degree on the quality of the relationship and the interactions between the family and the staff. The staff and the family may experience anger during their interactions with each other in response to their own reactions to the resident's illness, the health care system, or the different expectations and stresses the resident's complex health and psychosocial needs create. Staff members who cultivate personal awareness, practice mindful self-monitoring during interactions, explore the different causes of their anger toward family members, demonstrate specific communication skills, set clear boundaries, and seek personal support can overcome the challenges of these difficult conversations with the resident's family and begin to restore trust in the staff-resident-family relationship. Mindful self-monitoring is the ability to be in the moment, to be both participant and observer during interpersonal interactions, to adjust to nuances of information, behaviors, and feelings in oneself and others, and to integrate this with one's professional knowledge and experience.

Communication

Even if they are no longer able to understand the specific content of a message, cognitively impaired residents may be sensitive to body language and to tone of voice, especially when it conveys a criticism. The resident often senses a caregiver's frustration or anger and may become anxious or angry in response. Relaxed and smiling caregiver behavior during any communication can help calm the resident and thus improve that person's attention. The staff may need to modify their linguistic behavior (including body language and tone of voice) to accommodate the declining cognitive abilities of residents with dementia. The use of yes/no questions can facilitate communication with residents with advanced dementia by reducing the demands on them.

How the staff members speak and how the residents perceive that speech is also important. The goal of communication should be connecting with the residents rather than testing their memories. When staff members seek information from a resident and provide a meaningful context for the question, even questions that might be difficult to answer from a linguistic standpoint may be responded to successfully by a person with dementia. The clinician should avoid commanding, condescending, patronizing, or critical communicative behavior and instead be patient, respectful, and caring, using rephrasing statements and providing explanations. The staff should also avoid overaccommodating behaviors (e.g., simplified grammar and vocabulary, slow speech, withdrawal from conversation) or underaccommodating behaviors (avoiding communication with the resident). We discourage the use of pet names, diminutives (e.g., dear, sweetie, honey), and exaggerated intonation, although in certain contexts they may convey qualities of nurturing, endearment, intimacy, or solidarity (J. Small, Perry, and Lewis 2005).

Communication skills useful in responding to an angry resident or family member include a calm, slow tone of voice, an open posture, an apology when appropriate, reflections on the resident's or the family member's feelings ("You look upset, worried, angry, anxious"), validation ("I understand why you feel this way"), empathy ("I would also feel frustrated in this situation"), respect ("I respect and admire your dedication to your loved one's well-being"), support ("I'll be here if you want to talk later"), and a problem-solving approach ("Let's try to solve this problem together").

Effective communication with the residents' families is also important, as it can improve clinical processes, outcomes, and the quality of life of both the resident and the family (Bluestein and Bach 2007). Such communication involves different levels of physician involvement (e.g., from minimal involvement for the management of resistiveness to care to considerable involvement for palliative care decision making during a life-threatening emergency), and the involvement of different staff members (e.g., the resident is having a bad day and the nurse advises the family whether they should lengthen, shorten, or avoid a visit; the recreational therapist educates the family regarding the potential benefits of simulated presence therapy to address loneliness and discusses who should make a tape or video recording).

Resident-Oriented Strategies

Several resident-oriented strategies can be employed for the prevention and treatment of behavioral and psychological symptoms in LTC residents (table 13.4).

Meaningful Activities

A variety of structured (e.g., bingo, listening to live music) and unstructured activities (e.g., reading a book, listening to a book on a CD or tape, taking care of plants), if individualized, can greatly enhance a resident's sense of well-being. Many residents have been lifelong readers and retain their reading ability until the severe stages of dementia. Having a facility library with a collection of books from different classic and contemporary authors can facilitate this activity. Table 13.5 lists examples of meaningful activities for LTC populations, and table 13.6 lists activities family members can participate in with their loved one. Activities may have a powerful effect in engaging a resident if they are meaningful in the context of the resident's past occupation. For example, a former schoolteacher may be engaged by being made the lunchroom monitor.

One-on-One Strategies

Hearing and listening to the residents is crucial to high-quality care. Listening nurtures contentment and builds connections. Learning to elicit and listen to the residents' stories also serves as a cultural assessment tool. Every resident has one or more stories to tell, and these stories build bridges between the staff and the residents. The staff can help the residents cope with stress (physical, emotional, and environmental) by providing an outlet for their frustration by hearing the residents' expressions of distress. Enlisting another person (e.g., another resident, a volunteer) as a therapy buddy to involve a resident with behavioral and psychological symptoms in various activities (e.g., exercising together, dining together) and to provide daily support may be helpful. Conversations also help maintain the resident's language function.

Massage and Other Approaches Involving Therapeutic Touch

Most residents respond to tactile stimulation: a hug, an arm around the shoulder, a clasp of the hand, a back rub, or a hand massage. At many lev-

TABLE 13.5
Examples of meaningful activities for long-term care residents

Meaningful activities for residents with mild dementia, mild cognitive impairment, or intact cognition
  Participating in a book club
  Joining a discussion group (e.g., current events, sports, politics, science, history)
  Listening to a book or poetry reading
  Playing computer games
  Leading an exercise group for other residents
  Solving brain-teasers in a group setting (e.g., trivia challenges), working on puzzles individually
  Learning a (new) musical instrument
  Learning to sing
  Learning to dance
  Learning to plant new flowers or new plants and taking care of them
  Learning to cook new recipes and make new drinks
  Learning new artistry skills (e.g., making hand-painted yarn)
Meaningful activities for residents with moderate dementia
  Cooking, baking, kneading dough
  Gardening
  Washing, cleaning, helping with the dishes
  Singing in a group setting
  Playing a musical instrument
  Setting the table
  Reminiscing about previous vacations and trips
  Watching movies or travelogues
Meaningful activities for residents with severe dementia
  Folding towels
  Sealing envelopes
  Shredding paper
  Attending church
  Watching or listening to religious television shows, radio programs, religious music

els, residents need human touch. Massage therapy (e.g., back and shoulder massage) may reduce the anxiety and agitation related to pain. Combining massage and aromatherapy (e.g., hand massage with a lotion [lavender for soothing, citrus for activating]) may have an even better effect in calming an agitated resident.

Exercise and Physical Activity

Regular exercise and increased nonexercise physical activity play an important role in the maintenance of the emotional, cognitive, and functional well-being of LTC residents, and they may even decrease the rate of brain atrophy (Colcombe et al. 2006; Williams and Tappen 2007). An individualized, simple exercise program (one hour, two or more times weekly, of walking or of strength, balance, and flexibility training) may slow functional decline, decrease fall risk, and reduce symptoms of depression and agitation (Rolland et al. 2007a). We recommend extra flexibility training for men and extra strength training for women. Education in the health benefits of regular ex-

TABLE 13.6
Activities family and friends may engage in during visits to a loved one in long-term care

Eat in the facility, dine out, or go to a café

Walk with the resident or push the resident in a wheelchair

Give a hand massage, hugs and kisses, back rubs

Go for a car ride

Go for a nature walk

Watch birds and nature

Garden (e.g., water plants)

Bring and arrange flowers

Dance

Play ping-pong or any other game (e.g., board games, card games)

Play Wii games (e.g., golf, bowling)

Participate in creative activities (e.g., water-coloring, coloring by numbers)

Listen to music

Listen to live music played by a talented family member

Sing songs (e.g., religious hymns, Christmas carols, favorite songs [such as "You Are My Sunshine"])

Share jokes, read humorous passages, watch funny movies

Watch a television show or a movie (even if the resident seems to be not understanding the activity or not interested in the activity, as long as the visitor is enjoying the activity, at some level the resident will benefit from the companionship and from seeing the loved one's enjoyment)

Page through a memory book or a photo album and reminisce

Show the resident photos of recent travel by a family member (especially involving children, grandchildren, places that the resident has visited or liked)

Read cards or e-mails from family and friends

Read a passage from a religious text or listen to books on tape / CDs

Spend quiet time with the resident (physical presence is sufficient for the resident to experience companionship, e.g., the family member can read a book or a magazine while sitting next to the resident)

Listen, even when the resident's speech seems impossible to decipher

ercise may improve attendance and the likelihood of implementation by the staff. Most residents tolerate exercise well without adverse effects.

Exercise programs should involve aerobic activity (walking, swimming), strength training (using resistance bands [e.g., Thera-Bands endorsed by the American Physical Therapy Association], weights, or Pilates), flexibility (Pilates, yoga, and flexibility exercises), and balance training (tai chi and other balance exercises). The nursing home facility in the Evergreen Retirement Community in Oshkosh, Wisconsin, has an indoor swimming pool for the residents and the staff has found that a surprising number of their residents enjoy swimming, water aerobics, or just playing with water! Exercise programs, especially those with whole-body involvement rather than walking by itself, should be routinely available in all LTC facilities.

Music

Music intervention, particularly with live or preferred music, may reduce disruptive behaviors and improve moods in LTC residents (Madan 2005). Slow classical music (e.g., Bach, Vivaldi) has been found to calm agitated residents. Enjoying music is a superb way of maintaining one's connections to the past and to other people. People with dementia who can play a musical instrument (e.g., a piano) may not know what they ate twenty minutes ago, but at the piano they may recall, play, and sing dozens of songs by accessing their remote and implicit memory. Calming music (especially during mealtimes) may reduce agitation and improve oral intake. Drumming—in which the residents bang on drums, talk about what the sound reminds them of, or take each person's name, break it into syllables, and then beat each syllable on the drum—can be enjoyable and empowering. Group singing activities or "singing for the brain" programs not only can be fun, but also may have a positive impact in maintaining the residents' cognitive functioning. For many, music and dancing are a part of their culture. Soft music may help relieve tension and anxiety; energetic music may help lift a depressed mood. Religious music may elicit active participation from residents who are not responding to conventional music.

Nutrition

Hunger and thirst can often trigger agitation, and staff members who are attuned to the resident's needs can often abort a behavioral disturbance by offering food or a beverage of the resident's choice at the first sign of hunger or thirst. Group activities involving cooking (e.g., baking bread or cookies, popping popcorn) can get even difficult residents to participate and enjoy the activity.

Humor

Reading funny quotes aloud or asking a resident to read them, sharing cartoons, watching classic television or movie comedies, and sharing jokes (especially one-liners) can be done either in a formal group setting as a scheduled activity or incorporated into everyday care to enhance joy in the residents' lives. It is also important for clinicians to acknowledge and positively reinforce a resident's spontaneous use of humor to cope with daily strife.

Simulated Presence Therapy

Simulated presence therapy is a personalized approach that uses an audio or video recording of one side of a conversation with a family member talking about happy memories and important events, interposed with pauses for the resident's side of the conversation. Simulated presence therapy may help relieve the agitation and loneliness often manifesting as a wish to go home. An example of such a recording may be a daughter or son saying "Hi, Dad. I'm doing well and I hope you're doing well too. I can't wait to show you some photographs of your grandson Alex. I'll be seeing you soon. Love, your daughter Faith." A resident with short-term memory loss can hear or watch such calming messages dozens of time a day without recognizing the repetition.

Bright Light Therapy

Bright light therapy is done using a light therapy unit that is about 1 foot by 1.5 feet in surface area and uses white fluorescent light behind a plastic diffusing screen that filters out ultraviolet rays (Targum and Rosenthal 2008). We recommend exposure to bright light (minimum 2,500 lux; preferably 10,000 lux) for 30 to 90 minutes in the morning and/or evening for a therapeutic effect that may start within four days. The clinician should consider recommending bright light therapy during winter months (and, for some, in the fall and spring as well) for all residents with a history that suggests seasonal affective disorder (typically winter depression). Six percent of the U.S. population, primarily in northern climates, is affected by this disorder in its most marked form. Another 14 percent have a lesser form of seasonal mood changes, known as winter blues (Rosenthal 2006). Bright light therapy may also improve sleep for LTC residents with insomnia (especially if they have sleep phase advancement).

In this form of therapy, the resident is required to sit and perform some quiet activity in front of the light box while receiving light. For residents who will not sit in front of the light box, a uniformly high level of light in their surroundings may improve sleep as well as daytime agitation. Adverse effects of bright light therapy include eyestrain, headaches (which may manifest as agitation), and the risk of inducing hypomania or mania in residents with bipolar disorder. If a resident is unable to tolerate the light box treatment, the intensity of the treatment can be reduced by increasing the person's distance from the light box or changing the duration of the therapy. Some health insurance companies may cover the expense of a light therapy device if the indication is seasonal affective disorder.

Animal-Assisted Therapy

The use of animal-assisted therapy (also called *pet therapy*) and companion pet programs have become more common throughout the LTC system (Weinberg et al. 2004). Animal-assisted therapy, such as using a visiting or resident pet dog or cat, may reduce aggression, agitation, and loneliness, as well as promote social behavior in LTC residents (Filan and Llewellyn-Jones 2006; Banks, Willoughby, and Banks 2008). In addition to a human touch, many residents enjoy the touch of a pet, especially if they had pets earlier in their lives. Seeing a dog or cat walk up to them can elicit a positive response: they are suddenly present, captivated, and reaching down to pet the animal. Animal-assisted therapy gives the resident a chance to show love and bask in the memory of something warm. Physical touch, whether by a human or a furry animal, creates relaxation and a sense of connection. Withdrawn residents may smile and laugh, nonverbal residents may speak to and about the pet, and isolated residents may reminisce about a childhood pet.

The desire for and potential benefits of animal-assisted therapy strongly correlate with previous pet ownership. Any resident who has a strong life history of emotional intimacy with pets and wishes to have a pet should be offered animal-assisted therapy to prevent and treat loneliness and/or agitation. Local humane societies and animal shelters often have volunteers who take dogs, cats, puppies, and kittens to LTC facilities for free (although any donation is welcomed). These events can be scheduled as a regular recurring activity (e.g., weekly) or as a special event.

High-Tech Interventions

A variety of high-tech interventions may be tried to prevent and treat behavioral and psychological symptoms in LTC residents (table 13.7). Interactive robotic dogs may reduce loneliness in residents, and residents often become attached to these robots (Banks, Willoughby, and Banks 2008). Wii games have also become popular in LTC settings, and both the residents and the staff can enjoy these games. The safety and autonomy of the residents may improve with the use of technologies for managing the facility's domestic ambient environment (e.g., medical sensors, entertainment equipment, home automation systems) (Marsh et al. 2008).

TABLE 13.7
High-tech interventions and approaches

CD/tape player/iPod/MP3 player (to listen to music, books on tape, family conversations)

Big screen television (especially for residents with impaired vision or if a large group of residents are watching TV in a group setting)

DVD/VHS/Blu-ray player (to watch favorite family events that are videorecorded, favorite shows/movies/games/travel or cooking shows)

Computer with internet capability (e-mail; videophone communication with a distant family member; talking to family through the Internet [with or without using a viewcam]; legacy websites storing favorite pictures, movies, music, and family or other events)

Video games (e.g., Wii games by Nintendo)

Robotic animals (e.g., a robot cat that purrs each time the resident moves his or her hands over the cat's body)

Toy animals that are soft, can be warmed safely (e.g., in a microwave), and release soothing aromas (e.g., lavender)

Cognitive Rehabilitation

Cognitive rehabilitation is an individualized approach that uses psychosocial-environmental interventions to improve specific domains of cognitive function. The goal is not to enhance cognition, but to improve cognitive function in an everyday context (Dowd and Davidhizar 2003; Clare and Woods 2004; Kolanowski et al. 2008). Cognitive rehabilitation is tailored to the resident's level of cognitive impairment, starting with the easiest tasks and increasing in difficulty as success occurs with the easier tasks. Cognitive rehabilitation requires a high level of motivation from the residents and leadership from the facility's medical director, administrator, and director of nursing. Family involvement can help residents who hesitate to participate. Such a program is implemented with an interdisciplinary approach involving a recreational therapist, a speech therapist, or a neuropsychologist as team leader.

Cognitive rehabilitation may focus on several cognitive domains (e.g., attention, memory [episodic, semantic], speech, executive dysfunction) or on specific functions (e.g., using procedural memory, which is a memory of a prior experience without conscious reference to that experience [e.g., riding a bicycle, playing a musical instrument]). Residents with mild to moderate dementia often have a relatively intact procedural memory and can learn new skills or maintain existing skills by using this type of memory function. These activities have the potential not only to add fun to the residents' lives (e.g., learning to play table tennis [ping pong], maintaining skills at playing the piano or any musical instrument), but also to give the residents meaningful social roles (e.g., playing a musical instrument for a group of residents). Performing comedy routines for the staff with or without reading from cue cards, serving beverages, and greeting an audience as it arrives enhance and maintain social skills that are often preserved until the late stages of dementia. Special-care residents have dressed up as clowns to visit terminally ill residents. Taking part in a reading and discussion group (with books such as *The Birth of the Chocolate Chip Cookie* or *A Legend of Hollywood: Mickey Rooney*) is another intervention that can maintain cognition and improve mood through socialization and reminiscence. Many of the activities can be initiated by the family, professional caregivers, or volunteers (after a brief training). Other examples of cognitive rehabilitation include training residents with dementia to perform activities for residents with more advanced dementia, and making use of intergenerational groups (e.g., where residents with dementia work with preschoolers to teach them phonics and how to count).

Residents with mild to moderate dementia and topographical disorientation (i.e., an impaired ability to orient oneself in a real-life environment and navigate through it) may benefit from errorless-based techniques to improve their ability to find their own rooms or other commonly used rooms (e.g., the activities room, the dining room) and to prevent complications related to disorientation (e.g., a resident avoiding social contact or wandering into another resident's room) (Provencher et al. 2008). Errorless-based techniques involve correcting the resident just before he or she goes the wrong way, or asking the resident to go backwards a short distance from the target location and then to advance forward to the target location, gradually increasing the distance on subsequent trials until the resident can complete the whole route forward and repeat it.

Some residents who do not have dementia or a mild cognitive impairment, residents with only a mild cognitive impairment, and highly motivated residents with mild dementia may benefit from cognitive strategies to improve memory or slow memory decline (e.g., mnemonic strategies, spaced-retrieval training). Regularly engaging the residents in card games (e.g., Go Fish), puzzles (e.g., crossword puzzles, Sudoku, jigsaw puzzles), trivia games, and even computer games (e.g., FreeCell, a computer-based game similar to solitaire, or Brain Age by Nintendo) may also provide cognitive stimulation and slow cognitive decline. Cognitive rehabilitation strategies may enhance function even in residents with moderately severe dementia. For example, teaching residents how to scoop golf balls into a muffin tin (a Montessori technique) and repeating the activity may help those residents who have recently lost the ability to feed themselves regain that ability. Bright light has a modest benefit in improving cognitive symptoms of dementia and thus may enhance the benefits of cognitive rehabilitation (Riemersma-van der Lek et al. 2008).

Individual Psychotherapy

For motivated residents who are cognitively intact, residents with mild cognitive impairment, and residents in the early stages of dementia, the clinician should consider individual psychotherapy to treat anxiety and/or depressive disorders (e.g., adaptation to institutional life, bereavement, the stress of being diagnosed with cancer). When such services are available, the clinician should consider referral to a therapist for problem-solving therapy, or cognitive behavioral therapy to treat major depressive disorder, or supportive psychotherapy to treat a personality disorder or depression. Social workers are ideally suited to provide individual psychotherapy, as they have already established a rapport with the resident and the family and are aware of the resident's personal characteristics and the family's dynamics. Social workers should not just be filling out forms, but be freed to do therapy with the residents and their families.

Teaching breathing exercises or progressive relaxation to cognitively intact residents with anxiety symptoms may take only two to three minutes and should be considered a standard part of treatment for such residents. It is not uncommon for elderly people who have had early traumatic experiences to make it through adult life with minimal sequelae until their later years. Individual therapy can help these residents cope with the anxiety and depression related to such traumatic experiences. Working through past trauma by talking about emotions felt then and now may need to be done at a slower pace with an elderly person than with a younger person. Other interventions that may be helpful for cognitively intact residents with anxiety and depression include mindfulness-based stress reduction, interpersonal psychotherapy, and relaxation training (guided relaxation, guided imagery).

Reminiscence Therapy

Reminiscence therapy involves discussing past activities, events, and experiences with another person or with a group of people, usually with the aid of tangible prompts such as photographs, household and other familiar items from the past, or music or archival sound recordings. One form of reminiscence therapy involves life review, in which the person is guided chronologically through his or her life experiences, is encouraged to evaluate them, and may even produce a life-history book. Reminiscence therapy, although popular with the staff in LTC facilities for residents with dementia, has not been rigorously studied in this population. Preliminary evidence indicates that reminiscence therapy may enhance self-esteem, reduce social isolation and depression, and provide comfort for LTC residents (Pittiglio 2000). The clinician may consider life review for cognitively intact residents who have had many past accomplishments but currently are going through depression and existential problems (e.g., "What have I achieved in life?" or "What was the purpose of my life?").

Aromatherapy

Aromatherapy involves the use of essential oils to improve emotional well-being. This intervention has been found to be safe and effective for treating behavioral and psychological symptoms in LTC residents (Ballard et al. 2002). Recreational therapists are often skilled in using aromatherapy. Occasionally, contact dermatitis may occur as an adverse event. For residents with a poor olfactory function (e.g., many residents who have Alzheimer disease), this approach may not work.

Validation Therapy

Validation therapy was developed by Naomi Feil in 1963. The therapy is based on the general principle of validation—that is, the acceptance of the reality and personal truth of another person's experience—and incorporates a range of specific techniques (Feil 2002). For example, this therapy advocates validating the emotion that is expressed instead of trying to reorient the resident to reality. By not emphasizing the accuracy of facts, the caregiver is freed to express more empathy and find a meaningful point of connection. Preliminary data suggest that validation therapy may reduce the severity and frequency of behavioral and psychological symptoms in LTC residents (Tondi et al. 2007). Validation therapy is controversial and has not been accepted in the routine care of LTC residents. We support its use for residents with dementia who are experiencing emotional distress that is not thought to be due to underlying correctable medical conditions or medications.

Dance or Movement Therapy

For centuries, dance and rhythmic movement have been used in expressing and modifying emotions. Dance or movement therapy combines music, light exercise, and sensory stimulation, and it has been found to improve the cognitive, social, and emotional well-being of LTC residents with dementia (Hok-kanen et al. 2003).

Psychosocial-Environmental Interventions for Pain and Specific Behavioral and Psychological Symptoms

Aggression, sundowning, screaming, resistiveness to care, and pain are some of the most challenging conditions commonly encountered in LTC populations. The clinician may try a variety of psychosocial-environmental interventions to prevent and treat these common symptoms.

Aggression

Aggressive behaviors (both verbal and physical) by residents toward others are prevalent in LTC populations and can cause immense stress to caregivers. Most episodes of physical aggression occur during personal care (i.e., during an intrusion into the resident's personal space) and thus can be considered a defensive response (Bridges-Parlet, Knopman, and Thompson 1994). Verbal aggression and noncompliance with requests often precede physical aggression, and a return to normal behavior rapidly follows aggression. Caregivers need to be educated that aggression is an expression of the resident's unmet need, and they need to be trained to identify other common triggers besides intrusion into personal space (e.g., discomfort, pain, hunger, thirst, urinary tract infection, constipation, dehydration) that may result in any resident's becoming irritable or aggressive, as well as unique triggers for an individual resident (e.g., a resident who likes her furniture placed in a certain way and becomes angry if anyone changes the placement).

The staff need to be educated and trained to "listen" to nonverbal behaviors (e.g., clenched fists, an angry look) as well as verbal indicators of potential physical aggression (e.g., a resident telling the staff member "You better stop touching me or else I will hit you"). They also need to be trained to respond appropriately (e.g., leaving the resident alone [after ensuring his or her safety] and approaching that person at a later time). Depression and psychotic symptoms are also risk factors for aggressive behavior in residents with dementia. The injured residents have often (unknowingly) put themselves in harm's way by intruding into another resident's personal space, particularly one who is verbally aggressive and cognitively impaired (Shinoda-Tagawa et al. 2004). Interventions to prevent resident-to-resident aggression should focus on the behavior of the injured resident. Table 13.8 lists some simple strategies for dealing with a physically aggressive resident.

TABLE 13.8
Simple strategies for dealing with a physically aggressive resident

---

Allow at least a leg's length (or 3 to 4 feet) between you and the resident. For some residents, personal space requirements may be different.

Look for clenched fists, movement away from you, and expressions such as "Stay away from me" or "Get out of my face," which are indicators that the resident's personal space is violated. If so, move farther away.

Keep your body position slightly to the side of the resident, because the resident may interpret a face-to-face position as challenging or threatening.

Do not cross your arms over your chest, which sends an authoritative message. Position your hands loosely, one in the other, in front and slightly above the waist, with your elbows at your sides. This position will allow you to respond to a strike to the chest, face, and groin by blocking it with your arms.

Stand with your feet apart, one slightly behind the other, and your knees slightly bent. This posture gives you control over your center of gravity and allows for quick movement.

If the resident lunges toward you or tries to strike, do not hold his or her arm. Instead, block the blow and yield to the resident's force of movement as you step out of the way. This directs the momentum away from you as you move away. Ignore verbal insults, name calling, and so forth, and direct your concentration on the message behind the insult.

If grabbed, initially resist but then quickly give in. This causes the resident to momentarily relax his or her grip, or it throws him or her off balance enough for you to escape the grasp.

Plan what you will do as the level of aggression escalates. Teamwork and the decisiveness with which you move are critical.

Verbally aggressive and/or abusive behavior by a resident can be stressful for caregivers. It is important that the caregivers not take the aggressive behavior personally, put the behavior into context (e.g., the resident is probably in pain and, due to dementia, cannot use better ways to communicate or express frustration), not argue or try to reason, and, as necessary, consider seeking help from the resident's family or a veteran staff member.

Sundowning

Sundowning is a poorly defined term that is generally used to describe the escalation of confusion and agitation in the late afternoon and evening in people with dementia. The clinician should treat new-onset sundowning as delirium (e.g., treat the underlying cause [such as a UTI or adverse effects of a new medication—especially one with anticholinergic properties]). No specific medication has an antisundowning effect. Sundowning is best treated in the same way as agitation: by a systematic individualized approach to assess various potential causes (e.g., inappropriate medications, pain, depression, fatigue, a noisy or chaotic environment, boredom, sensory deprivation) and by appropriate treatment (e.g., an afternoon nap if fatigue is suspected; a multisensory room [Snoezelen] to address boredom and sensory deprivation).

Screaming

The treatment of screaming behavior is a treatment of its cause (e.g. undertreated pain or depression, loneliness, a need for staff help for toileting, hunger, an uncomfortable position, a hearing impairment, impatient predementia personality, visual hallucinations). Screaming behavior also causes considerable disruption of the social milieu in an LTC facility, as well as caregiver stress. Its treatment involves psychosocial-environmental interventions (e.g., soothing music, touch, a differential reinforcement system rewarding the resident's appropriate requests instead of his or her screaming behavior), with or without an appropriate pharmacological intervention (e.g., analgesic, antidepressant).

Resistiveness to Care

Possible causes of resistiveness to care include undertreated pain and/or depression, anxiety and paranoia, the resident's impression of being rushed or treated roughly, or the resident's fear of being dropped or treated poorly. Psychosocial-environmental interventions for resistiveness to care include having the staff member who has the best relationship with the resident provide that person's care or be present as a new staff member is taking over; having two staff members provide care (with one attempting to distract or reassure the resident, or to explain what is being done and why); dividing each task into small, successive steps; being patient and allowing ample time for care; allowing the resident to perform the parts of the task that he or she can still accomplish; stating instructions one step at a time; or attempting care at a later time. Pharmacological interventions may include analgesics and antidepressants.

Pain

Pain is common in LTC residents, and it responds to a variety of psychosocial-environmental interventions to a much greater extent than is often realized. Table 13.9 lists commonly used psychosocial-environmental interventions for pain management. Cold touch (e.g., ice packs) is particularly useful for neuropathic pain, and heat is particularly useful for muscle spasms.

> ⦂ **CLINICAL CASE** Mr. A, an 84-year-old man residing in an assisted living
> facility, complained of moderate to severe right knee pain that was not
> responding to 4 grams of acetaminophen per day; he could not tolerate

TABLE 13.9

Common psychosocial-environmental interventions to manage pain and pressure ulcers

---

Psychosocial-environmental interventions to manage pain

    Physical therapy, which is proven to be effective in reducing the pain and inflammation associated with any number of orthopedic problems (rotator cuff tendonitis, impingement syndrome, sprains and strains)

    Interventions to promote relaxation (soothing music, a calm environment, an unhurried approach, a soothing voice, breathing exercises, nature)

    Physical activity or exercise

    Cold touch

    Superficial heat

    Repositioning

    Massage (manual, through a massage chair)

    Cognitive behavioral therapy for cognitively intact residents

    Acupuncture

    Addressing the following misconceptions about pain in elderly people:

        Pain is a normal part of aging (it is not)

        Older adults are less sensitive to pain (they are not)

        Persons with advanced dementia do not experience pain (yes they do)

Psychosocial-environmental interventions to prevent and treat pressure ulcers

    Certified nursing assistants should check residents daily during personal care for changes in their skin

    Nurses should perform head-to-toe skin checks weekly for each resident

    Use specialty wound mattresses (e.g., constant-low-pressure mattresses and alternating-pressure mattresses), mattress replacements, and pressure-reducing support surfaces on beds (e.g., "padding pack"—a shrink-wrapped package of elbow pads, bolsters, and other padding)

    All residents who cannot reposition themselves should have their calves and heels on pillows at night

    All wheelchairs and geriatric chairs should have cushions

    Staff should turn bed-bound residents every two hours, and reposition residents in wheelchairs and geriatric chairs every hour

    Use moisture barriers routinely for incontinent residents

    Improve the fluid, protein, and calorie intakes for undernourished residents

---

NSAIDs. He declined a trial of low-dose tramadol or opioids after learning about their potential adverse effects. The physician recommended that Mr. A see an orthopedic surgeon for the possibility of steroid injections in his knee. Mr. A wanted to try acupuncture before knee injections, because his daughter strongly believed in this intervention. At this point Mr. A scored 16 on the MMSE and 15 on the 30-item GDS. He was given duloxetine 20 mg and he started going to a local center for integrative medicine that offered acupuncture. After four weeks he reported that his knee felt somewhat better, but that he was still depressed and did not like to go out of his room; he now scored 10 on the GDS. Duloxetine was increased to 40 mg daily, but Mr. A complained of insomnia and night sweats, so the dose was decreased to 30 mg daily. He continue the acupuncture. After four more weeks Mr. A reported that he was feeling "well," he had started attending activities, and he even expressing a wish to go fishing. He reported that his knee pain was dramatically improved with acupuncture. He exclaimed, "I can't believe acupuncture works!"

TEACHING POINTS Alternative treatment interventions such as acupuncture, if provided by a reputable center, may considerably help various medical conditions such as chronic pain, especially if the resident is interested in trying them. The treatment of depression with duloxetine may have also contributed to the good outcome.

Pressure Ulcers

Psychosocial-environmental interventions that are recommended to prevent and treat pressure ulcers involve a variety of approaches, from regular checks to pressure reduction, moisture barriers, nutrition, and movement (table 13.9). We recommend that every frail resident who leaves for a diagnostic test, appointment, or family visit lasting at least two hours (especially those using wheelchairs) receive a full skin check on returning to the LTC facility. Many LTC residents are in a wheelchair from four to eight hours a day. Pressure-reducing devices (e.g., cushions) and repositioning every hour should be routinely used for all residents in wheelchairs. Various specialty mattresses are available, but any type of wound mattress is better than a conventional mattress for the treatment of pressure ulcers.

Psychosocial-Environmental Interventions That Should Be Avoided

Psychosocial-environmental interventions that should be avoided include restraints, treating residents with advanced dementia like children, and employing reality-orientation therapy for residents with advanced dementia.

RESTRAINTS   Restraints are defined as "any device that limits an individual's freedom for voluntary movement" (Dawkins 1998). Various types of mechanical restraints include soft or leather ties for arms and legs, full-body vests, vests with long ties, hand mitts, pelvic ties, wheelchair bars, geri-chairs, and over-chair tables. We do not recommend using restraints for LTC residents for perceived safety reasons (e.g., to prevent falls or wandering), because the use of restraints is associated with increased agitation and, in some cases, with the occurrence or worsening of pressure sores, contractures, infections, incontinence, functional impairment, cardiac stress, accidental strangulation or injury, and death. The clinician should consider alternatives to restraints in order to improve safety for residents, and instead try environmental restructuring, increased staff involvement, an examination of the cause of the resident's behavior or disorientation, changes in lighting and the reduction of glare, the completion of a fall-risk assessment, and so forth.

A more important reason not to use restraints is to maintain the autonomy and dignity of LTC residents. The removal of restraints may often reduce agitation, and we recommend removing restraints for any resident who is demonstrating agitation. Environmental restraint, which some consider to be a safety measure, means the containment of individuals within specific rooms or units by methods such as locking doors and policing the use of space. Ethicists have questioned the utilitarian argument of maximizing the reduction of harm to residents and those around them through restraint. In efforts to overcome the current high use of restraints, person-centered care is the key first step, followed by evidence-based medical care and the appropriate use of psychosocial-environmental interventions.

TREATING RESIDENTS WITH ADVANCED DEMENTIA LIKE CHILDREN
It is not acceptable to treat residents with advanced dementia like children, that is, to infantilize them. The residents have lived a long life and have a wealth of experiences before they entered the LTC facility. We recommend paying homage to the residents' lives and achievements and treating them as elders whose wisdom and intellect has been hidden or imprisoned by dementia, but not lost. Every resident would like us not only to honor him or her, but also to support him or her in the spiritual and emotional journey being undertaken, especially when that person is in a diminished and fragile state.

REALITY-ORIENTATION THERAPY   We do not recommend repeatedly correcting a resident with cognitive impairment regarding the day of the week, the time of day, or the place where that person is living, as this may trigger frustration and lower the person's mood. However, the liberal use of calendars and reality-orientation boards (showing the date, the day of the week, the weather, and the name of the facility) may be useful. We also recommend activity boards showing facility activities and times.

Activities for Special Populations
Young Residents

One-quarter of all strokes occur in people under the age of 65, and some of these individuals may need temporary or permanent admission to LTC, due to the devastating effects of strokes on their physical and cognitive functions. Some 10 percent of dementias occur in people younger than 65, and a substantial proportion (25%–50%) of young-onset dementias may be frontotemporal dementia. Neurological disorders such as multiple sclerosis, traumatic brain injury, and spinal cord injury may result in LTC facilities seeing younger patients. The psychosocial needs of this population are different from those of the typical older LTC resident, who is a woman in her 80s with AD or mixed dementia (AD and VaD). We recommend that the younger population in LTC be offered activities appropriate to their age group (e.g., a different reminiscence group activity that involves events in the 1960s and 1970s rather than 1940s and 1950s).

Male Residents

In a typical LTC facility, women outnumber men by three or more to one. Men in LTC often experience isolation and a lack of male companionship. It may be helpful to establish a men's group or encourage men who are on the staff—including maintenance personnel—to spend a few minutes with these residents. Many of the facility's activities (e.g., making cookies or knitting) may not be suited to the interests or experiences of male residents. Thus the various activities offered to all residents should include those that are geared toward the interests of male residents (e.g., activities that involve tools [made of rubber or another safe synthetic material, rather than metal] or that are associated with hunting and fishing).

Resident with a Chronic Mental Illness

Many residents with a chronic mental illness may be reluctant to participate in activities in large groups (e.g., bingo), but they may thrive in one-on-one or small-group activities (involving two to four residents who are familiar to them) that are meaningful to them (e.g., putting letters in envelopes, shredding documents, cooking).

Residents with a Developmental Disability

Residents with a developmental disability may have been involved in workshops during much of the earlier part of their lives, places often featuring more complex activities that they were able to perform before the development of their dementia. Such residents may find great benefit in still having a workshop they can go to for activities (e.g., shredding documents, sorting papers).

Residents Who Are Relatively Cognitively Intact

Residents who are relatively cognitively intact may prefer activities that are intellectually stimulating (e.g., discussion groups on contemporary topics [politics, sports], book clubs, computer clubs). They may eschew activities such as bingo.

Innovative Programs and Approaches

A variety of innovative programs and approaches use psychosocial-environmental interventions to improve the residents' quality of life. One of the most important factors in LTC facilities that embrace one or more of these programs is having a physician (especially the medical director) and the administrator champion these programs. Also, keeping the staff informed about success stories related to the program and involving the residents' families are crucial elements if the program is to be sustainable.

The Eden Alternative (www.edenalt.org) has become well known for its approach to making LTC facilities more homelike by introducing plants, pets, and other environmental changes that remove institutional austerity. The philosophy of the Eden Alternative teaches that older people who enter an LTC facility should continue to grow and find meaning in life. Guiding the staff to respect these individuals as mature adults regardless of their cognitive or physical states is a goal of the Eden education program. In the language of Eden, residents are referred to as *elders*, and the staff is encouraged to see elders as wise.

Wellspring Innovative Solutions (www.lifespan-network.org/beacon _wellspring.asp) is a Beacon Institute culture-change program that enables LTC facilities to effect culture changes within their existing plan and wherever they are along the continuum of change. Wellspring primarily focuses on strengthening the clinical and managerial skills of staff members, empowering residents and frontline staff members, and creating a high quality of life for residents.

The Green House Project (www.ncbcapitalimpact.org), in Tupelo, Mississippi, is intended to deinstitutionalize LTC by eliminating large nursing home facilities and creating habilitative social settings. Its primary purpose is to serve as a place where older and disabled adults can receive assistance and support with activities of daily living and clinical care, without such assistance and care becoming the focus of their existence.

TimeSlips (www.timeslips.org), developed by Anne Basting in 1998, is a group storytelling process used in many LTC facilities nationwide. The process focuses on the imagination and creativity of the residents, rather than on memory and reminiscence. A group of residents, led by an individual trained in TimeSlips, write stories based on a picture they all look at.

The Montessori method is based on procedural—that is, implicit—memory, which is activated by repetitive muscle movements and emphasizes identifying each person's strengths and building an individualized program upon those strengths. Montessori exercises are based on taste, vision, hearing, smell, and touch. The key aspect of this method is to let the resident learn and experience things for him- or herself and to only guide the resident in doing so. Thus, by principle, all Montessori-based activities have to be meaningful, rather then just leisure activities or things to do. Cameron Camp has studied the use of Montessori-based activities in LTC populations and has found growing evidence that they improve the residents' emotional well-being and their quality of life. Montessori-based activities tap into different skills that are used on a daily basis. For example, arranging flowers emphasizes eye-hand coordination, physical movement, and care of the environment. Dishwashing is designed to continue and strengthen preserved skills required for ADLs. A reading roundtable is a group reading activity that focuses on social interaction and cognitive stimulation (Camp, Cohen-Mansfield, and Capezuti 2002). Resident-Assisted Montessori Programming, based on Montessori principles, is a novel approach in which residents with early to middle-stage dementia are trained to lead a reading activity for persons with more advanced dementia (Skrajner and Camp 2007). Montessori-based activity programming involving preschool children, in which persons with early dementia develop lessons for the youngsters, has also been found to be beneficial for both the residents and the visitors.

The Spark of Life program (www.dementiacareaustralia.com) is a planned playful-activity program developed by Jane Verity and specifically designed for people with dementia. Its focus is on the quality of the interaction rather than on the activity itself. Staff members trained in this approach use spontaneity, joy, humor, fun with words, and body language. Any playful activity, if it is not to be demeaning, has to be done in a respectful manner. The response of the person with dementia should be one of the key factors in deciding whether to continue a particular activity.

Snoezelen (a registered trademark of Rompa, in Chesterfield, England) is an activity program that uses multisensory stimulation to create a comfortable, safe environment. Sight, hearing, touch, taste, and smell are stimulated through the use of lighting effects, tactile surfaces, meditative music, and aromatic oils. This provides meaningful activity without the need for intellectual reasoning, and it results in the release of stress and frustration (Chitsey, Haight, and Jones 2002).

Residents with minimal or mild cognitive impairments may benefit from a program that teaches them to maintain brain function through brain-healthy nutrition (e.g., a Mediterranean diet, foods rich in omega-3 fatty acids, fruits, and vegetables), nutritional supplements (e.g., vitamin B_{12}, vitamin D, omega-3 capsules), emotional well-being strategies (stress management and mind-body interventions [such as breathing exercises, visualization, relaxation training, mindfulness-based stress reduction strategies]), an active lifestyle (physical exercise, brain exercises [such as puzzles, word searches, reading aloud], spirituality, socialization, and creative endeavors [painting, playing a musical instrument, dancing]). This program should also feature early, aggressive treatment of the risk factors for developing dementia (e.g., hypertension, diabetes, obesity, hyperlipidemia, metabolic syndrome, sleep apnea, smoking), including strategies for the secondary prevention of strokes. One goal of such a program is to prevent or postpone the onset of dementia both for cognitively intact residents with a long life expectancy and for residents with mild cognitive impairments. Another goal is to slow cognitive and functional declines for residents with mild dementia. Such a brain-and-memory fitness program can have cognitive rehabilitation (described earlier) as a major component for motivated residents. For other residents, a brain-and-memory fitness program can involve the implementation of any other aspect besides cognitive rehabilitation (e.g., exercise, nutritional strategies, creative activities) that a particular resident is interested in.

The Enriched Opportunities Program was devised by the Bradford Dementia Group, a part of the University of Bradford in the United Kingdom (Brooker and Woolley 2007). It consists of five key elements that work together to bring about a sustainable, activity-based model of care. These elements are specialist expertise (the staff role of Locksmith); individualized assessment and case work; an activity and occupation program; staff training; and management and leadership.

Overcoming Barriers to the Implementation of Interventions

Many of the interventions discussed above are time intensive. But this is no different from interventions to address medical issues such as urinary incontinence, in which carrying out evidence-based interventions (such as scheduled or prompted voiding) takes more time than cleaning up after an "accident." Also, the consequences of not adequately meeting the residents' psychosocial needs are an increase in their agitation, aggression, depressed moods, and anxiety, which, in turn, increases the staff's workload and often leads to the prescription of psychotropic medication. Psychotropics, in their turn, may cause daytime sedation, reduce oral intake, and cause falls and injuries, all of which further increase the staff's workload. Leadership, innovation, adequate staffing (in both quality and quantity), and training can overcome the barriers to time-intensive interventions. One significant hindrance to implementing high-quality, psychosocial-environmental interventions is a lack of adequate staffing in the evenings and on weekends. These are the times when traditionally things are quiet, but often a lack of adequate, structured activity programs during these periods is a significant risk factor for agitation and depression. Also, attendance at activity programs does not guarantee engagement. A lack of personal knowledge of a resident's interests and the absence of a good relationship with the resident are also barriers to engaging the resident in activity programs. Person-centered care, and determination and support from the administrative leaders of the facility, are keys to overcoming most of these barriers.

Assistive Devices

Staff members commonly encounter agitation during personal care, especially when they are lifting and transferring the residents. This agitation is usually an expression of the resident's emotional and physical discomfort. Discomfort can be greatly minimized by the use of appropriate assistive devices. Some of these devices (e.g., Merry Walkers) may also help promote the residents' dignity by allowing them to ambulate safely, while others (e.g., hip pads and hip protectors) may reduce complications from falls (e.g., hip fractures), although this benefit is debatable (Rubenstein 2008). Resident-handling tasks, including lifting and transferring, are physically demanding and unpredictable, and they are often performed under unfavorable conditions. Manually lifting physically dependent residents is a high-risk activity for both the staff and the resident. Inadequate space and poorly designed work environments also contribute to awkward positions when performing nursing care. We recommend the routine use of appropriate assistive devices (e.g., a Hoyer lift), as they may improve resident and staff safety, reduce agitation, and promote resident dignity.

Interdisciplinary Teams

Most behavioral and psychological symptoms are best treated by an interdisciplinary team. Table 13.10 delineates the members who constitute an ideal interdisciplinary team. The roles of some key team members are described below.

Recreational therapists are professionals whose training is much more rigorous and evidence based than that of many staff members who are given the title of "activity therapists." Recreational therapists use the framework from the American Therapeutic Recreation Association's *Dementia Practice Guidelines* regarding assessment, prescriptions, treatment, and outcome measurements. After performing a comprehensive assessment to identify background factors (e.g., cognitive ability) and proximal factors (e.g., psychosocial need states), recreational therapists use a host of tools and interventions (e.g., air mat therapy, a sensory stimulation box) to address behavioral problems in LTC residents.

Music therapists are trained in a four-year college program, followed by a six-month internship, and they are registered through the National Association for Music Therapy. Music therapists may lead a group music activity as part of a daily continuous activity schedule, as well as provide one-on-one

TABLE 13.10
Members of an ideal interdisciplinary team

Resident
Family member
Nursing assistant
Nurse
Recreational therapist
Music therapist
Art therapist
Activity therapist
Chaplain
Social worker
Registered dietitian
Physical therapist
Occupational therapist
Speech therapist
Housekeeping staff
Pharmacist
Primary care physician, psychiatrist, and physician extender (e.g., nurse practitioner, physician assistant)
Managers (e.g., director of nursing, administrator, supervisor)

music therapy for specific residents with depression and/or agitation who have been referred to the therapist by a physician, a nurse practitioner, or a physician assistant. Medicare and Medicaid may reimburse the cost of music therapy in LTC, but such decisions are made on a case-by-case basis.

Art therapists are registered through the American Art Therapy Association after completion of a master's-level program and 1,000 hours of supervised clinical experience beyond a graduate internship. Art therapists use a variety of media—including paint, ceramics, natural materials, and fabrics—to guide residents through everything from one-on-one painting sessions to group quilting projects.

The interdisciplinary team may need to try many interventions before identifying those that benefit a resident. For example, some residents may not like group activities, and some may not like music. Some residents may have enjoyed painting in the past but, as their dementia becomes severe, they no longer understand the function of a paintbrush, and what was a source of joy before may now become a source of confusion. Thus activities need to be individually tailored, as well as periodically modified to accommodate declining cognitive and functional abilities.

Conclusion

The portrait of people living in long-term care facilities needs to change from "exuberant life, gloomy descent" to "exuberant life, peaceful and contented descent." There is no reason for LTC residents not to experience the fullness of life. The connections of LTC residents (including those with dementia) with others and to their own past life can be sustained at a far higher level than is generally believed. The promotion of person-centered care and good practice for residents with behavioral and psychological symptoms of dementia may reduce the need for and use of antipsychotic and other psychotropic medications. Behavioral symptoms are complex. They require that caregivers understand the presumed causes of the symptoms and intervene appropriately, using evidence-based, caregiver-oriented, and resident-oriented techniques. Psychosocial-environmental interventions have the potential to dramatically improve the quality of life for LTC residents and their caregivers.

CHAPTER 14

An Ideal Long-Term Care Home

Be the light you wish to see in the world.

—Mahatma Gandhi

Visionary and determined people are reinventing long-term care facilities. These individuals believe that each of us, no matter how old, sick, frail, disabled, or forgetful, deserves to have a loving home—not a facility. These individuals have pioneered LTC homes to replace LTC facilities. Such LTC homes make the quality of life for their residents life affirming, create a culture that rekindles the human spirit, and mend the frayed social fabric of our current society (Morley and Flaherty 2002). Such transformational change is needed not only in LTC facilities, but also in the entire culture of aging. Societies based on market-driven economies have deeply embedded value systems that inherently favor economically productive younger people and marginalize nonproductive older people. Understanding the reasons for such an attitude suggests that education could play a crucial role in correcting it. Also, state-of-the-art LTC homes demonstrate that transformational change is not just a philosophy, but also a reality.

There are several remarkable LTC homes in the United States, led by people with vision and determination and staffed by compassionate, creative, and competent individuals. The residents and the staff members in these LTC homes have more friends among themselves than they have restrictions and rules to follow. LTC homes know that the single most important thing the residents and their caregivers (family and professional) value—more than good food, good medical care, or clean facilities—is the warmth of a caring relationship. LTC homes sustain their high-quality care through a relentless adherence to person-centered care. We need to give credit to homes that have adopted person-centered care, and we also need to create incentives and training for every home to begin its own journey toward person-centered care. An ideal LTC home not only becomes a home of choice in the community, but it also reduces staff turnover and the cost of health care (e.g., reduced hospitalizations at the end of life).

An ideal LTC home has several essential characteristics, as listed in table 14.1 (White 2005; Zimmerman et al. 2005). This list is long and daunting. Nevertheless, all of the elements are achievable. The psychological and spiritual challenges of facing a decline in one's health and having to live with strangers in an unfamiliar place are daunting for anyone, and especially for elderly people. In addition, a loss of independence, the fear of becoming a burden, no involvement in decision making, limited access to care (including palliative care), and negative attitudes by some of staff, especially when we feel vulnerable and lack power, may all fracture our sense of dignity (Chochinov 2007). An LTC home makes dignity-conserving care its core concept and works diligently to relieve the psychological and spiritual suffering of its residents.

Reports from the Institute of Medicine and many other sources are replete with data and stories about the poor quality of care in LTC facilities (Institute of Medicine 2003). It is a tragedy and a sad reflection on our society that, for many elderly persons, a social death occurs long before physical death, with a sense of isolation, disenfranchisement, and loss of control (Owen 2005). We have learned from the past 200 years of caring for older adults that pessimism and neglect, often spawned by poor financial reimbursements for health care, can lead to declining standards of care, poor outcomes, and a decreasing quality of life for people living in LTC facilities. Most of the successful changes in LTC up to this point have involved reducing the frequency of certain poor practices, rather than adopting new practices. It is the latter type of change that needs to begin now. Substantial improvements in the current quality of mental health care provided in LTC facilities must be made in order to improve the quality of life for the majority their residents (American Geriatrics Society and American Association for Geriatric Psychiatry 2003a).

LTC facilities must also embrace other systematic changes that will promote the quality of their residents' lives. These changes involve the concepts of culture change (with its corollary concept of innovative diffusion) and continuous quality improvement. Moreover, these changes are needed

TABLE 14.1
Key characteristics of an ideal long-term care home

Leadership characteristics
  A visionary leadership team that adopts the goal of making person-centered care routine rather
    than rare
  A leadership team that involves at least one physician with expertise in geriatrics (e.g., geriatrician,
    geriatric psychiatrist, certified advanced practice nurse in geriatrics)
  A medical director who has certification for nursing home medical directorship from the American
    Medical Directors Association
Quality of medical, psychiatric, vision, dental, and podiatric care
  High-quality, on-site medical, psychiatric, vision, dental, and podiatric care
  High level of availability and involvement of physicians and midlevel health care practitioners
    (nurse practitioners, physician assistants, clinical nurse specialists) with expertise in geriatrics
  Mental health care provided on site by a mental health care provider with expertise in geriatrics
    (e.g., geriatric psychiatrist)
  A high level of communication among physicians, midlevel health care practitioners, and the staff
  A culture of prevention
  Palliative care from the time a resident is admitted
  An interdisciplinary team approach
Psychosocial care
  Dignity-conserving care
  Loving relationships
  Routine spiritual care
  Acknowledgment and facilitation of the residents' need for sexual intimacy, regardless of their
    sexual orientation
  Cultural sensitivity
Resident's family
  Excellent psychosocial support for the resident's family
  A high level of family involvement in meeting the resident's psychosocial needs
  Family volunteerism at the long-term care home and thus integration into the milieu
Characteristics of the staff
  Adequate staffing levels to provide good-quality care for all residents at all times
  Ongoing training to improve staff skills in providing person-centered and evidence-based care for
    behavioral and psychological symptoms of dementia
  Staff members rigorously trained in dementia care, person-centered care, and palliative care
  Well-paid staff members
  Permanent assignments for the majority of (and preferably all) staff members, making it possible
    for them to form close relationships with the residents and their families
  An overarching care goal of making each day of the resident's stay as pleasant and meaningful as
    possible
  A culture in which staff members are expected and encouraged to show residents affection and
    spend time with them
  Much more respect and a greater voice in decision making given to nursing aides than is currently
    the case
  Excellent communication among staff members and between staff members and the family
Design
  Homelike, clean, and serene design for the facility
  Ample natural light and appropriate indoor lighting
  Wandering gardens and easy and safe access to the outdoors
  An individual room for each resident
  A high degree of accessibility to nature and natural surroundings
Activity programming
  High-quality, continuous activity programming that is commensurate with the cognitive abilities,
    interests, and talents of each resident

continued

TABLE 14.1 *continued*

Use of technology
  Electronic medical records
  Computerized physician order entry
  Free Wi-Fi access
Partnership with key organizations
  Alzheimer's Association
  American Medical Directors Association
  Bradford Dementia Group
  Aging and Disability Resource Centers
  Other organizations

at multiple levels: at the institutional level (concerning policy and training), at the unit level (regarding care procedures and follow-up), at the individual level (e.g., providing more scrutiny over the fit and function of hearing aids), and at the societal level (e.g., addressing the costs of designing an ideal LTC home and overall health care cost issues for the LTC population).

Culture Change

Culture change is a philosophy and a process that seeks to transform LTC facilities from restrictive institutions into vibrant and serene communities of older adults and the people who care for them. A key principle of culture change is that the residents and the staff will become empowered, self-determining decision makers. An organizational chart that embraces culture change does not flow from the top down, but rather is one that is likely to depict the resident in the center of a constellation of services that deliver direct and supportive care. Culture change should include providing an environment that reflects the comforts of home, including accommodations for married couples and residents with significant others, regardless of sexual orientation.

It is important to learn about the current culture in an LTC facility before embarking on culture change. This involves first taking time to listen to the residents and the staff. The leaders then need to understand and appreciate what they have heard in order to determine how to proceed. It is important to pace change, as it may take three to five years to revise the culture to become one that is highly person centered. One of the hardest things for a leadership team to do is to give up control. An outside consultant may be helpful in working periodically with the leadership team to help them relinquish some of their control as they continue to empower residents and staff.

Innovative Diffusion

More emphasis may be needed on the way change takes place within organizations. Innovative diffusion is the process by which change is adopted (Rogers 1995). The pace of change can be accelerated by paying attention to several dynamics, such as the relative advantage of the innovation, an investment in a trial period, the extent to which potential adopters can witness the positive outcomes of other users, communication with opinion leaders, the adaptability of the innovation itself, its compatibility with existing technology and systems of care, and the existence of a compatible infrastructure to support the innovation. Effective change requires careful planning, and ongoing support, coupled with one of the models of how to approach culture change, appear to be a feasible way of accomplishing this.

Models of Culture Change

A regenerative care model is based on the view that aging is a stage of life during which a person can still develop. This model is resident centered and seeks to increase the residents' autonomy and control. The notion of continued personal growth that is inherent in this model is supported by a management philosophy of allowing the residents control over their lives, continued learning, and a community focus. The model's learning circles involve residents expressing their opinions, preferences, concerns, and interests in certain activities and events.

A neighborhood model of culture change offers smaller units (eight to 20 residents), consistent staff assignments, separate dining and living room areas, and local (i.e., community) decision making. Typically, a neighborhood or community director (or manager or coordinator), selected or appointed from among the staff, facilitates the discussion and solicits input from each resident. The neighborhood staff can also attend the meeting.

Five Steps to Transform the Culture of a Long-Term Care Facility

1. Focus on senior leaders. The senior leadership team, which includes the board of trustees, administrators, the director of nursing, the medical director, and the mental health director (or the director of psychosocial well-being) needs to be inspirational and visionary, to be teachers and mentors to create an LTC home in which all residents have opportunities to thrive.

2. Communicate the message. Leaders need to take time to explain what they mean, and they need to mean what they say. For example, culture

change and person-centered care need to be defined and explained to all staff members to achieve the engagement of all stakeholders on a journey of transformation.

3. Use objective measures. Employ these measures to assess a successful person-centered care culture, and use the data as learning tools to achieve benchmark goals.

4. Tap into the leadership skills of all team members. Transformational leaders need to ask questions that will motivate the staff members to think critically about their roles and about how to solve problems that impede progress toward person-centered care.

5. Have patience. Creating an ideal LTC home takes time and effort. Time should be used as a resource to be managed strategically. Setting reasonable goals and making wise choices to accomplish a few crucial objectives (versus the many important ones) are some examples of how time can be optimized.

Continuous Quality Improvement

Continuous quality improvement is both a philosophy and an attitude. It involves analyzing capabilities and processes and improving them repeatedly to achieve its objective, which is customer satisfaction. It does not emphasize blame, but instead promotes innovation and focuses on a team approach to improving care that incorporates workers at every level of the organization. Continuous quality improvement is one of the primary means of upgrading the quality of health care in LTC facilities.

Any culture change should have a strong emphasis on continuous quality improvement, based on established indicators of quality (table 14.2). Continued development, innovation, and collaboration are also necessary to fully address the issues that influence the residents' mental health (White 2005). The implementation of quality improvement was found to be greater in nursing homes with an organized culture that emphasized innovation and teamwork. Employees of nursing homes that implement and demonstrate a greater degree of quality improvement may have greater job satisfaction and may be more likely to adopt specific clinical guidelines. Nursing homes in the United States can use their data (as reported in the On-Line Survey Certification and Reporting [OSCAR] and the Minimum Data Set Quality Indicator) to compare their facility with others in their region, their state, and the nation.

TABLE 14.2
*Indicators that can be tracked to measure continuous
quality improvement*

Reducing the occurrence of high-risk pressure ulcers
Reducing the use of physical restraints
Reducing the prescription of inappropriate medications
Improving the management of pain (physical and emotional)
Establishing individual targets for improving quality
Assessing resident and family satisfaction with the quality of care
Increasing staff retention
Improving the consistent assignment of staff members, so that the
    residents regularly receive care from the same caregiver

The Leadership Team

Leadership is required to develop and sustain an ideal LTC home. Each member of an ideal leadership team exudes kindness, humanity, and respect—the core values of providing care. The leadership team leads the charge to create a climate of organizational warmth in which optimism, trust, and generosity can thrive. Table 14.3 lists the characteristics of an ideal leadership team. Networking with experts, in-house leadership seminars, and peer mentoring help sustain leaders at all levels. To address the multiple components necessary for system-level change in a person-centered environment, Quality Partners of Rhode Island (www.riqualitypartners.org) developed the HATCh (Holistic Approach to Transformational Change) model, which encompasses improvement efforts in care practices, the LTC environment, workplace prac-

TABLE 14.3
Characteristics of an ideal leadership team

High ethical standards
Compassion (a deep awareness of the suffering of another coupled with a wish to relieve it)
Interdependence (i.e., reliance on one another for mutual support or sustenance)
Conscientiousness (i.e., a disposition to be organized, diligent, and goal oriented)
Openness (i.e., intellectual curiosity, imaginativeness)
A high priority given to one's own health (emotional, physical, and spiritual)
Belief in a holistic approach
The ability to lighten up, and to have a healthy sense of humor
An awareness of the difference between curing and healing
Knowledge of support systems, structures, and procedures that promote safety and reliability
Provision of intensive training for the staff during routine operations
Routine examinations to assess safety and reliability, and an analysis process for accidents and
    mistakes that incorporates organizational learning
Promotion of a culture of safety that is embedded in the organization

tices, leadership, the regulatory environment, and the community. We urge all leaders of LTC facilities to adopt the HATCh model.

The leadership team in an ideal LTC home needs to develop a culture of safety (Bonner et al. 2008). For example, the team should aggressively address elements of a resident-safety mindset by encouraging open communication and nonpunitive responses to errors and by building teamwork within units. Such an approach helps LTC homes avoid catastrophes in an environment in which normal accidents can be expected (because of complexity or other risk factors). The leadership team should periodically ask staff members about things they have learned as they provide care to the residents and what changes are needed to improve current practices. Learning and continuous improvement are inextricably linked in the evolution of a culture of safety.

Leadership work in any field, and especially in LTC, is rigorous but rewarding. Focusing on one's own health (physical, emotional, and spiritual) is crucial to a professionally and personally balanced life. Leaders who focus on self-care also serve as role models for staff members to do so. Leaders are encouraged to share their methods to prevent burnout (e.g., find meaning in your work, exercise, learn to say "No" when you are feeling stretched, make some time for yourself, have a hobby or a second passion [e.g., play a musical instrument]) with other staff members.

The leadership team itself needs to subscribe to, as well as to guide the staff members in following, several ethical principles of health care for residents (table 14.4). Having a connection to the LTC home, its residents, the staff, and other stakeholders is a key characteristic of the best administrators, medical directors, and others on the leadership team. Excellent leaders emphasize that every day presents opportunities to communicate, learn, teach, and praise fellow staff members.

TABLE 14.4
Ethical principles of health care for residents

Respect for dignity

Well-being

Participation: irrespective of their capacities, all residents are enabled to participate as much as possible in their own care

Equal consideration: caring for the caregivers (family and professional) is as important as caring for the residents

Nonabandonment

Moderation: care is provided in the least intrusive and least restrictive—yet fully adequate—manner

Proportionality: care is offered at a level of organizational capacity that is proportionate to the needs and concerns of the residents and their caregivers

Due to the limited availability of board-certified geriatricians (approximately 8,000) and board-certified geriatric psychiatrists (approximately 1,700), certified advanced practice nurses in geriatrics (approximately 3,500) should be given leadership roles (e.g., medical directorships) in LTC assisted living and nursing homes (Willging 2008).

High-Quality Health Care

High-quality health care (medical, psychiatric, dental, vision, podiatric) is an integral component of an ideal LTC home. Preventive medicine and a focus on physical, emotional, and spiritual well-being are core concepts of health care services in an ideal LTC home. This includes high-quality mental health care, involving the routine presence of a qualified mental health clinician in the LTC home, interdisciplinary and multidimensional services, and innovative approaches to blending training and education with consultation and feedback on clinical practices (Bartels, Moak, and Dums 2002). Table 14.5 lists some areas amenable to prevention efforts in LTC facilities (Davis, Smith, and Tyler 2005; Capezuti et al. 2007). For example, implementing a falls prevention program may involve identifying residents who are at high risk, performing fall-risk assessments, developing individual care plans, following up with the staff and the residents, and having a designated fall nurse spend half to a full day each week on the falls prevention and management program (Rask et al. 2007).

Health care providers are encouraged to partner with LTC homes and health care delivery organizations (e.g., local medical schools and universities) to develop evidence-based prevention programs. High-quality medical care makes use of and implements, whenever possible, the American Medical Directors Association's *Clinical Practice Guidelines* (www.amda.com). Examples of the conditions for which clinical practice guidelines are available include dementia, depression, falls and osteoporosis, delirium and acute problematic behavior, diabetes management, and pain management for LTC residents. Exercises, rehabilitative therapies, dental services, and chiropractic therapies should all be considered part of a comprehensive program that is clearly defined in the care plans.

High-quality health care can be best provided by an interdisciplinary team. Interdisciplinary teams employ communication, collaboration, cooperation, and coordination among disciplines to address a specific problem. Although financial barriers to interdisciplinary teams becoming a reality in LTC facilities are considerable in many settings, the establishment of an interdisciplin-

TABLE 14.5
Examples of prevention programs for long-term care homes

Prevention of pain (e.g., through aggressive treatment of acute pain, treatment of a vitamin D deficiency)

Prevention of pressure ulcers, or decubiti (e.g., through the prevention of nutritional deficiencies)

Prevention of falls and injuries (e.g., hip fractures, through a regular exercise program such as tai chi; routine screening for and treatment of osteoporosis)

Prevention from using restraints (e.g., through staff training in psychosocial-environmental interventions to manage problematic behaviors; availability of same-day, on-site assessment by a health care professional such as an advanced practice nurse)

Prevention of dehydration (e.g., through encouraging the frequent intake of fluid)

Prevention of constipation (e.g., through a prophylactic use of laxatives to prevent opioid-induced constipation)

Prevention of incontinence (e.g., through scheduled toileting and prompt voiding)

Prevention of dry skin (e.g., through the daily use of moisturizing lotion on high-risk areas)

Prevention of nutritional problems, such as a vitamin deficiency or protein-energy malnutrition (e.g., through the use of nutritional supplements)

Prevention of sarcopenia (e.g., through strength training)

Prevention of pneumonia (e.g., through the use of pneumococcal vaccines)

Prevention of dental problems (e.g., through periodic dental exams)

Prevention of vision impairments (e.g., through the correction of cataracts)

Prevention of hearing impairments (e.g., through a system-wide commitment to improve the use of hearing aids; staff training in the appropriate use of hearing aids; removal of ear wax)

Prevention of drug-induced cognitive decline, functional decline, and drug-induced behavioral and psychological symptoms (e.g., through avoiding the use of medications that are on the Beer's list)

Prevention of errors during the transition from a hospital to a long-term care facility and vice versa (e.g., through the use of standardized transfer forms [see www.amda.com for a copy of the universal transfer form])

Prevention of excess disability (e.g., through a better alignment between environmental demands and the preserved abilities of residents)

Prevention of depression (e.g., through exposure to adult day programs before admission to a long-term care facility; planned admission to the LTC facility rather than an unplanned admission)

Prevention of suicide (e.g., through a routine assessment for suicide risk at the time of admission to a long-term care home)

Prevention of insomnia (e.g., through increased exposure to bright light in the daytime)

Prevention of physical aggression by residents (e.g., through staff training to detect and treat the cause of agitation and verbal aggression before it escalates into physical aggression)

Prevention of unnecessary transfers to an emergency room or hospital (e.g., by treating pneumonia in the nursing home when appropriate; implementing palliative and hospice care options)

Prevention of a prolongation of the dying process that is not in keeping with the resident's wishes (e.g., by providing timely palliative and hospice care)

---

ary team should still be a goal in most facilities. Organizational leaders need to set expectations so that teamwork will occur, and they should support its careful development and ongoing maintenance. Team-building exercises and opportunities for team members to interact in a relaxed and open atmosphere are important. Creative solutions, such as a ten-minute huddle during which key staff members (CNA, nurse, social worker, and physician) meet to discuss a problem (e.g., persistent aggression), and then further communication and collaboration through telephone calls and e-mails, may be a practical way to work as an interdisciplinary team. The resident's nursing assistant or nurse can be the team leader and coordinator, as she or he is always there and knows the situation better than other team members.

Availability and Accessibility of Health Care Providers

In an ideal LTC home, health care providers (physicians, midlevel practitioners [e.g., nurse practitioners, physician assistants], pharmacists) are both available and accessible. Health care providers must focus on the care of the resident and advocate for the resident. They must be visible and available to the residents, their families, and the staff for questions related to resident care. They should also try to partner with the residents and their families in coping with health conditions, rather than managing the residents in an authoritarian, "I know what is best" manner. Health care providers who are willing to do what is right despite barriers posed by inadequate reimbursement and other system issues, and who are capable of crossing over to neighboring disciplines (e.g., palliative care, mental health), will be the future leaders of LTC.

The Psychosocial Well-Being Program

An ideal psychosocial well-being program adopts a resident-centered care model, provides continuous activity programming, and understands the residents' behavioral and psychological symptoms as expressions of their unmet biological, psychosocial, spiritual, cultural, and environmental needs.

- Biological: Reduce excess disability (e.g., pain, sensory impairment, psychiatric disorders [depression, psychotic symptoms]), reduce medication-related problems (medication errors, inappropriate medication, adverse drug events), and employ evidence-based care of medical and psychiatric disorders.
- Psychosocial: Know the residents, develop a trusting and caring relationship with the residents, and meet the residents' psychosocial needs through psychosocial interventions and environmental modifications.
- Spiritual: Meet the residents' spiritual needs.
- Cultural: Respect and encourage the expression of the residents' cultural beliefs and rituals.
- Environmental: Maintain clean facilities with plenty of natural sun-

light, make them esthetically pleasing, and provide ample opportunities to be with nature (wandering gardens and the like).

The Staff

Staff job satisfaction is a crucial component of an ideal LTC home. Increasing the time that staff members spend with residents is key to improving their job satisfaction (Tyler et al. 2006). Managers should strive for consistent staffing assignments, so that a staff member takes care of the same residents each day and gets to know those residents, their schedules, and their preferences. An emphasis on team effort and staff flexibility also helps sustain improvements in the quality of care. Health care providers must strive to deliver high-quality care, with the goal of a heightened quality of life for all residents. Attending to the welfare and ongoing training of staff members who have demonstrated a commitment to their jobs may lessen their tendency to become jaded over time or to seek job opportunities elsewhere. Staff members, especially CNAs, routinely experience abusive behavior from the residents, including, but not limited to, being yelled at, talked down to, called names, and cursed at, as well as being a target of rage reactions, physical aggression, and sexually disinhibited behavior (verbal and physical). This causes immense stress. Supporting the staff and providing high-quality training in dealing with these situations is an important aspect of person-centered care.

Table 14.6 lists examples of programs an LTC home may initiate (Furman et al. 2007). For example, safe patient handling (e.g., lifting, transferring) using a comprehensive patient-care ergonomic program results not only in fewer and less-severe injuries to caregivers, but also in less pain, less combativeness, and less depression in residents (Nelson et al. 2008). As another example, residents who have improved urinary continence are more engaged in activities, have a lower fall risk, and are more alert during the day.

Professional caregivers must seek to understand each resident's culture and then use that information to create an environment of healing around that resident. For example, ritual and ceremony can play an important role for residents with a Native American heritage. Cultural sensitivity training for the staff, the residents, and their families can assist LTC homes to provide an environment in which older lesbians and gay men do not need to be fearful or hide, but instead can experience the same quality of life as older adults in general (H. Cohen et al. 2008).

Developing productive relationships with state surveyors, promoting creativity in the residents, and recognizing that risk taking is a normal part

TABLE 14.6
Examples of initiatives and programs an ideal long-term care home may adopt

Know the residents
Detect and treat depression early
Prevent suicide
Detect and treat pain early
Implement a systematic, individualized intervention for the treatment of agitation
Employ a medication-safety or a medication-review team (geriatrician, geriatric psychiatrist, pharmacist, occupational therapist, nurse)
Institute a safe patient-handling program
Introduce mindfulness in routine care
Implement a program to extinguish caregiver burnout
Implement "dressing without stressing"
Discuss the goals of care

of adult life are important tasks for LTC staff. The consistent ethical thread throughout culture change is resident self-direction and resident (and staff) empowerment (Mitty 2005).

Barriers to Achieving an Ideal Long-Term Care Home

Providing high-quality care in LTC facilities presents considerable challenges. Complex medical problems, psychosocial issues and family dynamics, unrealistic expectations of the residents and their families, unrealistic expectations of the staff regarding the role of psychotropic medications to "fix" agitation, a high workforce turnover, stringent fiscal constraints, a frequently adversarial regulatory process, and heightened legal liability are just some of the challenges health care providers face. While seemingly paradoxical, higher administrative expenses (implying more management capacity) may reduce both staff turnover and staffing levels (Kash, Castle, and Phillips 2007). Employee recognition programs may improve staff satisfaction. Such programs routinely recognize the hard and creative work of members of an interdisciplinary team both individually and collectively.

A lack of adequate staffing (in quantity and quality) and a lack of high-quality staff training are also major barriers. According to the Centers for Medicare and Medicaid Services (CMS), nursing home residents, on average, receive a half-hour of care per day from a registered nurse, 48 minutes from a licensed practical nurse, and two hours and 18 minutes from an aide. Hands-on intensive training (e.g., provided by the Alzheimer's Association and by Dementia Care Mapping) is not routinely made available to the staff of LTC facilities.

The lack of research regarding LTC populations is another major barrier. The relevance of the DSM-IV-TR psychiatric diagnostic system to residents of LTC facilities is unclear. Epidemiological data on behavioral and psychological symptoms and psychiatric disorders in LTC populations are still preliminary. Well-designed, large, randomized controlled trials in LTC populations regarding pharmacological and psychosocial-environmental interventions are just beginning to shed light on the best interventions for behavioral and psychological symptoms. There are not many rigorous studies of palliative care in LTC, and those that have been done have been published only in the last few years. Before 2002, most published studies regarding palliative care in LTC residents were descriptive. Thus there is a crucial need for research on creative and innovative solutions aimed at improving the quality of end-of-life care in an LTC setting (Oliver, Porock, and Zweig 2004).

Racial inequalities are prevalent in health care services involving LTC populations. Unrecognized systematic and individual stereotyping may be a factor in racial inequity regarding the use of hospice care (e.g., African Americans use a hospice less than whites) (Greiner, Perera, and Ahluwalia 2003). Do Not Resuscitate orders are less common among blacks and Latinos than among whites. Latinos are less likely to have feeding tube restrictions than blacks and whites, and living wills are less prevalent among blacks (Dobalian 2006).

Age discrimination is another significant barrier. The design of treatment interventions should be based on a resident's needs and strengths. System problems exist, such as an overt or covert discouragement of reporting pain, or staffing schedules that do not allow for an efficient transfer of information from front-line providers to supervisors who can confirm the information and take action. One strategy to identify system problems is to ask a sample of residents who are cognitively intact what happens if they complain of pain or request pain medicine. Their answers can provide insight into the facility's informal and actual (as opposed to written) policies and procedures.

Financial disparities can significantly influence the care received in an LTC facility. Poor people are less likely to have living wills, and LTC facilities with a large Medicaid population may not have adequate resources to hire key team members such as recreational therapists, music therapists, and art therapists. High levels of community support and periodic fundraising drives may help reduce these financial barriers. San Francisco's multicultural Bethany Center, a 40-year-old Housing and Urban Development home for frail elderly residents, offers one of the best models for caring for the nation's 6.4 million dual-eligible Medicaid and Medicare elderly and for disabled people who have few financial resources but require intensive and expensive care. Inadequate reimbursement is another significant barrier to providing high-quality care to LTC populations. The government can play a key role in boosting the quality of care provided in LTC facilities in several ways, such as providing a higher reimbursement to professional caregivers for family meetings, extending the six-month limit for hospice care for residents with dementia, and raising the amount paid to LTC facilities for residents who are on Medicaid.

Helping Prospective Residents and Their Families Choose a Long-Term Care Facility

LTC facilities can help prospective residents and their families choose a facility by inviting them to come for both scheduled visits and informal unannounced visits, encouraging the families of current residents to give their candid opinions to prospective residents and their families, and training the staff to be professional and warm at all times in welcoming prospective residents and their families, as well as promptly addressing their concerns. Nursing homes should encourage prospective residents and their families to review their recent state inspection results, which are public documents that are available upon request. Nursing homes should encourage prospective residents and their families to review quality-improvement data on nursing homes (available online at www.medicare.gov). LTC facilities can also encourage prospective residents and their families to visit the Web pages of the American Association of Homes and Services for the Aging and the American Health Care Association, the umbrella organizations for most of the nursing homes in the United States.

Technology in Long-Term Care Homes

Electronic medical records and computerized physician order entry may, over time, greatly enhance the quality of care for LTC residents. Many LTC facilities are making creative uses of technology to implement evidence-based practices and maximize quality. Involving physicians in the planning process to implement technology is crucial for its success. Examples of such projects include using electronic records in addressing vitamin D deficiencies in residents and in gradually reducing doses of antipsychotic medications. Implementing clinical practice guidelines is another excellent use of technology to achieve and sustain an ideal LTC home. Using medication safety teams and implementing technology-driven practices may substantially reduce prevent-

AN IDEAL LONG-TERM CARE HOME   417

able adverse drug events in LTC populations (Vogelsmeier, Halbesleben, and Scott-Cawiezell 2008). An ideal LTC home may provide free wireless internet access to residents and visitors, as well as a computer room with free access to computers. This may also encourage adolescents, young children, and the grandchildren of residents to spend more time in the LTC home.

The Role of Nonprofit Organizations and the Government

An ideal LTC home forges a close relationship with the local chapter of the Alzheimer's Association. This organization's staff members provide state-of-the-art education and training on all aspects of dementia (from teaching the basics of what dementia is to providing personal care for people with advanced dementia). Staff members of the Alzheimer's Association also provide many services that are of benefit to residents (e.g., support groups for residents with mild dementia) and their families (e.g., support groups for caregivers).

The Bradford Dementia Group, a part of the University of Bradford in the United Kingdom, continually refines the dementia care mapping method developed by the originator of person-centered care, the late Tom Kitwood. Dementia care mapping is a method to evaluate and improve the care given to persons with dementia in formal care settings (e.g., LTC homes). Dementia care mapping is a complex tool, and training in this method is available only from trainers approved by the Bradford Dementia Group (e.g., Jentle Harts Consulting, www.jentleharts.com), who have undergone a rigorous preparation for this role.

Aging Disability and Resource Centers (ADRCs) are one-stop shops that supply vital information to elders in the community. They help consumers understand their options and learn about services, so that they can make informed decisions. The U.S. Agency on Aging and the CMS are partnering to fund ADRCs in more than 100 communities in 43 states. LTC homes can make informational brochures from ADRCs available to residents and their families.

Psychosocial well-being, palliative care, and end-of-life care for residents in LTC facilities should be seen as an urgent public health issue, and the government should provide funding for such services. Increased funding for psychosocial well-being, palliative care, and end-of-life care for residents in LTC facilities may reduce the government's overall costs for LTC, primarily by reducing inappropriate or unnecessary hospitalizations and futile care. Policy makers must continue to give a high priority to the quality and safety of LTC, which is perhaps as important a concern as Medicaid. Improving state surveyors' knowledge in diverse aspects of health care (e.g., feeding tubes, nutrition, and weight loss) is critically important in improving the quality of life for the residents and their families, as well as the staff, in LTC homes.

Many organizations are devoted to improving the quality of life for LTC residents (table 14.7). An ideal LTC home actively partners with such organizations. For example, Quality Partners of Rhode Island (www.riqualitypart ners.org), the national Nursing Home Quality Improvement Organization Support Center since 2001 (contracted by CMS), provides clinical support and quality-improvement materials to quality-improvement organizations throughout the United States (Ouslander, Patry, and Besdine 2007). Quality-improvement organizations work with nursing homes to set performance targets for quality measures using the CMS "Setting Targets—Achieving Results" Web site (www.nhqualitycampaign.org), using a new care process tool (the Nursing Home Improvement Feedback Tool), measuring resident and staff satisfaction, and reducing the turnover of CNAs. The Medicare quality-improvement support Web site (www.medqic.org) has a variety of tools that can be adapted for use by health care providers (including the medical directors of nursing homes). Organizations such as the American Association of Homes and Services for the Aging and the American Health Care Association provide resources and models to improve quality through culture change and systematic approaches to continuous quality improvement. Nursing homes are encouraged to sign up for the national campaign to improve the quality of nursing home care at www.nhqualitycampaign.org.

Preparing for the Residents of the Future

In the next 20 years, 78 million baby boomers will be entering their senior years. This baby boomer generation will be more knowledgeable, assertive, computer-savvy, and vocal consumers than the current generation of seniors (Kodner 1993). They will expect more preventive and well-being services, greater access to technology, and more sophisticated information from providers to help them make informed choices about treatment, care, and housing to best match their values and preferences. Baby boomers will want services based less on aging than on their interests, hobbies, and politics. An ideal LTC home will start addressing these needs now, because a growing number of current seniors have the take-charge attitude typical of baby boomers. In fact, a future LTC home may look completely different from current models, as baby boomers will be less inclined to follow age-segregated lifestyles. Holistic wellness programs (e.g., brain-and-memory fitness programs to delay

TABLE 14.7
Some organizations devoted to enhancing the quality of life for long-term care residents

Advancing Excellence in America's Nursing Homes

Alliance for Quality Nursing Home Care

American Association of Geriatric Psychiatry

American Association of Homes and Services for the Aging

American Association of Nurse Assessment Coordinators

American College of Health Care Administrators

American Geriatric Society

American Health Care Association

American Medical Directors Association

Centers for Medicare and Medicaid Services and its contractors (i.e., the Quality Improvement
   Organizations and their national support center [Quality Improvement Organization Support
   Center], managed by Quality Partners of Rhode Island)

Gerontological Society of America

Institute for Healthcare Improvement

International Psychogeriatric Association

National Citizens Coalition for Nursing Home Reform

National Commission for Quality Long-Term Care

Pioneer Network

the onset or slow the progression of dementia), preferably within a spa in an LTC home, may become more popular. Many cruise ships may be converted to continuing care retirement communities.

As baby boomers age, the need for LTC services will increase dramatically. In the future, there may not be enough LTC facilities to accommodate all of these people. Smart-home technology may enable many to age in place with emergency assistance, fall prevention/detection, reminder systems, medication administration, and assistance for those with hearing, visual, or cognitive impairments (Cheek, Nikpour, and Nowlin 2005). Smart-home technology will help older people by providing continuous monitoring and thus improve their psychosocial well-being. Future technology in LTC homes will support virtual teamwork, telehealth, disease management, and information sharing through the use of electronic medical records. As families spread out geographically, there will be a greater need for long-distance caregiving, which will benefit greatly from robotics and video- and Web-based communications.

Whatever the face of future LTC homes may be, more physicians and midlevel health care providers, preferably with expertise in geriatrics, will be needed to work in LTC settings. Future LTC homes, as well as many other health care settings, will use health-information technology that will be interoperable and implemented across all settings. Sooner or later, our society as a whole will need to grapple with the difficult issues both of meeting the health care needs of elderly people in the future and of distributive justice (i.e., how much of the country's limited resources should be allotted to what aspect of caring for frail elderly people [e.g., life-prolonging care versus palliative or preventive care]).

Conclusion

Restoring public confidence in long-term care is overdue. Vigorous efforts to establish an ideal LTC home should be a key step in achieving this. The paramount goals of professional caregivers in LTC homes are to maximize the residents' independence, ensure dignity, promote choice, create a sense of community, and be the driving force for quality and efficiency. All of these should be incorporated into both the mission and the vision of an LTC home. A top-down administrative style will have to be replaced by a team approach in which direction from consumers occupies the most important position in all of the facility's decision making. The ultimate goal is to make the aging process in LTC homes as healthy as it can be for everyone. In the future, LTC homes will be person-centered, technologically driven, and more tightly focused on prevention and wellness. However, even in the best LTC homes, there is always room for improvement. Creating an ideal LTC home is not a destination but a journey, and the time to act is now.

Abbreviations

AD	Alzheimer disease
ADLs	activities of daily living
ADRCs	Aging Disability and Resource Centers
AIDS	acquired immune-deficiency syndrome
AIMS	Abnormal Involuntary Movement Scale
aMCI	amnestic mild cognitive impairment
BEHAVE-AD	Behavioral Symptoms in Alzheimer's Disease
BMI	body mass index
BUN	blood urea nitrogen
BZs	benzodiazepines
CADASIL	cerebral autosomal dominant arteriopathy with subcortical infarcts and leuko-encephalopathy
CAM	Confusion Assessment Method
CBC	complete blood count
CBZ	carbamazepine
ChEI	cholinesterase inhibitor
CJD	Creutzfeldt-Jakob disease
CMAI	Cohen-Mansfield Agitation Inventory
CNA	certified nursing assistant
CMS	Centers for Medicare and Medicaid Services
COPD	chronic obstructive pulmonary disease
COWAT	Controlled Oral Word Association Test
COX-2	cyclooxygenase-2
CPAP	continuous positive airway pressure
CPR	cardiopulmonary resuscitation
CPS	Cognitive Performance Scale

CSDD	Cornell Scale for Depression in Dementia
CSF	cerebrospinal fluid
CT	computed tomography
DLB	dementia with Lewy bodies
DNH	Do Not Hospitalize
DNI	Do Not Intubate
DNR	Do Not Resuscitate
DSM-IV-TR	*Diagnostic and Statistical Manual of Mental Disorders*, 4th ed., text revision
ECT	electroconvulsive therapy
EdFED-Q	Edinburgh Feeding Evaluation in Dementia Questionnaire
EEG	electroencephalogram
EKG	electrocardiogram
EPS	extrapyramidal symptoms
ETOH	ethanol
FAQ	Functional Activity Questionnaire
FDA	U.S. Food and Drug Administration
FTA-ABS	fluorescent treponemal antibody absorption test
FTD	frontotemporal dementia
FTDfv	frontal lobe variant of frontotemporal dementia
FTDP-17	frontotemporal dementia with parkinsonism linked to chromosome 17
GAD	generalized anxiety disorder
GDS	Geriatric Depression Scale
GERD	gastroesophageal reflux disease
HAD	HIV-associated dementia
HATCh	Holistic Approach to Transformational Change
HD	Huntington disease
HIV	human immunodeficiency virus
IADLs	instrumental activities of daily living
LPN	licensed practical nurse
LTC	long-term care
MCI	mild cognitive impairment
MDD	major depressive disorder
MDS	Minimum Data Set
MM-CGI	Marwit-Meuser Caregiver Grief Inventory
MMSE	Mini-Mental State Examination
MNA	Mini Nutritional Assessment
MRI	magnetic resonance imaging
MRSA	methicillin-resistant *Staphylococcus aureus*

NMDA	N-methyl-D-aspartate
NPH	normal pressure hydrocephalus
NPI	Neuropsychiatric Inventory
NPI-NH	Neuropsychiatric Inventory-Nursing Home Version
NSAID	nonsteroidal anti-inflammatory drug
OBRA	Omnibus Budget Reconciliation Act
OCD	obsessive-compulsive disorder
OSA	obstructive sleep apnea
OSCAR	On-Line Survey Certification and Reporting
OXC	oxcarbazepine
PAINAD	Pain Assessment in Advanced Dementia
PCA	patient-controlled analgesia
PD	Parkinson disease
PDD	Parkinson disease dementia
PDPsy	persistent psychotic symptoms with Parkinson disease
PET	positron emission tomography
PHQ	Patient Health Questionnaire
PSMS	Physical Self-Maintenance Scale
PTSD	post-traumatic stress disorder
RBD	REM sleep behavior disorder
REM	rapid eye movement
RLS	restless leg syndrome
RN	registered nurse
SAM-e	S-adenosyl methionine
SLUMS	Saint Louis University Mental State Examination
SSRI	selective serotonin reuptake inhibitor
TCA	tricyclic antidepressant
TIA	transient ischemic attack
TMT	Trail Making Test
TSH	thyroid-stimulating hormone
UTI	urinary tract infection
VaD	vascular dementia
ZBI	Zarit Burden Inventory

Resources

Practice Guidelines

Rabins, P. V., D. Blacker, B. W. Rovner, et al. 2007. *Practice Guidelines for the Treatment of Patients with Alzheimer's Disease and Other Dementias*, 2nd ed. Arlington, VA: American Psychiatric Publishing.

www.amda.com: The Web site of the American Medical Directors Association, the organization of medical directors of nursing homes. Various clinical practice guidelines for the assessment and treatment of common clinical syndromes (e.g., depression, pain, falls, delirium, behavioral disturbances) and palliative care in nursing homes are available through this site.

Books for Family Caregivers to Understand Dementia-Related Issues (Nontechnical)

Mace, N. L., and P. V. Rabins. 2006. *The 36-Hour Day: A Family Guide to Caring for Persons with Alzheimer Disease, Other Dementias, and Memory Loss in Later Life*, 4th ed. Baltimore: Johns Hopkins University Press.

Bell, V., and D. Troxel. 2002. *A Dignified Life: The Best Friends Approach to Alzheimer's Care; A Guide for Family Caregivers*. Deerfield Beach, FL: Health Communication.

Glenner, J. A., J. M. Stehman, J. Davagnino, M. J. Galante, and M. L. Green. 2005. *When Your Loved One Has Dementia: A Simple Guide for Caregivers*. Baltimore: Johns Hopkins University Press. This is a good beginning book for a person who is learning to care for someone with dementia.

Peterson, R. (ed.). 2002. *Mayo Clinic on Alzheimer's Disease*. Rochester, MN: Mayo Clinic.

Books for Health Care Professionals

Purtilo, R. P., and H. ten Have (eds.). 2004. *Ethical Foundations of Palliative Care for Alzheimer Disease*. Baltimore: Johns Hopkins University Press.

Brawley, E. 1997. *Designing for Alzheimer's Disease: Strategies for Creating Better Care Environments*. New York: Wiley.

Lynn, J., J. L. Schuster, and A. Kabecnell. 2008. *Improving Care for the End of Life: A Sourcebook for Health Care Managers and Clinicians*. New York: Oxford University Press.

Books For Baby Boomers Who Are Helping Their Elderly Family Members

McCullough, D. 2008. *My Mother, Your Mother: Embracing "Slow Medicine"; The Compassionate Approach to Caring for Your Aging Loved Ones*. New York: Harper.

Books for Family Caregivers to Cope with a Loved One's Being in a Long-Term Care Facility

Canfield, J., M. V. Hansen, and L. Thieman. 2004. *Chicken Soup for the Caregiver's Soul*. Deerfield Beach, FL: Health Communication.

Byers, M., A. Guyer, and N. Willich. 2005. *"Your Mother Has Alzheimer's": Three Daughters Answer Their Father's Call*. Ponte Vedra Beach, FL: Cord.

Jacobs, B. J. 2006. *The Emotional Survival Guide for Caregivers: Looking After Yourself and Your Family while Helping an Aging Parent*. New York: Guilford.

Hays, T. 2005. *The Pleasure Was Mine*. New York: St. Martin's Press. [Fiction.]

Schor, J. 2008. *The Nursing Home Guide: A Doctor Reveals What You Need to Know about Long-Term Care*. New York: Berkley.

Tanner, Ira J. 1980. *Healing the Pain of Everyday Loss*. New York, Harper Collins.

Books for Skill-Based Activities for Residents in Long-Term Care Facilities

Decker, J. A. 1997. *Making the Moments Count: Leisure Activities for Caregiving Relationships*. Baltimore: Johns Hopkins University Press.

American Therapeutic Recreation Association. *Simple Pleasures: A Multi-Level Sensorimotor Intervention for Nursing Home Residents with Dementia*. www.atra-online.com.

Camp, C. J. *A Different Visit*. www.myersresearch.org.

Palliative Care in Long-Term Care Facilities

Improving Palliative Care in Nursing Homes. A document freely available at the Web site of the Center to Advance Palliative Care (www.capc.org). This site is also rich in other resources regarding palliative care in long-term care facilities.

Residents' Rights, and Abuse and Neglect

The Long-Term Care Ombudsman Program, administered by the U.S. Administration on Aging through the LTC ombudsmen, is one of the best resources to learn about residents' rights and good care practices. The Web site (www.aoa.gov) provides useful information related to resident's rights and addresses concerns related to abuse and neglect.

Spirituality in Long-Term Care

Shamy, E. 2003. *A Guide to the Spiritual Dimension of Care for People with Alzheimer's Disease and Related Dementia: More than Body, Brain, and Breath.* Philadelphia: Jessica Kingsley.

Creativity in Long-Term Care

Basting, A., and J. Killick. 2003. *The Arts and Dementia Care.* Brooklyn: National Center for Creative Aging. Available through the Web site www.creativeaging.org. This book provides information about how to initiate, develop, and sustain arts programs for people with dementia. Examples of Web sites that are excellent resources for engaging residents in long-term care facilities in creative activities include

www.ageandcommunity.org: Center on Age and Community;

www.timeslips.org: TimeSlips, a program for group storytelling;

www.kairosdance.org: the Dancing Heart program is a way of reaching people with dementia; and

www.songwritingworks.org: the Songwriting Works program enables people with dementia to write songs.

Web Resources for Family and Professional Caregivers

http://neuroandpsych.slu.edu/healthybrain/: The Web site of the Center for Healthy Brain Aging, Department of Neurology and Psychiatry, Division of Geriatric Medicine, Saint Louis University School of Medicine.

http://aging.slu.edu/newsletters/: The Web site for *Aging Successfully* newsletters from the Center for Successful Aging, Department of Internal Medicine, Division of Geriatric Medicine, Saint Louis University School of Medicine.

Professional Associations and Other Resource-Rich Web Sites

www.alz.org: The Web site of the Alzheimer's Association (telephone: 800-272-3900). The Alzheimer's Association covers every aspect of Alzheimer disease and related dementias as they relate to physicians, researchers, patients, and family caregivers at this comprehensive, easy-to-use Web site. In addition, the Association's Campaign for Quality Residential Care has published *Dementia Care Practice Recommendations for Assisted Living Residents and Nursing Homes.*

http://hartfordign.org/: The John A. Hartford Institute for Geriatric Nursing has an excellent Web site for a variety of resources and information involving several aspects of caring for older adults (such as assessment tools and best practices for dementia, delirium, pain, depression, and nutrition).

www.psych.org: The Web site of the American Psychiatric Association includes a recent position paper on the diagnosis and treatment of dementia.

www.ipa-online.org: The International Psychogeriatric Association has produced a Behavioral and Psychological Symptoms of Dementia (BPSD) information pack, and one for nurses is in development.

www.geronet.med.ucla.edu/centers/borun/: The Web site of the Borun Center of Gerontological Research at UCLA has protocols, guidelines, and support information on pain management.

www.healthinaging.org: The Web site of the American Geriatrics Society's Foundation for Health in Aging has a wealth of educational material on caring for elderly people in long-term care facilities. The Society's public education Web page provides several resources. A free, text-only version of its caregiving guide, *Eldercare at Home*, offers a problem-solving approach to managing common problems that caregivers face. A link to "FHA Tip Sheets" includes one that has advice on avoiding caregiver burnout. The Foundation also provides a free referral service, accessed from that same Web page or at 800-563-4916, to connect caregivers and older adults with geriatrics health care professionals in their areas.

www.aagpgpa.org: The Web site of the American Association for Geriatric Psychiatry has a position paper on end-of-life care and many other resources useful for long-term care psychiatry practices. See the section for health care professionals to find educational resources related to important issues in geriatric care, including family and caregiver counseling, access to psychiatric care, facts about mental health in geriatric patients, and more.

www.gmhfonline.org: The Geriatric Mental Health Foundation has an excellent Web site for finding local geriatric psychiatrists.

www.nia.nih.gov: The Web site of the National Institute on Aging's Alzheimer's Disease Education and Referral Center (ADEAR) has many resources for patients and their families regarding Alzheimer disease and other dementias.

www.aan.com/go/practice/guidelines/: The American Academy of Neurology has practice guidelines for dementia at this Web site.

www.aafp.org/online/en/home/clinical/clinicalrecs.html: The American Academy of Family Physicians has clinical practice guidelines for the current pharmacological management of dementia at this Web site.

www.agis.com: An online resource for family caregivers.

www.lbda.org: The Web site of the Lewy Body Dementia Association is an excellent source of information to understand clinical manifestations and treatment options for Lewy body dementia. It also has a list of resources for patient and caregiver support.

www.directcarealliance.org: This is a professional organization for certified nursing assistants. Various resources are available at this Web site to improve the education and training of CNAs working in long-term care facilities.

www.medqic.org: This Web site has a 152-page *Falls Management Program* manual that can be downloaded.

www.myinnerview.com: The Web site of My InnerView, a Wisconsin-based company that promotes an evidence-based approach to quality in long-term care.

www.musictherapy.org. The Web site of the American Music Therapy Association. Various resources and references regarding the potential benefits of music therapy for long-term care residents are available at this site.

www.patchadams.org: The Web site of the Gesundheit Institute, founded by physician-clown Patch Adams. This institute dedicates itself to laughter and holistic medicine.

www.worldlaughtertour.com: Laughter therapy.

www.snoezeleninfo.com: The Web site of FlagHouse, a leading Snozelen Multi-Sensory Environment (MSE) installer.

Dementia Care Mapping

www.brad.ac.uk/health/dementia/: The Web site of the Bradford Dementia Group, School of Health Studies, University of Bradford, Bradford, United Kingdom. This group was founded by the late Tom Kitwood. Dementia Care Mapping (DCM) was developed by Mr. Kitwood and is continually being refined with validity and reliability studies by the Bradford Dementia Group.

Jentle Harts Consulting: www.jentleharts.com. This is a good resource where long-term care facility personnel can get training in dementia care mapping.

References

Aalten, P., F. R. Verhey, M. Boziki, et al. 2007. Neuropsychiatric syndromes in dementia: Results from the European Alzheimer Disease Consortium, part 1. *Dementia and Geriatric Cognitive Disorders* 24:457–63.

Abrams, R., and J. Sadavoy. 2004. Personality disorders. In J. Sadovoy, L. F. Jarvik, G. T. Grossberg, and B. S. Meyers (eds.), *Comprehensive Textbook of Geriatric Psychiatry*, 3rd ed., pp. 701–22. New York: W. W. Norton.

Achterberg, W., A. M. Pot, A. Kerkstra, et al. 2006. Depressive symptoms in newly admitted nursing home residents. *International Journal of Geriatric Psychiatry* 21:1156–62.

Agronin, M. E. 2004. Somatoform disorders. In D. G. Blazer, D. C. Steffens, and E. W. Busse (eds.), *The American Psychiatric Publishing Textbook of Geriatric Psychiatry*, 3rd ed., 295–302. Washington, DC: American Psychiatric Publishing.

Agronin, M. E., and G. Maletta. 2000. Personality disorders in late life: Understanding and overcoming the gap in research. *American Journal of Geriatric Psychiatry* 8:4–18.

Albert, S. G., B. R. Nakra, G. T. Grossberg, et al. 1994. Drinking behavior and vasopressin responses to hyperosmolality in Alzheimer's disease. *International Psychogeriatrics* 6:79–86.

Alessi, C. A., J. L. Martin, A. P. Webber, et al. 2005. Randomized, controlled trial of a nonpharmacological intervention to improve abnormal sleep/wake patterns in nursing home residents. *Journal of the American Geriatrics Society* 53:803–10.

Alexopoulos, G. S., R. C. Abrams, R. C. Young, et al. 1988. Cornell Scale for Depression in Dementia. *Biological Psychiatry* 23:271–84.

Alexopoulos, G. S., B. S. Meyers, R. C. Young, et al. 1997. Vascular depression. *Archives of General Psychiatry* 54:915–22.

Alexopoulos, G. S., J. M. Silver, D. A. Kahn, et al. 1998. *The Expert Consensus Guideline Series: Treatment of Agitation in Older Persons with Dementia*. Minneapolis: McGraw-Hill.

Alexopoulos, G. S., D. V. Jeste, H. Chung, et al. 2005. *The Expert Consensus Guideline Series: Treatment of Dementia and Its Behavioral Disturbances*. Minneapolis: McGraw-Hill.

Allen, R. S., B. E. Thorn, S. E. Fisher, et al. 2003. Prescription and dosage of analgesic medication in relation to resident behaviors in the nursing home. *Journal of the American Geriatrics Society* 51:534–38.

Almeida, O., and S. Fenner. 2002. Bipolar disorder: Similarities and differences between patients with illness onset before and after 65 years of age. *International Psychogeriatrics* 14(3):311–22.

Alzheimer's Association. 2009. Alzheimer's disease facts and figures. *Alzheimer's and Dementia* 5:234–70.

Amella, E. J. 2004. Feeding and hydration issues for older adults with dementia. *Nursing Clinics of North America* 39:607–23.

American Diabetes Association. 2002. Position statement: Evidence-based nutrition principles and recommendations for the treatment and prevention of diabetes and related complications. *Diabetes Care* 25 (suppl. 1):S50–60.

American Geriatrics Society and American Association for Geriatric Psychiatry. 2003a. The American Geriatrics Society and American Association for Geriatric Psychiatry recommendations for policies in support of quality mental health care in U.S. nursing homes. *Journal of the American Geriatrics Society* 51:1299–1304.

———. 2003b. Consensus statement on improving the quality of mental health care in U.S. nursing homes: Management of depression and behavioral symptoms associated with dementia. *Journal of the American Geriatrics Society* 51:1287–98.

American Geriatrics Society Panel on Persistent Pain in Older Persons. 2002. The management of persistent pain in older adults. *Journal of the American Geriatrics Society* 50:S205–24.

American Health Care Association. 2001. *The Long Term Care Survey.* Washington, DC: American Health Care Association.

———. 2002. Results of the 2002 AHCA survey of nursing staff vacancy and turnover in nursing homes. www.ahcancal.org/research_data/ [accessed August 17, 2008].

American Medical Directors Association. 1999. *Clinical Practice Guideline on Chronic Pain Management in the Long-Term Care Setting.* www.amda.com/tools/guidelines.cfm.

American Psychiatric Association. 2004. *Diagnostic and Statistical Manual of Mental Disorders,* 4th ed., text revision. Washington, DC: American Psychiatric Press.

———. 2007. *Practice Guidelines for Treatment of Patients with Alzheimer's Disease and Other Dementias,* 2nd ed. www.psychiatryonline.com/pracGuide/pracGuideTopic_3.aspx.

Ancoli-Israel, S., M. R. Klauber, N. Butters, et al. 1991. Dementia in institutionalized elderly: Relations to sleep apnea. *Journal of the American Geriatrics Society* 3:258–63.

Andrews, G. J. 2006. Managing challenging behavior in dementia. *British Medical Journal* 332:741.

Aravanis, S. C., and American Medical Association. 1994. *Diagnostic and Treatment Guidelines on Elder Abuse and Neglect.* Chicago: American Medical Association.

Archer, N., R. G. Brown, S. J. Reeves, et al. 2007. Premorbid personality and behavioral and psychological symptoms in probable Alzheimer Disease. *American Journal of Geriatric Psychiatry* 15:202–13.

Archibald, C. 2006. Promoting hydration in patients with dementia in healthcare settings. *Nursing Stand* 20:49–52.

Armstrong, S. C., K. L. Cozza, and N. B. Sandson. 2003. Six patterns of drug-drug interactions. *Psychosomatics* 44:255–58.

Ashar, B. H., and A. Rowland-Seymour. 2008. Advising patients who use dietary supplements. *American Journal of Medicine* 121:91–97.

Assisted Living Federation of America. 2006. *Overview of Assisted Living: Facts and Trends*. Alexandria, VA: American Association of Homes and Services for the Aging.

Atkinson, R. M. 2004. Substance abuse. In J. Sadavoy, L. F. Jarvik, G. T. Grossberg, et al. (eds.), *Comprehensive Textbook of Geriatric Psychiatry*, 3rd ed., pp. 723–62. New York: W. W. Norton.

Atri, A., L. N. Shaughnessy, J. J. Locascio, et al. 2008. Long-term course and effectiveness of combination therapy in Alzheimer's disease. *Alzheimer Disease and Associated Disorders* 22:209–21.

Avorn, J., S. B. Soumerai, D. E. Everitt, et al. 1992. A randomized trial of a program to reduce the use of psychoactive drugs in nursing homes. *New England Journal of Medicine* 327:168–73.

Baer, W. M., and L. C. Hanson. 2000. Families' perception of the added value of hospice in the nursing home. *Journal of the American Geriatrics Society* 48:879–82.

Baik, H. W., and R. M. Russell. 1999. Vitamin B_{12} deficiency in the elderly. *Annual Review of Nutrition* 19:357–77.

Baker, H. 2007. Nutrition in the elderly: Nutritional aspects of chronic diseases. *Geriatrics* 62:21–25.

Bales, C. W., and G. Buhr. 2008. Is obesity bad for older persons? A systematic review of the pros and cons of weight reduction in later life. *Journal of the American Medical Directors Association* 9:302–12.

Ballantyne, J. C., and J. Mao. 2003. Opioid therapy for chronic pain. *New England Journal of Medicine* 349:1943–53.

Ballard, C. G., C. Bannister, M. Solis, et al. 1996. The prevalence, associations and symptoms of depression amongst dementia sufferers. *Journal of Affective Disorder* 36:135–44.

Ballard, C. G., J. Fossey, R. Chithramohan, et al. 2001. Quality of care in private sector and NHS facilities for people with dementia: Cross sectional survey. *British Medical Journal* 323:426–27.

Ballard, C. G., J. T. O'Brien, K. Reichelt, et al. 2002. Aromatherapy as a safe and effective treatment for the management of agitation in severe dementia: The results of a double-blind, placebo-controlled trial with Melissa. *Journal of Clinical Psychiatry* 63:553–58.

Ballard, C. G., A. Thomas, J. Fossey, et al. 2004. A 3-month, randomized, placebo-controlled, neuroleptic discontinuation study in 100 people with dementia: The Neuropsychiatric Inventory Median Cutoff is a predictor of clinical outcome. *Journal of Clinical Psychiatry* 65:114–19.

Bandelow, B., D. Wedekind, and T. Leon. 2007. Pregabalin for the treatment of generalized anxiety disorder: A novel pharmacologic intervention. *Expert Review of Neurotherapeutics* 7:769–81.

Banks, M. R., L. M. Willoughby, and W. A. Banks. 2008. Animal-assisted therapy and loneliness in nursing homes: Use of robotic versus living dogs. *Journal of the American Medical Directors Association* 9:173–77.

Barker, W. W., C. A. Luis, A. Kashuba, et al. 2002. Relative frequencies of Alzheimer disease, Lewy body, vascular and frontotemporal dementia, and hippocampal sclerosis in the State of Florida Brain Bank. *Alzheimer Disease and Associated Disorders* 16:203–12.

Barrett, A. M. 2005. Is it Alzheimer's disease or something else? *Postgraduate Medicine* 117:47–53.

Bartels, S. J., G. S. Moak, and A. R. Dums. 2002. Models of mental health services in nursing homes: A review of the literature. *Psychiatric Services* 53:1390–96.

Baum, L. W. 2005. Sex, hormones, and Alzheimer's disease. *Journals of Gerontology, Series A: Biological Sciences and Medical Sciences* 60A:736–43.

Baumgarten, M., J. A. Hanley, C. Infante-Rivard, et al. 1994. Health of family members caring for elderly persons with dementia: A longitudinal study. *Annals of Internal Medicine* 120:126–32.

Bedard, M., D. W. Molloy, L. Squire, et al. 2001. The Zarit Burden Interview: A new short version and screening version. *Gerontologist* 41:652–57.

Beekman, A. T., E. de Beurs, A. J. van Balkom, et al. 2000. Anxiety and depression in later life: Co-occurrence and commonality of risk factors. *American Journal of Psychiatry* 157:89–95.

Beitman, B. D., M. Kushner, and G. T. Grossberg. 1991. Late onset panic disorder: Evidence from a study of patients with chest pain and normal cardiac evaluations. *International Journal of Psychiatry and Medicine* 21:29–35.

Belle, S. H., L. Brugio, R. Burns, et al. 2006. Enhancing the quality of life of dementia caregivers from different ethnic or racial groups. *Annals of Internal Medicine* 145:727–38.

Berger, J. T. 2000. Sexuality and intimacy in the nursing home: A romantic couple of mixed cognitive capacities. *Journal of Clinical Ethics* 11:309–13.

Best-Martini, B., and K. A. Botenhagen-DiGenova. 2003. *Exercise for Frail Elders*. Champaign, IL: Human Kinetics Publishers.

Bigos, K. L., B. G. Pollock, K. C. Coley, et al. 2008. Sex, race, and smoking impact olanzapine exposure. *Journal of Clinical Pharmacology* 48:157–65.

Bishop, T. F., and R. S. Morrison. 2007. Geriatric palliative care—part 1: Pain and symptom management. *Clinical Geriatrics* 15:25–32.

Bjelakovic, G., D. Nikolova, L. L. Gluud, et al. 2007. Mortality in randomized trials of antioxidant supplements for primary and secondary prevention: Systematic review and meta-analysis. *Journal of the American Medical Association* 297:842–57.

Black, D. W., C. H. Baumgard, and S. E. Bell. 1995. A 16- to 45-year follow-up of 71 men with antisocial personality disorder. *Comprehensive Psychiatry* 36:130–40.

Blazer, D. G. 2002. *Depression in Late Life*. New York: Wiley.

Blazer, D. G., and C. F. Hybels. 2005. Origins of depression in later life. *Psychological Medicine* 35:1241–52.

Blazer, D. G., C. F. Hybels, and J. C. Hays. 2004. Demography and epidemiology of psychiatric disorders in late life. In D. G. Blazer, D. C. Steffens, and E. W. Busse (eds.), *The American Psychiatric Publishing Textbook of Geriatric Psychiatry*, 3rd ed., pp. 17–36. Washington, DC: American Psychiatric Press.

Bluestein, D., and P. L. Bach. 2007. Working with families in long-term care. *Journal of the American Medical Directors Association* 8:265–70.

Boeve, B. F., M. H. Silber, and T. J. Ferman. 1998. REM sleep behavior disorder and degenerative dementia: An association likely reflecting Lewy body disease. *Neurology* 51:363–70.

———. 2002. Current management of sleep disturbances in dementia. *Current Neurological and Neuroscience Report* 2:169–77.

Bonner, A. F., N. G. Castle, S. Perera, et al. 2008. Patient safety culture: A review of the nursing home literature and recommendations for practice. *Annals of Long-Term Care* 16:18–22.

Borroni, B., C. Agosti, and A. Padovani. 2008. Behavioral and psychological symptoms in dementia with Lewy-bodies (DLB): Frequency and relationship with disease severity and motor impairment. *Archives of Gerontology and Geriatrics* 46:101–6.

Bosek, M. S., E. Lowry, D. A. Lindeman, et al. 2003. Promoting a good death for persons with dementia in nursing facilities: Family caregivers' perspectives. *JONAS Health Law Ethics Regulation* 5:34–41.

Bourdel-Marchasson, I., S. Vincent, C. Germain, et al. 2004. Delirium symptoms and low dietary intake in older inpatients are independent predictors of institutionalization: A 1-year prospective population-based study. *Journals of Gerontology, Series A: Biological and Medical Sciences* 59A:M350–54.

Bowie, C. R., C. Fallon, and P. D. Harvey. 2006. Convergence of clinical staff ratings and research ratings to assess patients with schizophrenia in nursing homes. *Psychiatric Services* 57:838–43.

Boxer, A. L., and B. L. Miller. 2005. Clinical features of frontotemporal dementia. *Alzheimer Disease and Associated Disorders* 19 (suppl. 3):27–30.

Braden, B. I., and N. Bergstrom. 1989. Clinical utility of the Braden Scale for predicting pressure sore risk. *Decubitus* 2:44–51.

Brandt, H. E., L. Deliens, M. E. Ooms, et al. 2005. Symptoms, signs, problems, and diseases of terminally ill nursing home patients: A nationwide observational study in the Netherlands. *Archives of Internal Medicine* 165:314–20.

Bridges-Parlet, S., D. Knopman, and T. Thompson. 1994. A descriptive study of physically aggressive behavior in dementia by direct observation. *Journal of the American Geriatrics Society* 42:192–97.

Briesacher, B. A., R. Limcangco, L. Simoni-Wastila, et al. 2005. The quality of antipsychotic drug prescribing in nursing homes. *Archives of Internal Medicine* 165:1280–85.

Broadway, J., and J. Mintzer. 2007. The many faces of psychosis in the elderly. *Current Opinion in Psychiatry* 20:551–58.

Brodaty, H., and G. Luscombe. 1996. Depression in persons with dementia. *International Psychogeriatrics* 8:609–22.

Brooker, D. J., and R. J. Woolley. 2007. Enriching opportunities for people living with dementia: The development of a blueprint for a sustainable activity-based model. *Aging and Mental Health* 11:371–83.

Brooks, J. O. III, and J. C. Hoblyn. 2005. Secondary mania in older adults. *American Journal of Psychiatry* 162:2033–38.

Brown, L. C., S. R. Majumdar, and J. A. Johnson. 2008. Type of antidepressant therapy and risk of type 2 diabetes in people with depression. *Diabetes Research and Clinical Practice* 79:61–67.

Bureau of Labor Statistics. 2008. *Workplace Injuries and Illnesses in 2007.* www.bls.gov/news/release/pdf/osh.pdf.

Burns, A., A. Gallagley, and J. Byrne. 2004. Delirium. *Journal of Neurology, Neurosurgery and Psychiatry* 75:362–67.

Butters, J. A., J. T. Becker, M. D. Zmuda, et al. 2000. Changes in cognitive functioning following treatment of late-life depression. *American Journal of Psychiatry* 157:1949–54.

Buysse, D. J. 2008. Chronic insomnia. *American Journal of Psychiatry* 165:678–86.

Cairney, J., L. McCabe, S. Veldhuizen, et al. 2007. Epidemiology of social phobia in later life. *American Journal of Geriatric Psychiatry* 15:224–33.

Camicioli, R., and L. Licis. 2004. Motor impairment predicts falls in specialized Alzheimer care units. *Alzheimer Disease and Associated Disorders* 18:214–18.

Camp, C. J., J. Cohen-Mansfield, and E. A. Capezuti. 2002. Use of nonpharmacologic interventions among nursing home residents with dementia. *Psychiatric Services* 53:1397–1401.

Cano, C., K. D. Hennesey, J. Warren, et al. 1997. Medicare Part A utilization and expenditures for psychiatric services, 1995. *Health Care Finance Review* 18:177–93.

Capezuti, E., L. M. Wagner, B. L. Brush, et al. 2007. Consequences of an intervention to reduce restrictive side rail use in nursing homes. *Journal of the American Geriatrics Society* 55:334–41.

Carney, M. T., F. S. Kahan, and B. E. C. Paris. 2003. Elder abuse: Is every bruise a sign of abuse? *Mount Sinai Journal of Medicine* 70:69–74.

Carter, M. W. 2003. Factors associated with ambulatory care-sensitive hospitalizations among nursing home residents. *Journal of Aging and Health* 15:295–331.

Carter, M. W., and F. W. Porell. 2005. Vulnerable populations at risk of potentially avoidable hospitalizations: The case of nursing home residents with Alzheimer's disease. *American Journal of Alzheimer's Disease and Other Dementia* 20:349–58.

Casarett, D. J., K. B. Hirschman, and M. R. Henry. 2001. Does hospice have a role in nursing home care at the end of life? *Journal of the American Geriatrics Society* 49:1493–98.

Caselli, R. J., and R. Yaari. 2007/2008. Medical management of frontotemporal dementia. *American Journal of Alzheimer's Disease and Other Dementias* 22:489–98.

Caselli, R. J., T. G. Beach, R. Yaari, et al. 2006. Alzheimer's disease a century later. *Journal of Clinical Psychiatry* 67:1784–1800.

Chan, D. K. Y., D. J. Cordato, and E. O'Rourke. 2008. Management for motor and non-motor complications in late Parkinson's disease. *Geriatrics* 63:22–27.

Chancellor, M. B., and F. de Miguel. 2007. Treatment of overactive bladder: Selective use of anticholinergic agents with low drug-drug interaction potential. *Geriatrics* 62:15–24.

Chandra, V., N. E. Barucha, and B. S. Schoenberg. 1986. Conditions associated with Alzheimer's disease at death: Case-control study. *Neurology* 36:209–11.

Charles, C., A. Gafni, and T. Whelan. 1999. Decision-making in the physician-patient encounter: Revisiting the shared treatment decision-making model. *Social Science and Medicine* 49:651–61.

Cheek, P., L. Nikpour, and H. D. Nowlin. 2005. Aging well with smart technology. *Nursing Administrative Quarterly* 29:329–38.

Chen, J. Y., Y. Stern, M. Sano, et al. 1991. Cumulative risks of developing extrapyramidal signs, psychosis, or myoclonus in the course of Alzheimer's disease. *Archives of Neurology* 48:1141–43.

Chew, M. L., B. H. Mulsant, B. G. Pollock, et al. 2008. Anticholinergic activity of 107 medications commonly used by older adults. *Journal of the American Geriatrics Society* 56(7):1333–41.

Chibnall, J. T., and R. C. Tait. 2001. Pain assessment in cognitively impaired and unimpaired older adults: A comparison of four scales. *Pain* 92:173–86.

Chibnall, J. T., R. C. Tait, B. Harman, et al. 2005. Effect of acetaminophen on behavior, well-being and psychotropic medication use in nursing home residents with moderate to severe dementia. *Journal of the American Geriatrics Society* 53:1921–29.

Chitsey, A. M., B. K. Haight, and M. M. Jones. 2002. Snoezelen: A multisensory environmental intervention. *Journal of Gerontological Nursing* 28:41–49.

Chochinov, H. M. 2007. Dignity and the essence of medicine: The A, B, C, and D of dignity conserving care. *British Medical Journal* 335:184–87.

Chochinov, H. M., K. G. Wilson, M. Enns, et al. 1994. Prevalence of depression in the terminally ill: Effects of diagnostic criteria and symptom threshold judgments. *American Journal of Psychiatry* 151:537–40.

Christmas, C. 2006. Medical care of the hip fracture patient. *Clinical Geriatrics* 14(4):40–45.

Cipher, D. J., P. A. Clifford, and K. D. Roper. 2006. Behavioral manifestations of pain in the demented elderly. *Journal of the American Medical Directors Association* 7:355–65.

Clare, L., and R. Woods. 2004. Cognitive training and cognitive rehabilitation for people with early stage Alzheimer's disease: A review. *Neuropsychological Rehabilitation* 4:385–401.

Clarfield, A. M. 2003. The decreasing prevalence of reversible dementias: An updated meta-analysis. *Archives of Internal Medicine* 63:2219–29.

Cohen, C. I., K. Hyland, and D. Kimhy. 2003. The utility of mandatory depression screening of dementia patients in nursing homes. *American Journal of Psychiatry* 160:2012–17.

Cohen, C. I., I. Vahia, P. Reyes, et al. 2008. Schizophrenia in later life: Clinical symptoms and social well-being. *Psychiatric Services* 59:232–34.

Cohen, H. L., L. C. Curry, D. Jenkins, et al. 2008. Older lesbians and gay men: Long-term care issues. *Annals of Long-Term Care: Clinical Care and Aging* 16:33–38.

Cohen-Mansfield, J. 1986. Agitated behaviors in the elderly II: Preliminary results in the cognitively deteriorated. *Journal of the American Geriatrics Society* 34:722–27.

Cohen-Mansfield, J., A. Libin, and M. S. Marx. 2007. Nonpharmacological treatment of agitation: A controlled trial of systematic individualized intervention. *Journals of Gerontology, Series A: Biological Sciences and Medical Sciences* 62A:908–16.

Cohen-Mansfield, J., M. S. Marx, and A. S. Rosenthal. 1989. A description of agitation in a nursing home. *Journal of Gerontology* 44:M77–84.

Cohen-Mansfield, J., S. Lipson, P. Werner, et al. 1999. *Archives of Internal Medicine* 159: 1733–40.

Colcombe, S. J., K. I. Erickson, P. E. Scalf, et al. 2006. Aerobic exercise training increases brain volume in aging humans. *Journals of Gerontology, Series A: Biological Sciences and Medical Sciences* 61A:1166–70.

Cole, M. G. 2004. Delirium in elderly patients. *American Journal of Geriatric Psychiatry* 12:7–21.

Cole, M. G., J. McCusker, N. Dendukuri, et al. 2003. The prognostic significance of subsyndromal delirium in elderly medical inpatients. *Journal of the American Geriatrics Society* 51:754–60.

Collerton, D., D. Burn, I. McKeith, et al. 2003. Systematic review and meta-analysis show that dementia with Lewy bodies is a visual-perceptual and attentional-executive dementia. *Dementia and Geriatric Cognitive Disorder* 16:229–37.

Collopy, B., P. Boyle, and B. Jennings. 1991. New directions in nursing home ethics. *Hastings Center Report* 2 (suppl.):S1–15.

Conwell, Y., J. M. Lyness, O. Duberstein, et al. 2002. Risk factors for suicide in later life. *Biological Psychiatry* 52(3):193–204.

Cooper, J. W., M. H. Freeman, C. L. Cook, et al. 2007. Assessment of psychotropic and psychoactive drug loads and falls in nursing facility residents. *Consultant Pharmacist* 22:483–89.

Cowles, M. C. 2006. *Nursing Home Statistical Yearbook, 2005*. McMinnville, OR: Cowles Research Group.

Cummings, J. L. 2005. Neuropsychiatric and behavioral alterations and their management in moderate to severe Alzheimer's disease. *Neurology* 65 (suppl. 3):S18–24.

Cummings, J. L., and G. Cole. 2002. Alzheimer disease. *Journal of the American Medical Association* 287:2335–38.

Cummings, J. L., L. Schneider, P. N. Tariot, et al. 2004. Reduction of behavioral disturbances and caregiver distress by galantamine in patients with Alzheimer's disease. *American Journal of Psychiatry* 161:532–38.

Dada, F., S. Sethi, and G. T. Grossberg. 2001. Generalized anxiety disorder in the elderly. *Psychiatric Clinics of North America* 24:155–64.

D'Agata, E., and S. L. Mitchell. 2008. Patterns of antimicrobial use among nursing home residents with advanced dementia. *Archives of Internal Medicine* 168:357–62.

Davis, M. N., S. T. Smith, and S. Tyler. 2005. Improving transition and communication between acute care and long-term care: A system for better continuity of care. *Annals of Long-Term Care* 13:25–32.

Dawkins, V. H. 1998. Restraints and the elderly with mental illness: Ethical issues and moral reasoning. *Journal of Psychosocial Nursing* 36(10):22–27.

Day, K., D. Carreon, and C. Stump. 2000. The therapeutic design of environments for people with dementia: A review of the empirical research. *Gerontologist* 40:397–416.

Della, S. S., H. Spinnler, and A. Venneri. 2004. Walking difficulties in patients with Alzheimer's disease might originate from gait apraxia. *Journal of Neurology, Neurosurgery and Psychiatry* 75:196–201.

Desai, A. K. 2003. Use of psychopharmacologic agents in the elderly. *Clinics in Geriatric Medicine* 19:697–719.

———. 2004. Psychotropic side effects of commonly prescribed medications in the elderly. *Primary Psychiatry* 11:27–34.

Desai, A. K., and G. T. Grossberg. 2001. Recognition and management of behavioral disturbances in dementia. *Primary Care Companion Journal of Clinical Psychiatry* 3:93–109.

———. 2003a. Buspirone in Alzheimer's disease. *Expert Review in Neurotherapeutics* 3:19–28.

———. 2003c. Herbals and botanicals in geriatric psychiatry. *American Journal of Geriatric Psychiatry* 11:498–506.

———. 2005. Diagnosis and treatment of Alzheimer's disease. *Neurology* 64:S34–39.

Deutsch, L. H., F. W. Bylsma, B. W. Rovner, et al. 1991. Psychosis and physical aggression in probable Alzheimer's disease. *American Journal of Psychiatry* 148:1159–63.

Devanand, D. P., M. S. Nobler, T. Singer, et al. 1994. Is dysthymia a different disorder in the elderly? *American Journal of Psychiatry* 151:1592–99.

Dharmarajan, T. S., M. R. Kanagala, P. Murakonda, et al. 2008. Do acid-lowering agents affect vitamin B_{12} status in older adults? *Journal of the American Medical Directors Association* 9:162–67.

Diez, J. J. 2002. Hypothyroidism in patients older than 55 years: An analysis of the etiology and assessment of the effectiveness of therapy. *Journals of Gerontology, Series A: Biological Sciences and Medical Sciences* 57A:M315–20.

Dimant, J. 2001. Medication errors and adverse drug events in nursing homes: Problems, causes, regulations, and proposed solutions. *Journal of the American Medical Directors Association* 2:81–93.

Dobalian, A. 2006. Advance care planning documents in nursing facilities: Results from a nationally representative survey. *Archives of Gerontology and Geriatrics* 43:193–212.

Doghramji, K. 2006. When patients can't sleep: Updated guide to workup and hypnotic therapy. *Current Psychiatry* 5:49–60.

Donohue, W. A., J. L. Dibble, and L. B. Schiamberg. 2008. A social capital approach to the prevention of elder mistreatment. *Journal of Elder Abuse and Neglect* 20:1–23.

Doody, R. S., J. C. Stevens, C. Beck, et al. 2001. Practice parameter: Management of dementia (an evidence-based review). *Neurology* 56:1154–66.

Doraiswamy, P. M., J. Leon, J. L. Cummings, et al. 2002. Prevalence and impact of medical comorbidity in Alzheimer's disease. *Journals of Gerontology, Series A: Biological Sciences and Medical Sciences* 57A:M173–77.

Douglas, I. J., and L. Smeeth. 2008. Exposure to antipsychotics and risk of stroke: Self-controlled case series study. *British Medical Journal* 337:a1227.

Dowd, S. B., and R. Davidhizar. 2003. Can mental and physical activities such as chess and gardening help in the prevention and treatment of Alzheimer's? Healthy aging through stimulation of the mind. *Journal of Practical Nursing* 53:11–13.

Dowling, G. A., R. L. Burr, E. J. Van Someren, et al. 2007. Melatonin and bright light treatment for rest-activity disruption in institutionalized patients with Alzheimer's disease. *Journal of the American Geriatrics Society* 56:239–46.

Draper, B., H. Brodaty, L. F. Low, et al. 2002. Self-destructive behaviors in nursing home residents. *Journal of the American Geriatrics Society* 50:354–58.

Eeles, E., and K. Rockwood. 2008. Delirium in the long-term care setting: Clinical and research challenges. *Journal of the American Medical Directors Association* 9:157–61.

Elklit, A., and M. O'Connor. 2005. Post-traumatic stress disorder in a Danish population of elderly bereaved. *Scandinavian Journal of Psychology* 46:439–45.

Elliot, R. 2003. Executive functions and their disorders. *British Medical Bulletin* 65:49–59.

Emre, M., D. Aarsland, A. Albanese, et al. 2004. Rivastigmine for dementia associated with Parkinson's disease. *New England Journal of Medicine* 351:2509–18.

Espinoza, S., and L. P. Fried. 2007. Risk factors for frailty in older adults. *Clinical Geriatrics* 15(6):37–44.

Evans, B. C., and N. L. Crogan. 2005. Using the FoodEx-LTC to assess institutional food service practices through nursing home residents' perspectives on nutrition care. *Journals of Gerontology, Series A: Biological Sciences and Medical Sciences* 60A:125–28.

Evans, W. J., J. E. Morley, J. Argiles, et al. 2008. Cachexia: A new definition. *Clinical Nutrition* 27(6):793–99.

Fann, J. R. 2000. The epidemiology of delirium: A review of studies and methodological issues. *Seminars in Clinical Neuropsychiatry* 5:64–74.

Farrell, K. R., and L. Ganzini. 1995. Misdiagnosing delirium as depression in medically ill elderly patients. *Archives of Internal Medicine* 155:2459–64.

Feil, N. 2002. *The Validation Breakthrough: Simple Techniques for Communicating with People with Alzheimer's-Type Dementia*, 2nd ed. Baltimore: Health Professions Press.

Feinberg, M. 1993. The problems of anticholinergic adverse effects in older patients. *Drugs and Aging* 3:335–48.

Feinsod, F. M., S. A. Levenson, K. Rapp, et al. 2004. Dehydration in frail, older residents in longterm care facilities. *Journal of the American Medical Directors Association* 5(2):S35–41.

Feldman, H. H., and M. Woodward. 2005. The staging and assessment of moderate to severe Alzheimer disease. *Neurology* 65(3):S10–17.

Felix, H. C. 2008. Obesity, disability, and nursing home admission. *Annals of Long-Term Care* 16:33–36.

Ferman, T. J., and B. F. Boeve. 2007. Dementia with Lewy bodies. *Neurological Clinics* 25:741–60.

Fernandez, H. H., M. E. Trieschmann, and M. S. Okun. 2004. Rebound psychosis: Effect of discontinuation of antipsychotics in Parkinson's disease. *Movement Disorders* 20:104–15.

Ferrell, B. A. 2004. The management of pain in long-term care. *Clinical Journal of Pain* 20:240–43.

Ferretti, L., S. M. McCurry, R. Logsdon, et al. 2001. Anxiety and Alzheimer's disease. *Journal of Geriatric Psychiatry and Neurology* 14:52–58.

Fick, D. M., J. W. Cooper, W. E. Wade, et al. 2003. Updating the Beer's criteria for potentially inappropriate medication use in older adults: Results of a U.S. consensus panel of experts. *Archives of Internal Medicine* 163:2716–24.

Filan, S. L., and R. H. Llewellyn-Jones. 2006. Animal-assisted therapy for dementia: A review of the literature. *International Psychogeriatrics* 18:597–611.

Finucane, T. E., C. Christmas, and B. A. Leff. 2007. Tube feeding in dementia: How incentives undermine health care quality and patient safety. *Journal of the American Medical Directors Association* 8:205–8.

Flaherty, J. H., and J. E. Morley. 2004. Delirium: A call to improve current standards of care. *Journals of Gerontology, Series A: Biological Sciences and Medical Sciences* 59A:341–43.

Fleming, D. 2007. Addressing ethical issues in the nursing home. *Missouri Medicine* 104:387–91.

Flint, A. J. 1998. Management of anxiety in late life. *Journal of Geriatric Psychiatry and Neurology* 11:194–200.

———. 2005. Generalized anxiety disorder in elderly patients: Epidemiology, diagnosis and treatment options. *Drugs and Aging* 22:101–14.

Flint, A. J., and N. Gagnon. 2003. Diagnosis and management of panic disorder in older patients. *Drugs and Aging* 20:881–91.

Fossey, J., C. Ballard, E. Juszczak, et al. 2006. Effect of enhanced psychosocial care on antipsychotic use in nursing home residents with severe dementia: Cluster randomized trial. *British Medical Journal* 332:756–58.

Fox, P. A., P. Raina, and A. R. Jadad. 1999. Prevalence and treatment of pain in older adults in nursing homes and other long-term care institutions: A systematic review. *Canadian Medical Association Journal* 160:329–33.

French, D. D., R. Campbell, A. Spehar, et al. 2005. Outpatient medications and hip fractures in the U.S.: A national veterans study. *Drugs and Aging* 22:877–85.

Friedlander, A. H., M. E. Mahler, and J. A. Yagiela. 2006. Restless leg syndrome: Manifestations, treatment and dental implications. *Journal of the American Dental Association* 137:755–61.

Fujikawa, T., S. Yamawaki, and Y. Touhouda. 1995. Silent cerebral infections in patients with late-onset mania. *Stroke* 26:946–49.

Furman, C. D., S. E. Kelly, K. Knapp, et al. 2007. Eliciting goals of care in a nursing home. *Journal of the American Medical Directors Association* 8:e35–41.

Ganzini, L. 2007. Care of patients with delirium at the end of life. *Annals of Long-Term Care* 15:35–40.

Ganzini, L., L. Volicer, W. A. Nelson, et al. 2004. Ten myths about decision-making capacity. *Journal of the American Medical Directors Association* 5:263–67.

Garfinkel, D., S. Zur-Gil, and J. Ben-Israel. 2007. The war against polypharmacy: A new cost-effective geriatric-palliative approach for improving drug therapy in disabled elderly people. *International Medical Association Journal* 9:430–34.

Gasper, M. C., B. R. Ott, and K. L. Lapane. 2005. Is donepezil therapy associated with reduced mortality in nursing home residents with dementia? *American Journal of Geriatric Psychiatry* 3:1–7.

Gates, D., E. Fitzwater, S. Telintelo, et al. 2004. Preventing assaults by nursing home residents: Nursing assistants' knowledge and confidence: A pilot study. *Journal of the American Medical Directors Association* 5:S17–21.

Gaugler, J. E., A. B. Edwards, E. E. Femia, et al. 2000. Predictors of institutionalization of cognitively impaired elders: Family help and the timing of placement. *Journals of Gerontology, Series B: Psychological Sciences and Social Sciences* 55B:P247–55.

Gehrman, P. R., J. L. Martin, T. Shochat, et al. 2003. Sleep-disordered breathing and agitation in institutionalized adults with Alzheimer's disease. *American Journal of Geriatric Psychiatry* 11:426–33.

George, L. 1991. Cognitive impairment. In L. N. Robins and D. A. Regier (eds.), *Psychiatric Disorders in America: The Epidemiologic Catchment Area Study*, pp. 291–327. New York: Free Press.

Gibbs, L. M., and L. Young. 2007. The medical director's role: Neglect in long-term care. *Journal of the American Medical Directors Association* 8:194–96.

Gilchrest, B. A. 1996. A review of skin ageing and its medical therapy. *British Journal of Dermatology* 135:867–75.

Gildengers, A., M. Butters, K. Seligman, et al. 2004. Cognitive functioning in late-life bipolar disorder. *American Journal of Psychiatry* 161(4):736–38.

Gill, S. S., S. E. Bronskill, S. L. Normand, et al. 2007. Antipsychotic drug use and mortality in older adults with dementia. *Annals of Internal Medicine* 146:775–86.

Gill, T. M., E. A. Gahbauer, H. G. Allore, et al. 2006. Transitions between frailty states among community-dwelling older persons. *Archives of Internal Medicine* 166:418–23.

Gilley, D. W., R. S. Wilson, L. A. Beckett, et al. 1997. Psychotic symptoms and physically aggressive behavior in Alzheimer's disease. *Journal of the American Geriatrics Society* 45:1074–79.

Gillick, M. R., and A. E. Volandes. 2008. The standard of caring: Why do we still use feeding tubes in patients with advanced dementia? *Journal of the American Medical Directors Association* 9:364–67.

Gleason, O. C. 2003. Delirium. *American Family Physician* 67:1027–34.

Goldman, J. S., J. Adamson, A. Karydas, et al. 2007/2008. New genes, new dilemmas: FTLD genetics and its implications for families. *American Journal of Alzheimer's Disease and Other Dementias* 22:507–15.

Gosney, M. A., M. F. Hammond, A. Shenkin, et al. 2008. Effect of micronutrient supplementation on mood in nursing home residents. *Gerontology* 54(5):292–99.

Gostin, L. O. 1995. Informed consent, cultural sensitivity, and respect for persons. *Journal of the American Medical Association* 274:844–45.

Greenwood, C. E., C. Tam, M. Chan, et al. 2005. Behavioral disturbances, not cognitive deterioration, are associated with altered food selection in seniors with Alzheimer's disease. *Journals of Gerontology, Series A: Biological Sciences and Medical Sciences* 60A:499–505.

Greiner, K. A., S. Perera, and J. S. Ahluwalia. 2003. Hospice usage by minorities in the last year of life: Results from the National Mortality Follow-Back Survey. *Journal of the American Geriatrics Society* 51:970–78.

Griffiths, J., G. Fortune, V. Barber, et al. 2007. The prevalence of post-traumatic stress disorder in survivors of ICU treatment: A systematic review. *Intensive Care in Medicine* 33:1506–18.

Grossberg, G. T., and A. K. Desai. 2003a. Late-life psychoses. In A. M. Mellow (ed.), *Geriatric Psychiatry*, pp. 75–110. Washington, DC: American Psychiatric Publishing.

———. 2003b. Management of Alzheimer's disease. *Journals of Gerontology, Series A: Biological Sciences and Medical Sciences* 58A:M331–53.

———. 2006. Cognition in Alzheimer's disease and related disorders. In C. G. Kruse, H. Y. Meltzer, C. Sennef, et al. (eds.), *Thinking about Cognition: Concepts, Targets and Therapeutics*, pp. 19–38. Washington, DC: IOS Press.

Grossberg, G. T., and B. Fox. 2007. *The Essential Herb-Drug-Vitamin Interaction Guide: The Safe Way to Use Medications and Supplements Together.* New York: Broadway Books.

Grossberg, G. T., and J. Manepalli. 1995. The older patient with psychotic symptoms. *Psychiatric Services* 46:55–59.

Gruber-Baldini, A. L., M. Boustani, P. D. Sloane, et al. 2004. Behavioral symptoms in residential care / assisted living facilities: Prevalence, risk factors, and medication management. *Journal of the American Geriatrics Society* 52:1610–17.

Guay, D. R. P. 2008. Inappropriate sexual behaviors in cognitively impaired older individuals. *American Journal of Geriatric Pharmacotherapy* 6:269–88.

Gurwitz, J. H., T. S. Field, J. Avorn, et al. 2005. Incidence and preventability of adverse drug events in nursing homes. *American Journal of Medicine* 118:251–58.

Gwyther, L. P. 1998. Social issues of the Alzheimer's patient and family. *American Journal of Medicine* 104:17S–21S.

———. 2000. Family issues in dementia: Finding a new normal. *Neurological Clinics* 18:993–1010.

Hajjar, R. R., and H. K. Kamel. 2004a. Sexuality in the nursing home, part 1: Attitudes and barriers to sexual expression. *Journal of the American Medical Directors Association* S43–47.

———. 2004b. Sexuality in the nursing home, part 2: Managing abnormal behavior. *Journal of the American Medical Directors Association* S49–52.

Hall, P., C. Schroder, and L. Weaver. 2002. The last 48 hours of life in long-term care: A focused chart audit. *Journal of the American Geriatrics Society* 50:501–6.

Hallam, B. J., N. D. Silverberg, A. K. LaMarre, et al. 2007. Clinical presentation of prodromal frontotemporal dementia. *American Journal of Alzheimer's Disease and Other Dementias* 22:456–67.

Hallberg, I. R., G. Holst, A. Nordmark, et al. 1995. Cooperation during morning care between nurses and severely demented institutionalized patients. *Clinical Nursing Research* 4:78–104.

Hammer, R. M. 1999. The lived experience of being at home: A phenomenological investigation. *Journal of Gerontological Nursing* 25:10–18.

Hancock, J. H., G. Livingston, and M. Orrell. 2006. Quality of life of people with dementia in residential care homes. *British Journal of Psychiatry* 158:460–64.

Hansberry, M. R., E. Chen, and M. J. Gorbien. 2005. Dementia and elder abuse. *Clinics in Geriatric Medicine* 21:315–32.

Harjivan, C., and A. Lyles. 2002. Improved medication use in long-term care: Building on the consultant pharmacist's drug regimen review. *American Journal of Managed Care* 8:318–26.

Hayley, D. C., C. K. Cassel, L. Snyder, et al. 1996. Ethical and legal issues in nursing home care. *Archives of Internal Medicine* 156:249–56.

Hening, W. A. 2007. Current guidelines and standards of practice for restless leg syndrome. *American Journal of Medicine* 120:S22–27.

Herr, K. A., P. R. Mobily, F. J. Kohout, et al. 1998. Evaluation of the faces pain scale for use with the elderly. *Clinical Journal of Pain* 14:29–38.

Herr, K. A., K. F. Spratt, L. Garand, et al. 2007. Evaluation of the Iowa Pain Thermometer and other selected pain intensity scales in younger and older adult cohorts using controlled clinical pain: A preliminary study. *Pain Medicine* 8:585–600.

Herrmann, N., and K. L. Lanctot. 2007. Pharmacologic management of neuropsychiatric symptoms of Alzheimer disease. *Canadian Journal of Psychiatry* 52:630–46.

Herrmann, N., D. Kidron, K. I. Shulman, et al. 1998. Clock tests in depression, Alzheimer's disease, and elderly controls. *International Journal of Psychiatry and Medicine* 28:437–47.

Higgins, A., P. Barker, and C. M. Begley. 2004. Hypersexuality and dementia: Dealing with inappropriate sexual expression. *British Journal of Nursing* 13:1330–34.

Hokkanen, L., L. Rantala, A. M. Remes, et al. 2003. Dance/movement therapeutic methods in management of dementia. *Journal of the American Geriatrics Society* 51:576–78.

Holmes, H. M., G. A. Sachs, J. W. Shega, et al. 2008. Integrating palliative medicine into the care of persons with advanced dementia: Identifying appropriate medication use. *Journal of the American Geriatrics Society* 56:1306–11.

Hommet, C., K. Mondon, V. Camus, et al. 2008. Epilepsy and dementia in the elderly. *Dementia and Geriatric Cognitive Disorder* 25:293–300.

House Committee on Government Reform. 2001. *Abuse of Residents Is a Major Problem in U.S. Nursing Homes.* Special Investigations Division, minority staff report prepared for Representative Henry Waxman. Washington, DC: Government Printing Office.

Hoverman, C., L. R. Shugarman, D. Saliba, et al. 2008. Use of postacute care by nursing home residents hospitalized for stroke or hip fracture: How prevalent and to what end? *Journal of the American Geriatrics Society* 56(8):1490–96.

Howard, R. J., E. Jusczak, C. G. Ballard, et al. 2007. Donepezil for the treatment of agitation in Alzheimer's disease. *New England Journal of Medicine* 357:1382–92.

Huey, E. D., K. T. Putman, and J. Grafman. 2006. A systematic review of neurotransmitter deficits and treatments in frontotemporal dementia. *Neurology* 66:17–22.

Hughes, C. M., K. L. Lapane, V. Mor, et al. 2000. The impact of legislation on psychotropic drug use in nursing homes: A cross-national perspective. *Journal of the American Geriatrics Society* 48:931–37.

Husebo, B. S., L. I. Strand, R. Moe-Nilssen, et al. 2008. Who suffers most? Dementia and pain in nursing home patients: A cross-sectional study. *Journal of the American Medical Directors Association* 9:427–33.

Hybels, C. F., D. G. Blazer, and D. C. Steffens. 2006. Partial remission: A common outcome in older adults treated for major depression. *Geriatrics* 61:22–26.

Inouye, S. K. 2000. Assessment and management of delirium in hospitalized older patients. *Annals of Long-Term Care: Clinical Care and Aging* 8:53–59.

———. 2006. Delirium in older persons. *New England Journal of Medicine* 354:1157–65.

Inouye, S. K., and L. Ferrucci. 2006. Elucidating the pathophysiology of delirium and the interrelationship of delirium and dementia. *Journals of Gerontology, Series A: Biological Sciences and Medical Sciences* 61A:1277–80.

Inouye, S. K., C. H. van Dyck, C. A. Alessi, et al. 1990. Clarifying confusion: The Confusion Assessment method; A new method for detection of delirium. *Annals of Internal Medicine* 113:941–48.

Inouye, S. K., S. T. Bogardus Jr., P. A. Charpentier, et al. 1999. A multicomponent intervention to prevent delirium in hospitalized older patients. *New England Medical Journal* 340:669–76.

Inouye, S. K., M. D. Foreman, L. C. Mion, et al. 2001. Nurses' recognition of delirium and its symptoms: Comparison of nurse and researcher ratings. *Archives of Internal Medicine* 161:2467–73.

Institute of Medicine. 2003. Improving the quality of long-term care. www.iom.edu.

Irvine, A. B., M. Bourgeois, M. Billow, et al. 2007. Internet training for nurse aides to prevent resident aggression. *Journal of the American Medical Directors Association* 8:519–26.

Jayawardena, K. M., and S. Liao. 2006. Elder abuse at the end of life. *Journal of Palliative Medicine* 9:127–36.

Jeste, D. V., M. P. Caligiuri, J. S. Paulsen, et al. 1995. Risk of tardive dyskinesia in older patients: A prospective longitudinal study of 266 outpatients. *Archives of General Psychiatry* 52:756–65.

Jeste, D. V., G. S. Alexopoulos, S. J. Bartels, et al. 1999. Consensus statement on the upcoming crisis in geriatric mental health: Research agenda for the next two decades. *Archives of General Psychiatry* 56:848–53.

Johnston, D. 2000. A series of cases of dementia presenting with PTSD symptoms in World War II combat veterans. *Journal of the American Geriatrics Society* 48:70–72.

Jones, K., R. Fink, L. Clark, et al. 2005. Nursing home barriers to effective pain management: Why nursing home residents may not seek pain medication. *Journal of the American Medical Directors Association* 6:10–17.

Jones, R. N., E. R. Marcantonio, and T. Rabinowitz. 2003. Prevalence and correlates of recognized depression in U.S. nursing homes. *Journal of the American Geriatrics Society* 51:1404–9.

Jongenelis, K., A. M. Pot, A. M. Eisses, et al. 2004. Prevalence and risk indicators of depression in elderly nursing home patients: The AGED study. *Journal of Affective Disorders* 83:135–42.

Josephs, K. A. 2007. Capgras syndrome and its relationship to neurodegenerative disease. *Archives of Neurology* 64:1762–66.

Jost, B. C., and G. T. Grossberg. 1996. The evolution of psychiatric symptoms in Alzheimer's disease: A natural history study. *Journal of the American Geriatrics Society* 44:1978–81.

Kakuma, R., G. G. du Fort, L. Arsenault, et al. 2003. Delirium in older emergency department patients discharged home: Effect on survival. *Journal of the American Geriatrics Society* 51:443–50.

Kallenbach, L. E., and S. K. Rigler. 2006. Identification and management of depression in nursing facility residents. *Journal of the American Medical Directors Association* 7(7):448–55.

Kapo, J., L. J. Morrison, and S. Liao. 2007. Palliative care for the older adult. *Journal of Palliative Medicine* 10:185–209.

Kash, B. A., N. G. Castle, and C. D. Phillips. 2007. Nursing home spending, staffing, and turnover. *Health Care Management Review* 32:253–62.

Katz, I. R. 1998. Diagnosis and treatment of depression in patients with Alzheimer's disease and
other dementias. *Journal of Clinical Psychiatry* 59 (suppl. 9):S38–44.

Katz, S., T. D. Down, H. R. Cash, et al. 1970. Progress in the development of the index of ADL.
Gerontologist 10:20–30.

Kawas, C. H. 2003. Early Alzheimer's disease. *New England Journal of Medicine* 349:1056–63.

Kayser-Jones, J. 2000. Improving the nutritional care of nursing home residents. *Nursing Homes*
49:56–59.

Keeney, C. E., J. A. Scharfenberger, J. G. O'Brien, et al. 2008. Initiating and sustaining a standardized pain management program in long-term care facilities. *Journal of the American Medical
Directors Association* 9:347–53.

Kennedy, R. L., K. Chokkalingham, and R. Srinivasan. 2004. Obesity in the elderly: Who should
we be treating, and why, and how? *Current Opinion in Clinical Nutrition and Metabolism Care*
7:3–9.

Khouzam, H. R., and R. Emes. 2007. Late life psychosis: Assessment and general treatment strategies. *Comprehensive Therapeutics* 33:127–43.

Kiely, D. K., M. A. Bergmann, K. M. Murphy, et al. 2003. Delirium among newly admitted postacute facility patients: Prevalence, symptoms, and severity. *Journals of Gerontology, Series A:
Biological Sciences and Medical Sciences* 58A:M441–45.

Kiely, D. K., R. N. Jones, M. A. Bergmann, et al. 2006. Association between delirium resolution
and functional recovery among newly admitted postacute facility patients. *Journals of Gerontology, Series A: Biological Sciences and Medical Sciences* 61A:204–8.

Kihlgren, M., I. G. Lindsten, A. Norberg, et al. 1992. The content of the oral daily reports at a
long-term ward before and after staff training in integrity promoting care. *Scandinavian Journal of Caring Science* 6:105–12.

Kimball, A. B., D. Gladman, J. M. Gelfand, et al. 2008. National Psoriasis Foundation clinical
consensus on psoriasis comorbidities and recommendations for screening. *Journal of the
American Academy of Dermatology* 58:1031–42.

Kirby, M., and B. A. Lawlor. 1995. Biologic markers and neurochemical correlates of agitation
and psychosis in dementia. *Journal of Geriatric Psychiatry and Neurology* 8:S2–7.

Kitwood, T. 1997. *Dementia Reconsidered: The Person Comes First.* Buckingham, England: Open
University Press.

Knight, R. 2006. Creutzfeldt-Jakob disease: A rare cause of dementia in elderly persons. *Clinical
Infectious Disease* 43:340–46.

Knopman, D. S., B. F. Boeve, and R. C. Petersen. 2003. Essentials of the proper diagnoses of mild
cognitive impairment, dementia, and major subtypes of dementia. *Mayo Clinics Proceedings*
78:1290–1308.

Knopman, D. S., J. E. Parisi, B. F. Boeve, et al. 2003. Vascular dementia in a population-based
autopsy study. *Archives of Neurology* 60:569–75.

Kodner, D. L. 1993. Long-term care, 2010: Speculations and implications. *Journal of Long Term
Care Administration* 21:82–86.

Koenig, H. G. 1999. The healing power of faith. *Annals of Long-Term Care* 7:381–84.

Kohn, R., R. J. Westlake, S. A. Rasmussen, et al. 1997. Clinical features of obsessive-compulsive disorder in elderly patients. *American Journal of Geriatric Psychiatry* 5:211–15.

Kolanowski, A. M., L. Buettner, D. M. Fick, et al. 2008. Instituting cognitive rehabilitation in post-acute care. *Annals of Long-Term Care* 16:40–46.

Konetzka, R. T., W. Spector, and M. R. Limcangco. 2008. Reducing hospitalizations from long-term care settings. *Medical Care Research Review* 65:40–66.

Kopetz, S., C. D. Steele, J. Brandt, et al. 2000. Characteristics and outcomes of dementia residents in an assisted living facility. *International Journal of Geriatric Psychiatry* 15:586–93.

Krishnan, K. R. R., J. C. Hays, L. A. Tupler, et al. 1995. Clinical and phenomenological correlates of late-onset and early-onset depression. *American Journal of Psychiatry* 152:785–88.

Kumar, S., M. Bhatia, and M. Behari. 2002. Sleep disorders in Parkinson's disease. *Movement Disorders* 17:775–81.

Lachs, M. S., and L. Pillemer. 2004. Elder abuse. *Lancet* 364:1263–72.

Lacy, B. E., and M. S. Cole. 2004. Constipation in older adults. *Clinical Geriatrics* 12:44–54.

Lancet. 2003. The coming crisis of long-term care. *Lancet* 361:1755.

Lanctot, K. L., T. S. Best, N. Mittmann, et al. 1998. Efficacy and safety of narcoleptics in behavioral disorders associated with dementia. *Journal of Clinical Psychiatry* 59:550–61.

Landes, A. M., S. D. Sperry, M. E. Strauss, et al. 2001. Apathy in Alzheimer's disease. *Journal of the American Geriatric Society* 49:1700–1707.

Landreville, P., A. Bedard, R. Verreault, et al. 2006. Non-pharmacological interventions for aggressive behavior in older adults living in long-term care facilities. *International Psychogeriatrics* 18:47–73.

Langkamp-Henken, B., S. M. Wood, K. A. Herrlinger-Garcia, et al. 2006. Nutritional formula improved immune profiles of seniors living in nursing homes. *Journal of the American Geriatrics Society* 54:1861–70.

Lantz, M. S. 2007.Wandering in dementia. *Clinical Geriatrics* 15:21–24.

Lapane, K. L., and L. Resnik. 2005. Obesity in nursing homes: An escalating problem. *Journal of the American Geriatrics Society* 53:1386–91.

Larson, E. 2000. An 80-year-old man with memory loss. *Journal of the American Medical Association* 283:1046–53.

Lau, D. T., J. D. Kasper, D. E. Potter, et al. 2004. Potentially inappropriate medication prescriptions among elderly nursing home residents: Their scope and associated resident and facility characteristics. *Health Services Research* 39:1257–76.

———. 2005. Hospitalization and death associated with potentially inappropriate medication prescriptions among elderly nursing home residents. *Archives of Internal Medicine* 165:68–74.

Lavretsky, H. 2003. Therapy of depression in dementia. *Expert Review of Neurotherapeutics* 3:631–39.

Lawlor, B. A. 1996. Environmental and social aspects of behavioral disturbances in dementia. *International Psychogeriatrics* 8:S259–62.

Lee, H. B., and C. G. Lyketsos. 2004. Diagnosis and clinical management of depression in mild cognitive impairment. *Psychiatric Annals* 34:273–80.

Lee, H. B., J. A. Hanner, J. L. Yokley, et al. 2007. Clozapine for treatment-resistant agitation in dementia. *Journal of Geriatric Psychiatry and Neurology* 20:178–82.

Lee, J., J. Monette, N. Sourial, et al. 2007. The use of a cholinesterase inhibitor review committee in long-term care. *Journal of the American Medical Directors Association* 8:243–47.

Lefebvre-Chapiro, S., and the Doloplus-2 Group. 2001. The Doloplus-2 scale: Evaluating pain in the elderly. *European Journal of Palliative Care* 8:191–94.

Lenze, E. J., B. H. Mulsant, J. Mohlman, et al. 2005. Generalized anxiety disorder in later life: Lifetime course and comorbidity with major depressive disorder. *American Journal of Geriatric Psychiatry* 13:77–80.

Leonard, R., M. E. Tinetti, H. G. Allore, et al. 2006. Potentially modifiable resident characteristics that are associated with physical or verbal aggression among nursing home residents with dementia. *Archives of Internal Medicine* 166:1295–1300.

Leroi, I., Q. M. Samus, A. Rosenblatt, et al. 2007. A comparison of small and large assisted living facilities for the diagnosis and care of dementia: The Maryland Assisted Living Study. *International Journal of Geriatric Psychiatry* 22:224–32.

Le Roux, H., M. Gatz, and J. L. Wetherell. 2005. Age at onset of generalized anxiety disorder in older adults. *American Journal of Geriatric Psychiatry* 13:23–30.

Levin, C. A., W. Wei, A. Akincigil, et al. 2007. Prevalence and treatment of diagnosed depression among elderly nursing home residents in Ohio. *Journal of the American Medical Directors Association* 8:585–94.

Levine, J. M. 2003. Elder neglect and abuse: A primer for primary care physicians. *Geriatrics* 58:37–40.

Lindbloom, E. J., J. Brandt, L. D. Hough, et al. 2007. Elder mistreatment in the nursing home: A systematic review. *Journal of the American Medical Directors Association* 8:610–16.

Lindstrom, K., A. Ekedahl, A. Carlsten, et al. 2007. Can selective serotonin inhibitor drugs in elderly patients in nursing homes be reduced? *Scandinavian Journal of Primary Health Care* 25:3–8.

Liu, B. A., A. McGeer, M. A. McArthur, et al. 2007. Effect of multivitamin and mineral supplementation on episodes of infection in nursing home residents: A randomized, placebo-controlled study. *Journal of the American Geriatric Society* 55:35–42.

Livingston, G., K. Johnston, C. Katona, et al. 2005. Systematic review of psychological approaches to the management of neuropsychiatric symptoms of dementia. *American Journal of Psychiatry* 162:1996–2021.

Llewellyn-Jones, R. H., and J. Snowdon. 2007. Depression in nursing homes: Ensuring adequate treatment. *CNS Drugs* 21:627–40.

Llorente, M. D., D. W. Oslin, and J. Malphurs. 2006. Substance use disorders in the elderly. In M. E. Agronin and G. J. Maletta (eds.), *Principles and Practice of Geriatric Psychiatry*, pp. 471–88. New York: Lippincott Williams & Wilkins.

Lunney, J. R., J. Lynn, D. J. Foley, et al. 2003. Patterns of functional decline at the end of life. *Journal of the American Medical Association* 289:2387–92.

Lustbader, W. 2000. Thoughts on the meaning of frailty: Reasons to grow old; Meaning in later life. *Generations* (Winter):21–24.

Lyketsos, C. G., and P. V. Rabins. 2005. Antipsychotic drugs in dementia: What should be made of the risks? *Journal of the American Medical Association* 294:1963–65.

Lyketsos, C. G., C. Steele, E. Galik, et al. 1999a. Physical aggression in dementia patients and its relationship to depression. *American Journal of Psychiatry* 156:66–71.

Lyketsos, C. G., L. L. Veiel, A. Baker, et al. 1999b. A randomized, controlled trial of bright light therapy for agitated behaviors in dementia patients residing in long-term care. *International Journal of Geriatric Psychiatry* 14:520–25.

Lyketsos, C. G., M. Steinberg, J. T. Tschanz, et al. 2000. Mental and behavioral disturbances in dementia: Findings from the Cache County Study on Memory in Aging. *American Journal of Psychiatry* 157:708–14.

Lyketsos, C. G., O. Lopez, B. Jones, et al. 2002. Prevalence of neuropsychiatric symptoms in dementia and mild cognitive impairment: Results from the Cardiovascular Health Study. *Journal of the American Medical Association* 2888:1475–83.

Lyketsos, C. G., C. C. Colenda, C. Beck, et al. 2006. Position statement of the American Association for Geriatric Psychiatry regarding principles of care for patients with dementia resulting from Alzheimer's disease. *American Journal of Geriatric Psychiatry* 14:561–72.

Lyons, W. L. 2006. Delirium in postacute and long-term care. *Journal of the American Medical Directors Association* 7:254–61.

Mackinnon, A., J. McCallum, G. Andrews, et al. 1998. The Center for Epidemiological Studies Depression Scale in older samples in Indonesia, North Korea, Myanmar, Sri Lanka, and Thailand. *Journal of Gerontology, Series B: Psychological Sciences and Social Sciences* 53B:P343–52.

MacLean, D. S. 1999. Preventing abuse and neglect in long-term care, part 1: Legal and political aspects. *Annals of Long-Term Care* 7:452–58.

Madan, S. 2005. Music intervention for disruptive behaviors in long-term care residents with dementia. *Annals of Long-Term Care: Clinical Care and Aging* 13(12):33–36.

Magaziner, J., P. German, S. I. Zimmerman, et al. 2000. The prevalence of dementia in a statewide sample of new nursing home admissions aged 65 and older: Diagnosis by expert panel. *Gerontologist* 40:663–72.

Mahgoub, N., and M. Serby. 2007. Charles Bonnet syndrome: Long-term outcome of treatment. *Psychiatric Annals* 37:579–80.

Mahoney, F. I., and D. W. Barthel. 1965. Functional evaluation: The Barthel index. *Maryland State Medical Journal* 14:61–65.

Manepalli, J., A. K. Desai, and P. Sharma. 2009. Psychosocial-environmental treatments for Alzheimer's disease. *Primary Psychiatry* 16(6):39–47.

Manfredi, P. L., B. Breuer, S. Wallenstein, et al. 2003. Opioid treatment for agitation in patients with advanced dementia. *International Journal of Geriatric Psychiatry* 18:700–705.

Mansdorf, I. J., M. Harrington, J. Lund, et al. 2008. Neuropsychological testing in skilled nursing facilities: The failure to confirm diagnoses of dementia. *Journal of the American Medical Directors Association* 9:271–74.

Margallo-Lana, M., A. Swann, J. O'Brien, et al. 2001. Prevalence and pharmacological management of behavioral and psychological symptoms amongst dementia sufferers living in care environments. *International Journal of Geriatric Psychiatry* 16:39–44.

Marin, R. S., B. S. Fogel, J. Hawkins, et al. 1995. Apathy: A treatable syndrome. *Journal of Neuropsychiatry and Clinical Neurosciences* 7:23–30.

Marsh, A., C. Biniaris, D. Vergados, et al. 2008. An assisted-living home architecture with integrated healthcare services for elderly people. *Studies of Health Technology Information* 137:93–103.

Martens, P. J., R. Fransoo, E. Burland, et al. 2007. Prevalence of mental illness and its impact on the use of home care and nursing homes: A population-based study of older adults in Manitoba. *Canadian Journal of Psychiatry* 52:581–90.

Martin, J. L., and S. Ancoli-Israel. 2008. Sleep disturbances in long-term care. *Clinics in Geriatric Medicine* 24:39–50.

Martin, J. L., A. K. Mory, and C. A. Alessi. 2005. Nighttime oxygen desaturation and symptoms of sleep-disordered breathing in long-stay nursing home residents. *Journals of Gerontology, Series A: Biological Sciences and Medical Sciences* 60A:104–8.

Martin, J. L., A. P. Webber, T. Alam, et al. 2006. Daytime sleeping, sleep disturbance, and circadian rhythms in the nursing home. *American Journal of Geriatric Psychiatry* 14:121–29.

Martin, J. L., M. R. Marler, J. O. Harker, et al. 2007. A multicomponent nonpharmacological intervention improves activity rhythms among nursing home residents with disrupted sleep/wake patterns. *Journals of Gerontology, Series A: Biological Sciences and Medical Sciences* 62A:67–72.

Marwit, S. J., and T. M. Meuser. 2002. Development and initial validation of an inventory to assess grief in caregivers of persons with Alzheimer's disease. *Gerontologist* 42:751–65.

Mathews, F. E., and T. Dening. 2002. Prevalence of dementia in institutional care. *Lancet* 360:225–26.

McAlpine, D. D. 2003. Patterns of care for persons 65 years and older with schizophrenia. In C. I. Cohen (ed.), *Schizophrenia in Later Life*, pp. 3–18. Washington, DC: American Psychiatric Publishing.

McCarney, R., P. Fisher, S. Iliffe, et al. 2008. Ginkgo biloba for mild to moderate dementia in a community setting: A pragmatic, randomized, parallel group, double-blind, placebo-controlled trial. *International Journal of Geriatric Psychiatry* 23(12):1222–30.

McCarty, E. F., and C. Drebing. 2001. Delirium in older adults: Assessment and clinical management. *Journal of Geriatric Psychiatry* 34:183–95.

McGivney, S. A., M. Mulvihill, and B. Taylor. 1994. Validating the GDS depression screen in the nursing home. *Journal of the American Geriatrics Society* 42:490–92.

McKeith, I. G., D. J. Burns, C. G. Ballard, et al. 2003. Dementia with Lewy bodies. *Seminars in Clinical Neuropsychiatry* 8:46–57.

McKeith, I. G., D. W. Dickson, J. Lowe, et al. 2005. Consortium on DLB: Diagnosis and management of dementia with Lewy bodies; Third report of the DLB consortium. *Neurology* 65:1863–72.

McNeil, J. K. 1999. Neuropsychological characteristics of the dementia syndrome of depression: Onset, resolution, and three-year follow-up. *Clinical Neuropsychology* 13:136–46.

Mechanic, D., and D. D. McAlpine. 2000. Use of nursing homes in the care of persons with severe mental illness, 1985 to 1995. *Psychiatric Services* 51:354–58.

Meeks, T. W., S. A. Ropacki, and D. V. Jeste. 2006. The neurobiology of neuropsychiatric syndromes in dementia. *Current Opinion in Psychiatry* 19:581–86.

Mega, M. S., J. L. Cummings, T. Fiorello, et al. 1996. The spectrum of behavioral changes in Alzheimer's disease. *Neurology* 46:130–35.

Mendelson, W. B. 2005. A review of the evidence for the efficacy and safety of trazodone in insomnia. *Journal of Clinical Psychiatry* 66(4):469–76.

Mendez, M. F., and G. Lim. 2003. Seizures in elderly patients with dementia: Epidemiology and management. *Drugs and Aging* 20:791–803.

Mendez, M. F., M. Cherrier, K. M. Perryman, et al. 1996. Frontotemporal dementia versus Alzheimer's disease: Differential cognitive features. *Neurology* 47:1189–94.

Mendez, M. F., J. S. Shapira, R. J. Woods, et al. 2008. Psychotic symptoms in frontotemporal dementia: Prevalence and review. *Dementia and Geriatric Cognitive Disorders* 25:206–11.

Merlino, G., A. Piani, P. Dolso, et al. 2006. Sleep disorders in patients with end-stage renal disease undergoing dialysis therapy. *Nephrology Dialysis, Transplantation* 21:184–90.

Messinger-Rapport, B., J. E. Morley, D. R. Thomas, et al. 2007. Intensive session: New approaches to medical issues in long-term care. *Journal of the American Medical Directors Association* 8:421–33.

Miller, S. C., J. M. Teno, and V. Mor. 2004. Hospice and palliative care in nursing homes. *Clinics in Geriatric Medicine* 20:717–34.

Milligan, S. A., and A. L. Chesson. 2002. Restless leg syndrome in the older adult: Diagnosis and management. *Drugs and Aging* 19:741–51.

Mitchell, S. L. 1999. Extrapyramidal features in Alzheimer's disease. *Age and Aging* 28:401–9.

———. 2007. A 93-year-old man with advanced dementia and eating problems. *Journal of the American Medical Association* 298:2527–36.

Mitchell, S. L., D. K. Kiely, M. B. Hamel, et al. 2004. Estimating prognosis for nursing home residents with advanced dementia. *Journal of the American Medical Association* 291:2734–40.

Mittelman, M. S., D. L. Roth, D. W. Coon, et al. 2004. Sustained benefit of supportive intervention for depressive symptoms in caregivers of patients with Alzheimer's disease. *American Journal of Psychiatry* 161:850–56.

Mittelman, M. S., W. E. Haley, O. J. Clay, et al. 2006. Improving caregiver well-being delays nursing home placement of patients with Alzheimer disease. *Neurology* 67:1592–99.

Mitty, E. L. 2004. Assisted living: Aging in place and palliative care. *Geriatric Nursing* 25:149–56.

———. 2005. Culture change in nursing homes: An ethical perspective. *Annals of Long-Term Care* 13:47–51.

Miyasaki, J. M., K. Shannon, V. Voon, et al. 2006. Practice parameter: Evaluation and treatment of depression, psychosis, and dementia in Parkinson disease (an evidence-based review); Report of the Quality Standards Subcommittee of the American Academy of Neurology. *Neurology* 66:996–1002.

Mizrahi, R., S. E. Starkstein, R. Jorge, et al. 2006. Phenomenology and clinical correlates of delusions in Alzheimer disease. *American Journal of Geriatric Psychiatry* 14:573–81.

Moellentin, D., C. Picone, and E. Leadbetter. 2008. Memantine-induced myoclonus and delirium exacerbated by trimethoprim. *Annals of Pharmacotherapy* 42:443–47.

Morley, J. E. 2001. Decreased food intake with aging. *Journals of Gerontology, Series A: Biological Sciences and Medical Sciences* 56A (suppl. 2):81–88.

———. 2007. Should all long-term care residents receive vitamin D? *Journal of the American Medical Directors Association* 8:69–70.

———. 2008. Managing persons with dementia in the nursing home: High touch trumps high tech. *Journal of the American Medical Directors Association* 6:139–46.

Morley, J. E., and J. H. Flaherty. 2002. Putting the "home" back in nursing home. *Journals of Gerontology, Series A: Biological Sciences and Medical Sciences* 57A:M419–21.

Morley, J. E., J. Flood, and A. J. Silver. 1992. Effects of peripheral hormones on memory and ingestive behaviors. *Psychoneuroendocrinology* 17:391–99.

Morley, J. E., and D. R. Thomas. 2008. Cachexia: New advances in the management of wasting diseases. *Journal of the American Medical Directors Association* 9:205–10.

Morley, J. E., M. T. Haren, Y. Rolland, et al. 2006. Frailty. *Medical Clinics of North America* 90:837–47.

Morrison, R. S., and A. L. Siu. 2000. Survival in end-stage dementia following acute illness. *Journal of the American Medical Association* 284:47–52.

Morse, J. Q., and T. R. Lynch. 2000. Personality disorders in late life. *Current Psychiatry Report* 2:24–31.

Mulsant, B. H., and M. Ganguli. 1999. Epidemiology and diagnosis of depression in late life. *Journal of Clinical Psychiatry* 60 (suppl. 20):9–15.

National Center for Health Statistics. 2009. *National Nursing Home Survey 2004.* Hyattsville, MD: U.S. Department of Health and Human Services, Centers for Disease Control and Prevention.

National Institute on Aging and Duke University. 2004. *National Long-Term Care Survey.* www .nltcs.aas.duke.edu.

National Institute on Alcohol Abuse and Alcoholism. 1995. Diagnostic criteria for alcohol abuse. *Alcohol Alert* 30:1–6.

Nelson, A., J. Collins, K. Siddharthan, et al. 2008. Link between safe patient handling and patient outcomes in long-term care. *Rehabilitation Nursing* 33:33–43.

Nishtala, P. S., A. J. McLachlan, J. S. Bell, et al. 2008. Psychotropic prescribing in long-term care facilities: Impact of medication reviews and educational interventions. *American Journal of Geriatric Psychiatry* 16:621–32.

Noell-Waggoner, E. 2004. Lighting solutions for contemporary problems of older adults. *Journal of Psychosocial Nursing* 42(7):14–20.

Norberg, A. 1996. Perspectives of an institution-based research nurse. *International Psychogeriatrics* 8 (suppl. 3):459–64.

Norman, R. A. 2008. Common skin conditions in geriatric dermatology. *Annals of Long-Term Care: Clinical Care and Aging* 16:40–45.

Nygaard, H. A., and M. Jarland. 2005. Are nursing home patients with dementia diagnosis at increased risk for inadequate pain treatment? *International Journal of Geriatric Psychiatry* 20:730–37.

O'Brien, J. A., and J. J. Caro. 2001. Alzheimer's disease and other dementia in nursing homes: Levels of management and cost. *International Psychogeriatrics* 13:347–58.

O'Donnell, B. F. 2007. Cognitive impairment in schizophrenia: A life span perspective. *American Journal of Alzheimer's Disease and Other Dementias* 22:398–405.

O'Donnell, B. F., D. A. Drachman, H. J. Barnes, et al. 1992. Incontinence and troublesome behaviors predict institutionalization in dementia. *Journal of Geriatric Psychiatry and Neurology* 5:45–52.

Office of the Inspector General. 2001. *Psychotropic Drug Use in Nursing Homes.* Report no. OEI 02-00-00490. Washington, DC: U.S. Department of Health and Human Services.

Oliver, D. P., D. Porock, and S. Zweig. 2004. End-of-life care in U.S. nursing homes: A review of the evidence. *Journal of the American Medical Directors Association* 5:147–55.

Onofrj, M., A. Thomas, and L. Bonanni. 2007. New approaches to understanding hallucinations in Parkinson's disease: Phenomenology and possible origins. *Expert Review of Neurotherapeutics* 7:1731–50.

Orr, W. B. 2004. Apathy in the older adult. *Geriatrics* 59(7):34–36.

Oslin, D. W. 2005. Evidence-based treatment of geriatric substance abuse. *Psychiatric Clinics of North America* 28:897–911.

Ostling, S., and I. Skoog. 2002. Psychotic symptoms and paranoid ideation in a non-demented population-based sample of the very old. *Archives of General Psychiatry* 59:53–59.

Ott, B. R., and K. L. Lapane. 2002. Tacrine therapy is associated with reduced mortality in nursing home residents with dementia. *Journal of the American Geriatrics Society* 50:35–40.

Ouslander, J. G., G. Patry, and R. W. Besdine. 2007. Quality improvement in nursing homes: A call to action. *Journal of the American Medical Directors Association* 3:138–41.

Overshott, R., J. Byrne, and A. Burns. 2004. Nonpharmacological and pharmacological interventions for symptoms in Alzheimer's disease. *Expert Review of Neurotherapeutics* 4:809–21.

Owen, T. (ed.). 2005. *Dying in Older Age: Reflections and Experiences from an Older Person's Perspective*. London: Help the Aged and Sheffield University. www.helptheaged.org.uk.

Pact, V., and T. Giduz. 1999. Mirtazapine treats resting tremor, essential tremor and levodopa-induced dyskinesias. *Neurology* 53:1154.

Palop, J. J., and L. Mucke. 2009. Epilepsy and cognitive impairments in Alzheimer's disease. *Archives of Neurology* 66(4):435–40.

Paniagua, M. A., and E. W. Paniagua. 2008. The demented elder with insomnia. *Clinics in Geriatric Medicine* 24:69–81.

Paulsen, J. S., D. P. Salmon, L. J. Thal, et al. 2000. Incidence of and risk factors for hallucinations and delusions in patients with probable AD. *Neurology* 54:1965–71.

Payne, J. L., J-M. E. Sheppard, M. Steinberg, et al. 2002. Incidence, prevalence, and outcomes of depression in residents of a long-term care facility with dementia. *International Journal of Geriatric Psychiatry* 17:247–53.

Pepersack, T., J. Garbusinski, J. Robberecht, et al. 1999. Clinical relevance of thiamine status amongst hospitalized elderly patients. *Gerontology* 45:96–101.

Perlis, R. H., E. Brown, R. W. Baker, et al. 2006. Clinical features of bipolar depression versus major depressive disorder in large multicenter trials. *American Journal of Psychiatry* 163:225–31.

Perneczky, R., S. Wagenpfeil, K. Komossa, et al. 2006. Mapping scores onto stages: Mini-Mental State Examination and clinical dementia rating. *American Journal of Geriatric Psychiatry* 14(2):139–44.

Petersen, R. C., G. E. Smith, S. C. Waring, et al. 1999. Mild cognitive impairment: Clinical characterization and outcome. *Archives of Neurology* 56:303–8.

Pfeffer, R. I., T. T. Kurosaki, C. H. Harrah, et al. 1992. Measurement of functional activities in older adults in the community. *Journal of Gerontology* 37:323–29.

Pittiglio, L. 2000. Use of reminiscence therapy in patients with Alzheimer's disease. *Lippincott's Case Management* 5:216–20.

Poewe, W. 2006. The natural history of Parkinson's disease. *Journal of Neurology* 253 (suppl. 7):V112–16.

Poewe, W., and K. Seppi. 2001. Treatment options for depression and psychosis in Parkinson's disease. *Journal of Neurology* 248 (suppl. 3):12–21.

Pollock, B. G., B. H. Mulsant, J. Rosen, et al. 2007. A double-blind comparison of citalopram and risperidone for the treatment of behavioral and psychotic symptoms associated with dementia. *American Journal of Geriatric Psychiatry* 15:942–52.

Post, S. G. 2000. Commentary on "Sexuality and intimacy in the nursing home." *Journal of Clinical Ethics* (Winter):314–17.

Post, S. G., and P. J. Whitehouse. 1999. Spirituality, religion, and Alzheimer's disease. *Journal of Health Care Chaplaincy* 8:45–57.

Provencher, V., N. Bier, T. Audet, et al. 2008. Errorless-based techniques can improve route finding in early Alzheimer's disease: A case study. *American Journal of Alzheimer's Disease and Other Dementias* 23:47–56.

Purandare, N., A. Burns, S. Craig, et al. 2001. Depressive symptoms in patients with Alzheimer's disease. *International Journal of Geriatric Psychiatry* 16:960–64.

Rabinowitz, T., J. P. Hirdes, and I. Desjardins. 2006. Somatoform disorders in late life. In M. E. Agronin and G. J. Maletta (eds.), *Principles and Practice of Geriatric Psychiatry*, pp. 489–504. New York: Lippincott Williams & Wilkins.

Rabins, P. V., D. Blacker, B. W. Rovner, et al. 2007. *Treatment of Patients with Alzheimer's Disease and Other Dementias*, 2nd ed. American Psychiatric Association Practice Guidelines. www.psychiatryonline.com/pracGuide/pracGuideTopic_3.aspx [accessed August 31, 2009].

Rahman, A. N., and S. F. Simmons. 2005. Individualizing nutritional care with between-meal snacks for nursing home residents. *Journal of the American Medical Directors Association* 6(3):215–18.

Ramadan, M. I., S. F. Werder, and S. H. Preskorn. 2006. Protect against drug-drug interactions with anxiolytics. *Current Psychiatry* 5:21–28.

Rao, V., and C. G. Lyketsos. 2000. The benefits and risks of ECT for patients with degenerative dementia who also suffer from depression. *International Journal of Geriatric Psychiatry* 15:729–35.

Rao, V., J. Spiro, Q. M. Samus, et al. 2008. Insomnia and daytime sleepiness in people with dementia residing in assisted living: Findings from the Maryland Assisted Living Study. *International Journal of Geriatric Psychiatry* 23:199–206.

Rask, K., P. A. Parmelee, J. A. Taylor, et al. 2007. Implementation and evaluation of a nursing home fall management program. *Journal of the American Geriatrics Society* 55:342–49.

Ratnavalli, E., C. Brayne, K. Dawson, et al. 2002. The prevalence of frontotemporal dementia. *Neurology* 58:1615–21.

Ravina, B., K. Marder, H. H. Fernandez, et al. 2007. Diagnostic criteria for psychosis in Parkinson's disease: Report of an NINDS, NIMH work group. *Movement Disorders* 22:1061–68.

Ray, W. A., J. A. Taylor, K. G. Meador, et al. 1993. Reducing antipsychotic drug use in nursing homes: A controlled trial of provider education. *Archives of Internal Medicine* 153:713–21.

Reisberg, B., J. Borenstein, S. P. Salob, et al. 1987. Behavioral symptoms in Alzheimer's disease: Phenomenology and treatment. *Journal of Clinical Psychiatry* 48 (suppl. 5):9–15.

Rektorova, I., I. Rektor, M. Bares, et al. 2003. Pramipexole and pergolide in the treatment of depression in Parkinson's disease: A national multicenter prospective randomized study. *European Journal of Neurology* 10:399–406.

Reyes-Ortiz, C. A. 2001. Neglect and self-neglect of the elderly in long-term care. *Annals of Long-Term Care* 9:21–24.

Reynolds, C. F. III, M. A. Dew, B. G. Pollock, et al. 2006. Maintenance treatment of major depression in old age. *New England Journal of Medicine* 354:1130–38.

Richard, I. H. 2005. Anxiety disorders in Parkinson's disease. *Advances in Neurology* 96:42–55.

Ricker, J. H., and B. N. Axelrod. 1994. Analysis of an oral paradigm for the trail making test. *Assessment* 1(1):47–51.

Riemersma-van der Lek, R. F., D. F. Swaab, J. Twisk, et al. 2008. Effect of bright light and melatonin on cognitive and noncognitive function in elderly residents of group care facilities. *Journal of the American Medical Association* 299:2642–55.

Robertson, R. G., and M. Montagnini. 2004. Geriatric failure to thrive. *American Family Physician* 70:343–50.

Rochon, P. A., S. L. Normand, T. Gomes, et al. 2008. Antipsychotic therapy and short-term serious events in older adults with dementia. *Archives of Internal Medicine* 168:1090–96.

Rogers, E. M. 1995. *Diffusion of Innovations*, 4th ed. New York: Free Press.

Rolland, Y., F. Pillard, A. Klapouszczak, et al. 2007a. Exercise program for nursing home residents with Alzheimer's disease: A 1-year randomized, controlled trial. *Journal of the American Geriatrics Society* 55(2):158–65.

Rolland, Y., S. Andrieu, C. Cantet, et al. 2007b. Wandering behavior and Alzheimer disease: The REAL.FR prospective study. *Alzheimer Disease and Associated Disorders* 21:31–38.

Rosen, H. J., and J. Cummings. 2007. A real reason for patients with pseudobulbar affect to smile. *Annals of Neurology* 61:92–96.

Rosen, T., M. S. Lachs, A. J. Bharucha, et al. 2008. Resident-to-resident aggression in long-term care facilities: Insights from focus groups of nursing home residents and staff. *Journal of the American Geriatrics Society* 56(8):1398–1408.

Rosenblatt, A., Q. M. Samus, C. D. Steele, et al. 2004. The Maryland Assisted Living Study: Prevalence, recognition, and treatment of dementia and other psychiatric disorders in the assisted living population of central Maryland. *Journal of the American Geriatrics Society* 52:1618–25.

Rosenthal, N. E. 2006. *Winter Blues: Everything You Need to Know to Beat Seasonal Affective Disorder*. New York: Guilford Press.

Ross, G. W., and J. D. Bowen. 2002. The diagnosis and differential diagnosis of dementia. *Medical Clinics of North America* 86:455–76.

Roubenoff, R. 2000. Sarcopenia and its implications for the elderly. *European Journal of Clinical Nutrition* 54:S40–47.

Rubenstein, L. Z. 2008. Hip protectors in long-term care: Another confirmatory trial. *Journal of the American Medical Directors Association* 9:289–90.

Rueve, M. E., and R. S. Welton. 2008. Violence and mental illness. *Psychiatry* 5:35–48.

Russell, R. M., H. Rasmussen, and A. H. Lichtenstein. 1999. Modified food guide pyramid for people over seventy years of age. *Journal of Nutrition* 129:751–53.

Sachs, G. A., J. W. Shega, and D. Cox-Hayley. 2004. Barriers to excellent end-of-life care for patients with dementia. *Journal of General Internal Medicine* 19:1057–63.

Sajatovic, M., F. C. Blow, R. Ignacio, et al. 2004. Age-related modifiers of clinical presentation and health services use among veterans with bipolar disorder. *Psychiatric Services* 55(9):1014–21.

Saliba, D. 2008. PHQ-9 use in nursing home residents. Presented at the annual meeting of the American Geriatrics Society, April 30–May 4, Washington, DC.

Salzman, C. 2004. Late-life anxiety disorders. *Psychopharmacology Bulletin* 38 (suppl. 1):25–30.

Sandson, N. B. 2007. *Drug-Drug Interaction Primer: A Compendium of Case Vignettes for the Practicing Clinician.* Washington, DC: American Psychiatric Publishing.

Scarmeas, N., J. Brandt, D. Blacker, et al. 2007. Disruptive behavior as a predictor in Alzheimer disease. *Archives of Neurology* 64:1755–61.

Scherder, E. J. A., and A. Bouma. 2000. Visual analogue scales for pain assessment in Alzheimer's disease. *Gerontology* 46:47–53.

Schneeweiss, S., S. Setogouchi, A. Brookhart, et al. 2007. Risk of death associated with the use of conventional versus atypical antipsychotic drugs among elderly patients. *Canadian Medical Association Journal* 176:627–32.

Schneider, L. S., K. S. Dagerman, and P. Insel. 2005. Risk of death with atypical antipsychotic drug treatment for dementia: Meta-analysis of randomized placebo-controlled trials. *Journal of the American Medical Association* 294:1934–43.

Schneider, L. S., P. N. Tariot, K. S. Dagerman, et al. 2006. Effectiveness of atypical antipsychotic drugs in patients with Alzheimer's disease. *New England Journal of Medicine* 355:1525–38.

Schonfeld, L., B. King-Kallimanis, L. M. Brown, et al. 2007. Wanderers with cognitive impairment in Department of Veterans Affairs nursing home care units. *Journal of the American Geriatrics Society* 55:692–99.

Schultz, S. K., V. L. Ellingrod, C. Turvey, et al. 2003. The influence of cognitive impairment and behavioral dysregulation on daily functioning in the nursing home setting. *American Journal of Psychiatry* 160:582–84.

Schulz, R., R. Hebert, and K. Boerner. 2008. Bereavement after caregiving. *Geriatrics* 63:20–22.

Schulz, R., S. H. Belle, S. J. Czaja, et al. 2004. Long-term care placement of dementia patients and caregiver health and well-being. *Journal of the American Medical Association* 292:961–67.

Schweitzer, I., V. Tuckwell, J. O'Brien, et al. 2002. Is late-onset depression a prodrome to dementia? *International Journal of Geriatric Psychiatry* 17:997–1005.

Scott, I. U., O. D. Schein, W. Feuer, et al. 2001. Visual hallucinations in patients with retinal disease. *American Journal of Ophthalmology* 131:590–98.

Sehl, M. E., A. Naeim, and S. L. Charette. 2008. Macrocytosis in the elderly. *Clinical Geriatrics* 2:36–42.

Seidlitz, L. 2001. Personality factors in mental disorders in later life. *American Journal of Geriatric Psychiatry* 9:8–21.

Seitz, D. P., S. S. Gill, and L. T. van Zyl. 2007. Antipsychotics in the treatment of delirium: A systematic review. *Journal of Clinical Psychiatry* 68:11–21.

Selwood, A., K. Johnston, C. Katona, et al. 2007. Systematic review of the effect of psychological interventions in family caregivers of people with dementia. *Journal of Affective Disorders* 101:75–89.

Sherder, E., J. Oosterman, D. Swaab, et al. 2005. Recent developments in pain in dementia. *British Medical Journal* 330:461–64.

Shinoda-Tagawa, T., R. Leonard, J. Pontikas, et al. 2004. Resident-to-resident violent incidents in nursing homes. *Journal of the American Medical Association* 291:591–98.

Siddiqi, N., R. Stockdale, A. M. Britton, et al. 2007. Interventions for preventing delirium in hospitalized patients. *Cochrane Database of Systematic Reviews* 2. doi:10.1002/14651858. CD005563.pub2.

Sink, K. M., K. F. Holden, and K. Yaffe. 2005. Pharmacological treatment of neuropsychiatric symptoms of dementia: A review of the evidence. *Journal of the American Medical Association* 293:596–608.

Sink, K. M., J. Thomas III, H. Xu, et al. 2008. Dual use of bladder anticholinergics and cholinesterase inhibitors: Long-term functional and cognitive outcomes. *Journal of the American Geriatrics Society* 56:847–53.

Skapik, J. L., and G. J. Treisman. 2007. HIV, psychiatric comorbidity and aging. *Clinical Geriatrics* 15:26–36.

Skoog, G., and I. Skoog. 1999. A 40-year follow-up of patients with obsessive-compulsive disorder. *Archives of General Psychiatry* 56:121–27.

Skrajner, M. J., and C. J. Camp. 2007. Resident-Assisted Montessori Programming (RAMP): Use of a small group reading activity run by persons with dementia in adult day health care and long-term care settings. *American Journal of Alzheimer's Disease and Other Disorders* 22:27–32.

Sloane, P. D., S. Zimmerman, A. L. Gruber-Baldini, et al. 2005. Health and functional outcomes and health care utilization of persons with dementia in residential care and assisted living facilities: Comparison with nursing homes. *Gerontologist* 45:124–32.

Small, G. W. 2002. What we need to know about age-related memory loss. *British Medical Journal* 324:1502–5.

Small, G. W., P. V. Rabins, P. P. Barry, et al. 1997. Diagnosis and treatment of Alzheimer's disease and related disorders: Consensus statement of the American Association for Geriatric Psychiatry, the Alzheimer's Association, and the American Geriatrics Society. *Journal of the American Medical Association* 278:1363–71.

Small, J. A., J. Perry, and J. Lewis. 2005. Perceptions of family caregivers' psychosocial behavior when communicating with spouses who have Alzheimer's disease. *American Journal of Alzheimer's Disease and Other Dementias* 20:281–89.

Smith, M., L. A. Gerdner, G. R. Hall, et al. 2004. History, development, and future of the progressively lowered stress threshold: A conceptual model for dementia care. *Journal of the American Geriatrics Society* 52:1755–60.

Smoyak, S. A. 2005. Independence, dignity and choice in assisted living. *Journal of Psychosocial Nursing* 43(3):16–19.

Snowden, M., K. Sato, and P. Roy-Byrne. 2003. Assessment and treatment of nursing home residents with depression or behavioral symptoms associated with dementia: A review of the literature. *Journal of the American Geriatrics Society* 51:1305–17.

Sorrell, J. M. 2007. Caring for the caregivers. *Journal of Psychosocial Nursing and Mental Health Services* 45:17–20.

Spector, W., T. Shaffer, D. E. B. Potter, et al. 2007. Risk factors associated with the occurrence of fractures in U.S. nursing homes: Resident and facility characteristics and prescription medications. *Journal of the American Geriatrics Society* 55:327–33.

Sperry, L. 2006. Working with spiritual issues of the elderly and their caregivers. *Psychiatric Annals* 36:185–93.

Spiro, A., P. P. Schurr, and C. M. Aldwin. 1994. Combat-related post-traumatic stress disorder symptoms in older men. *Psychological Aging* 9:17–26.

Spitzer, R., K. Kroenke, and J. Williams. 1999. Validation and utility of a self-report version of PRIME-MD: The PHQ Primary Care Study. *Journal of the American Medical Association* 282:1737–44.

Spreen, F. O., and A. L. Benton. 1977. *Manual of Instructions for the Neurosensory Center Comprehensive Examination for Aphasia.* Victoria, BC: University of Victoria.

St. George, R. J., K. Delbaere, P. Williams, et al. 2008. Sleep quality and falls in older people living in self- and assisted-care villages. *Gerontology* 55(2):162–68.

Stadeford, A. 1984. *Bereavement: Complicated Grief; Facing Death.* London: Heinnemann Medical Books.

Starkstein, S. E., R. Jorge, R. Mizrahi, et al. 2005. The construct of minor and major depression in Alzheimer's disease. *American Journal of Psychiatry* 162:2086–93.

Stefanacci, R. 2006. Why doesn't CMS understand the LTC difference? *Clinical Geriatrics* 14:10–12.

Steinberg, M., J.-M. Sheppard, J. T. Tschanz, et al. 2003. The incidence of mental and behavioral disturbances in dementia: The Cache County study. *Journal of Neuropsychiatry and Clinical Neurosciences* 15:340–45.

Stewart, J. T. 2006. The frontal/subcortical dementias: Common dementing illnesses associated with prominent and disturbing behavioral changes. *Geriatrics* 61:23–27.

Stroebe, M., H. Schut, and W. Stroebe. 2007. Health outcomes of bereavement. *Lancet* 370:1960–73.

Strub, R. 2003. Vascular dementia. *Southern Medical Journal* 96:363–66.

Struck, B. D., and K. M. Ross. 2006. Health promotion in older adults: Prescribing exercise for the frail and home bound. *Geriatrics* 61:22–27.

Sultzer, D. L., S. M. Davis, P. N. Tariot, et al. 2008. Clinical symptom responses to atypical antipsychotic medications in Alzheimer's disease: Phase 1 outcomes from the CATIE-AD Effectiveness Trial. *American Journal of Psychiatry* 165:844–54.

Suominen, K., M. Henriksson, E. Isometsa, et al. 2003. A psychological autopsy study. *International Journal of Geriatric Psychiatry* 18:1095–1101.

Swanberg, M. M. 2007. Memantine for behavioral disturbances in frontotemporal dementia: A case series. *Alzheimer Disease and Associated Disorders* 38:164–66.

Sweet, R. A., V. L. Nimgaonkar, B. Devlin, et al. 2002. Increased familial risk of the psychotic phenotype of Alzheimer disease. *Neurology* 58:907–11.

Tait, R. C., and J. T. Chibnall. 2008. Under-treatment of pain in dementia: Assessment is key. *Journal of the American Medical Directors Association* 7:372–74.

Targum, S. D., and N. Rosenthal. 2008. Seasonal affective disorder. *Psychiatry* 5:31–33.

Tariot, P. N., C. A. Podgorski, L. Blazina, et al. 1993. Mental disorders in the nursing home: Another perspective. *American Journal of Psychiatry* 150:1063–69.

Tariq, S. H., N. Tumosa, J. T. Chibnall, et al. 2006. The Saint Louis University Mental Status (SLUMS) Examination for detecting mild cognitive impairment and dementia is more sensitive than the Mini-Mental State Examination (MMSE): A pilot study. *American Journal of Geriatric Psychiatry* 14:900–910.

Teigland, C. 2007. Use of antidepressants in LTC residents. Presented at the 15th Annual Alzheimer's Association Dementia Care Conference, August 26–29, Chicago, Illinois.

Tellis-Nayak, V. 2007. A person-centered workplace: The foundation for person-centered caregiving in long-term care. *Journal of the American Medical Directors Association* 8:46–54.

Teno, J., G. Kabumoto, T. Wetle, et al. 2004. Daily pain that was excruciating at some time in the previous week: Prevalence, characteristics, and outcomes in nursing home residents. *Journal of the American Geriatrics Society* 52:762–67.

Thakur, M., and D. G. Blazer. 2008. Depression in long-term care. *Journal of the American Medical Directors Association* 9:82–87.

Thomas, A., L. Bonanni, and M. Onofrj. 2007. Symptomatic REM sleep behaviour disorder. *Neurological Sciences* 28:S21–36.

Thomas, A. M., and S. R. Gambert. 2008. Hazards from the health food store—part I. *Clinical Geriatrics* 16:35–42.

Thomas, D. R. 2004. Vitamins in health and aging. *Clinics in Geriatric Medicine* 20:259–74.

Thomas, D. R., and J. E. Morley. 2006. Nursing home care. In M. S. J. Pathy, A. J. Sinclair, and J. E. Morley (eds.), *Principles and Practice of Geriatric Medicine*, 4th ed., vol. 2, pp. 1817–26. Chichester, West Sussex, England: John Wiley & Sons.

Thomas, D. R., W. Ashmen, J. E. Morley, et al. 2000. Nutritional management in long-term care: Development of a clinical guideline. *Journals of Gerontology, Series A: Biological Sciences and Medical Sciences* 55A:M725–34.

Thomas, D. R., C. D. Zdrowski, M. M. Wilson, et al. 2002. Malnutrition in subacute care. *American Journal of Clinical Nutrition* 75:308–13.

Thomas, D. R., T. R. Cote, L. Lawhorne, et al. 2008. Understanding clinical dehydration and its treatment. *Journal of the American Medical Directors Association* 9:292–301.

Thomas, P., P. Ingrand, F. Lalloue, et al. 2004. Reasons of informal caregivers for institutionalizing dementia patients previously living at home: The Pixel study. *International Journal of Geriatric Psychiatry* 19:127–218.

Tiraboschi, P., L. A. Hansen, M. Alford, et al. 2002. Early and widespread cholinergic losses differentiate dementia Lewy bodies from Alzheimer disease. *Archives of General Psychiatry* 59:946–51.

Tondi, L., L. Ribani, M. Bottazzi, et al. 2007. Validation therapy (VT) in nursing home: A case-control study. *Archives of Gerontology and Geriatrics* 44 (suppl. 1):407–11.

Tune, L. E. 2001. Anticholinergic effects of medications in the elderly patients. *Journal of Clinical Psychiatry* 62 (suppl. 21):11–14.

Turvey, C. L., C. Carney, S. Arndt, et al. 1999. Conjugal loss and syndromal depression in a sample of elders aged 70 years and older. *American Journal of Psychiatry* 156:1596–1601.

Tyler, D. A., V. A. Parker, R. L. Engle, et al. 2006. An exploration of job design in long-term care facilities and its effect on nursing employee satisfaction. *Health Care Management Review* 31:137–44.

Ulfvarson, J., J. Adami, R. Wredling, et al. 2003. Controlled withdrawal of selective serotonin reuptake inhibitor drugs in elderly patients in nursing homes with no indication of depression. *European Journal of Clinical Pharmacology* 59:735–40.

U.S. Census Bureau. 2007. *American Community Survey.* www.census.gov/acs/www/Products/ [accessed August 17, 2008].

Vaillant, G. E. 2002. *Aging Well*. Boston: Little, Brown.

Vance, J. 2008. Proceedings of the AMDA Assisted Living Consensus Conference, Washington DC, October 24, 2006. *Journal of the American Medical Directors Association* 9:378–82.

van der Flier, W. M., S. Staekenborg, Y. A. Pijnenburg, et al. 2007. Apolipoprotein E genotype influences presence and severity of delusions and aggressive behavior in Alzheimer disease. *Dementia and Geriatric Cognitive Disorder* 23:42–46.

van der Wurff, F. B., M. L. Stek, W. J. G. Hoogendijk, et al. 2003. The efficacy and safety of ECT in depressed older adults: A literature review. *International Journal of Geriatric Psychiatry* 18:894–904.

Vellas, B., H. Villars, G. Abellan, et al. 2006. Overview of the MNA(R): Its history and challenges. *Journal of Nutritional Health Aging* 10:456–65.

Vida, S., R. C. Monks, and P. D. Rosiers. 2002. Prevalence and correlates of elder abuse and neglect in a geriatric psychiatry service. *Canadian Journal of Psychiatry* 47:459–67.

Villareal, D. T., C. M. Apovian, R. Kushner, et al. 2005. Obesity in older adults: Technical review and position statement of the American Society for Nutrition and NAASO, The Obesity Society. *Obesity Research* 13:1849–63.

Vitiello, M. V., and S. Borson. 2001. Sleep disturbances in patients with Alzheimer's disease: Epidemiology, pathophysiology and treatment. *CNS Drugs* 15:777–96.

Vogelsmeier, A. A., J. R. B. Halbesleben, and J. R. Scott-Cawiezell. 2008. Technology implementation and workarounds in the nursing home. *Journal of the American Medical Informatics Association* 15:114–19.

Volicer, L., and A. C. Hurley. 1997. Comorbidity in Alzheimer's disease. *Journal of Mental Health and Aging* 3:5–17.

———. 2003. Management of behavioral symptoms in progressive degenerative dementias. *Journals of Gerontology, Series A: Biological Sciences and Medical Sciences* 58A:M837–45.

Volicer, L., J. Simard, J. H. Pupa, et al. 2006. Effects of continuous activity programming on behavioral symptoms of dementia. *Journal of the American Medical Directors Association* 7:426–31.

Volicer, L., L. DeRuvo, K. Hyer, et al. 2008. Development of a scale to measure quality of visits with relatives with dementia. *Journal of the American Medical Directors Association* 9(5):327–31.

Voyer, P., J. McCusker, M. G. Cole, et al. 2006 Influence of prior cognitive impairment on the severity of delirium symptoms among older patients. *Journal of Neuroscience Nursing* 38:90–101.

Wang, H. X., A. Wahlin, H. Basun, et al. 2001. Vitamin B_{12} and folate in relation to the development of Alzheimer's disease. *Neurology* 56:1188–94.

Wang, P. S., S. Schneeweiss, J. Avorn, et al. 2005. Risk of death in elderly users of conventional versus atypical antipsychotic medications. *New England Journal of Medicine* 353:2335–41.

Warden, V., A. C. Hurley, and L. Volicer. 2003. Development and psychometric evaluation of the pain assessment in advanced dementia. *Journal of the American Medical Directors Association* 4:9–15.

Watson, L. C., S. Lehmann, L. Mayer, et al. 2006. Depression in assisted living is common and related to physical burden. *American Journal of Geriatric Psychiatry* 14:876–83.

Watson, R., and L. J. Dreary. 1997. A longitudinal study of feeding difficulty and nursing intervention in elderly patients with dementia. *Journal of Advanced Nursing* 26:25–32.

Webster, J., and G. T. Grossberg. 1998. Late-life onset of psychotic symptoms. *American Journal of Geriatric Psychiatry* 6:223–27.

Weinberg, A. D., B. C. Fuchs, J. K. Pals, et al. 2004. Pet therapy/companion programs in nursing facilities: Policies, procedures, potential complications, and clinical issues. *Annals of Long-Term Care* 12:36–40.

Weintraub, D., and H. I. Hurtig. 2007. Presentation and management of psychosis in Parkinson's disease and dementia with Lewy bodies. *American Journal of Psychiatry* 164:1491–98.

Westerberg, C. E., K. A. Paller, S. Weintraub, et al. 2006. When memory does not fail: Familiarity-based recognition in mild cognitive impairment and Alzheimer's disease. *Neuropsychology* 20:193–205.

White, H. K. 2005. Promoting quality care in the nursing home. *Annals of Long-Term Care* 13:26–33.

Whitmer, R. A. 2007. The epidemiology of adiposity and dementia. *Current Alzheimer Research* 4:117–22.

Whitmer, R. A., D. R. Gustafson, E. Barrett-Connor, et al. 2008. Central obesity and increased risk of dementia more than three decades later. *Neurology Online.* doi:10.1212/01.wnl .0000306313.89165.efv1.

Willging, P. R. 2008. Medical direction and the future of assisted living. *Annals of Long-Term Care* 16:29–31.

Williams, C. L., and R. M. Tappen. 2007. Effect of exercise on mood in nursing home residents with Alzheimer's disease. *American Journal of Alzheimer's Disease and Other Dementias* 22:389–97.

Wilson, R. S., J. J. McCann, Y. Li, et al. 2007. Nursing home placement, day care use, and cognitive decline in Alzheimer's disease. *American Journal of Psychiatry* 164:910–15.

Wolfson, C., D. B. Wolfson, M. Asgharian, et al. 2001. A reevaluation of the duration of survival after the onset of dementia. *New England Journal of Medicine* 344:1111–16.

Won, A. B., K. L. Lapane, S. Vallow, et al. 2004. Persistent nonmalignant pain and analgesic prescribing patterns in elderly nursing home residents. *Journal of the American Geriatrics Society* 52:867–74.

Wood, S., J. L. Cummings, M. Hsu, et al. 2000. The use of the Neuropsychiatric Inventory in nursing home residents. *American Journal of Geriatric Psychiatry* 8:75–83.

Work Group on Alzheimer's Disease and Other Dementias. 2007. Practice guideline for the treatment of patients with Alzheimer's disease and other dementias, 2nd ed. Supplement to the *American Journal of Psychiatry* 164(12):A48 [pp. 1–56].

Wright, R. M. 2007. Use of osteoporosis medications in older nursing facility residents. *Journal of the American Medical Directors Association* 8:453–57.

Yasui-Furukori, N., and S. Kaneko. 2006. Digitalis intoxication induced by paroxetine co-administration. *Lancet* 367:788.

Yeh, S., S. Lovitt, and M. W. Schuster. 2007. Pharmacological treatment of geriatric cachexia: Evidence and safety in perspective. *Journal of the American Medical Directors Association* 8:363–77.

Yesavage, J. A., T. L. Brink, T. L. Rose, et al. 1983. Development and validation of a geriatric depression scale: A preliminary report. *Journal of Psychiatric Research* 17:37–49.

Young, H. M., S. L. Gray, W. C. McCormick, et al. 2008. Types, prevalence, and potential clinical significance of medication administration errors in assisted living. *Journal of the American Geriatrics Society* 56:1199–1205.

Zanni, G. R. 2006. Long-term care: Changing demographics, changing residents. *Consultant Pharmacist* 21:18–28.

Zapka, J. G., W. Hennessy, R. E. Carter, et al. 2006. End-of-life communication and hospital nurses: An educational pilot. *Journal of Cardiovascular Nursing* 21:223–31.

Zarit, S. H., K. E. Reever, and J. Bach-Peterson. 1980. Relatives of the impaired elderly: Correlates of feelings of burden. *Gerontologist* 20:649–55.

Zeisel, J., N. M. Silverstein, J. Hyde, et al. 2003. Environmental correlates to behavioral health outcomes in Alzheimer's special care units. *Gerontologist* 43:697–711.

Zhang, B., A. El-Jawahri, and H. G. Prigerson. 2006. Update on bereavement research: Evidence-based guideline for the diagnosis and treatment of complicated bereavement. *Journal of Palliative Medicine* 9:1188–1203.

Zimmerman, S., P. D. Sloan, C. S. Williams, et al. 2005. Dementia care and quality of life in assisted living and nursing homes. *Gerontologist* 45:133–46.

Zimring, S. D. 2006. Health care decision-making capacity: A legal perspective for long-term care providers. *Journal of the American Medical Directors Association* 7:322–26.

Zisook, S., and K. S. Kendler. 2007. Is bereavement-related depression different than non-bereavement-related depression? *Psychological Medicine* 37:779–94.

Zubenko, G. S., W. N. Zubenko, S. McPherson, et al. 2003. A collaborative study of the emergence and clinical features of the Major Depressive syndrome of Alzheimer's disease. *American Journal of Psychiatry* 160:857–66.

Zuidema, S. U., E. Derksen, F. R. Verhey, et al. 2007. Prevalence of neuropsychiatric symptoms in a large sample of Dutch nursing home patients with dementia. *International Journal of Geriatric Psychiatry* 22:632–38.

Zweig, S. C., R. L. Kruse, and E. F. Binder. 2004. Effect of do-not-resuscitate orders on hospitalization of nursing home residents evaluated for lower respiratory infections. *Journal of the American Geriatrics Society* 52:51–58.

Index

cognitive rehabilitation, 385–87
cognitive stimulation, 88
Cohen-Mansfield Agitation Inventory (CMAI), 40, 178
communication: with families, 22, 378–79; with residents, 22, 102, 128–29, 276, 376, 377–78, 394
community-based services, 14
community involvement, 363
complementary and alternative treatments, 146
confidentiality, 102
Confusion Assessment Method (CAM), 39
constipation, 107, 124, 309
Cornell Scale for Depression in Dementia (CSDD), 40, 43, 74, 124, 127
corticosteroids, 205t, 283
COX-2 inhibitors, 310, 311
creativity, 273–74, 355
Creutzfeldt-Jacob disease (CJD), 67
cultural differences: assessment of, 17; care and, 12–13, 297; communication and, 22, 102, 128–29, 276; ethics and, 258; sensitivity to, 164, 264, 362, 412, 413
culture change, 405–7

dance therapy, 88, 388–89
decision making capacity, 101–3
deficiency, micronutrient, 239t, 239–42
dehydration, 43, 107, 229, 237–38, 246, 248, 263; assessment of, 30, 34–35, 43, 238; prevention of, 233
delirium: anxiety in, 206–7; causes of, 107, 108, 108t; cellular-level processes in, 106; complications and, 115; dementia and, 113, 119, 120; diagnosis of, 39, 47t, 107–15; drug-induced, 304; end-of-life, 121, 282–83; medical causes of, 229t, 309; prevalence of, 7–9, 8t, 106, 267; prevention of, 120, 121t; prognosis for, 119–20, 277; with psychotic symptoms, 184–85; risk factors for, 107, 108t; subacute, 106; subsyndromal, 109; subtypes, 106–7; treatment of, 111–15, 116–20
delusional disorder, 173–74
delusions: biological factors in, 79; defined, 163; disorders causing, 56, 78, 124, 136,

163, 166–67, 169–70, 175–77, 182, 183, 185
dementia, 50–105; abuse and neglect in, 255; antipsychotics and, 118; assessment of, 21, 37–38, 39, 42, 45–46, 45t; in AZ, staging of, 38, 86; behavior models for, 369–73; causes of, irreversible, 51t, 51–68; causes of, reversible, 51t, 68–70, 76–77; decision-making capacity in, 101–3; and dehydration, 238; delirium and, 113, 119, 120; diagnosis of, 71–78, 110–11, 131–32; early-onset, 50, 63, 395; educating family about, 373–75; end-stage markers for, 278; and medical comorbidities, 92–93, 308–19; nutritional disorders in, 245–47; personality changes in, 219; prevalence of, 1, 3–4, 50; prognosis for, 276–77; PTSD and, 198; research ethics and, 259–60; risk factors and, 74, 398; routine screenings for, 43; semantic, 63, 64; sleep disorders in, 78, 79, 211–12, 214; staff training in, 376; symptoms of, 50, 56, 78–84, 89–91, 148–51, 320; triggers for LTC admission and, 78; under-diagnosis of, 112–13. *See also specific entries under dementia*
dementia, treatment of, 84–92; and aging in place, 101; appropriate, 51; caregiver support and, 103–4; care mapping and, 417; effectiveness of, 104–5; ethics of, 409t; goals for, 84, 85t, 92, 93; palliative care and, 45, 91–92; patient's right to, 104; patient values and, 90–91; psychosocial-environmental interventions and, 88–91; quality of life and, 85, 92–93; response assessment and, 89; STAR approach to, 89–90, 95; in terminal stage, 88, 268, 269t, 280–91
Dementia Practice Guidelines (ATRA), 400
dementia syndrome of depression, 73, 74, 78, 79, 130–32, 139–40
dementia with anxiety disorder, 201–4
dementia with delirium, 110, 113, 119, 120
dementia with Lewy bodies (DLB), 58–60; comorbid conditions and, 67, 79, 131, 246; diagnosis of, 58–59, 59t, 110, 178; psychosis in, 79, 176–77; treatment of, 85

About the Authors

Abhilash K. Desai, M.D., is associate professor and director of the Center for Healthy Brain Aging in the Division of Geriatric Psychiatry, Department of Neurology and Psychiatry, at Saint Louis University School of Medicine in Saint Louis, Missouri. He received an H.S.C. from Jaihind College and an M.D. from Seth G. S. Medical College, both in Bombay, India.

From 2004 to 2008, Dr. Desai served as medical director of the Alzheimer's Center of Excellence, ThedaCare Behavioral Health, in Appleton, Wisconsin, which received the Outstanding Organization Award from the Wisconsin Alzheimer's Association in 2007. He received the Best Performance by a Community Member award from the Wisconsin Association of Homes and Services for the Aging, Inc. He was named one of the Volunteers of the Year in 2001 by the Alzheimer's Association, Saint Louis chapter.

Dr. Desai's practice involves promoting the well-being and relieving the suffering both of residents living in assisted living homes and nursing homes and of their family members.

George T. Grossberg, M.D., is the Samuel W. Fordyce Professor and director of the Division of Geriatric Psychiatry in the Department of Psychiatry at Saint Louis University School of Medicine in Saint Louis, Missouri. He received a B.A. from Yeshiva University and an M.D. from Saint Louis University.

Dr. Grossberg is a former president of the American Association of Geriatric Psychiatry and of the International Psychogeriatric Association. He is a recipient of the Missouri Adult Day Care Association Outstanding Physician Award for supporting programs that allow seniors to continue living independently or at home with their families, as well as of the Fleishman-Hillard Award for career contributions to geriatrics.

Dr. Grossberg is coauthor of *The Essential Herb-Drug-Vitamin Interaction Guide* (2007). He has edited eight textbooks and written more than 400 articles, chapters, and abstracts. He currently serves as section editor of geriatric psychiatry for *Current Psychiatry* and is on the editorial boards of *Demencia Hoy*, the *International Journal of Alzheimer's Disease*, and the *Journal of the American Medical Directors Association*.

Dr. Grossberg has served as a consultant on nursing homes to the U.S. Department of Justice, Civil Rights Division; chaired the development of "Clinical Practice Guidelines for the Treatment of Depression in the Nursing Home" for the American Medical Directors Association; and developed educational guidelines on Alzheimer disease for the American Academy of Family Practice. He is a consultant to the pharmaceutical industry in developing protocols for central nervous system disorders in elderly people and is involved in a variety of basic as well as clinical research projects, all with a focus on behavioral disturbances in dementia.